The Dao of Madness

The Dao of Madness

Mental Illness and Self-Cultivation in Early Chinese Philosophy and Medicine

ALEXUS MCLEOD

OXFORD
UNIVERSITY PRESS

OXFORD
UNIVERSITY PRESS

Oxford University Press is a department of the University of Oxford. It furthers the University's objective of excellence in research, scholarship, and education by publishing worldwide. Oxford is a registered trade mark of Oxford University Press in the UK and certain other countries.

Published in the United States of America by Oxford University Press
198 Madison Avenue, New York, NY 10016, United States of America.

Library of Congress Cataloging-in-Publication Data
Names: McLeod, Alexus, author.
Title: The dao of madness : mental illness and self-cultivation in early Chinese philosophy and medicine / Alexus McLeod.
Description: New York, NY : Oxford University Press, [2021] |
Includes bibliographical references and index.
Identifiers: LCCN 2021008094 (print) | LCCN 2021008095 (ebook) |
ISBN 9780197505915 (hardback) | ISBN 9780197505946 (online) |
ISBN 9780197505922 (updf) | ISBN 9780197505939 (epub)
Subjects: LCSH: Mental health—China. | Mental illness—China. |
Mental health services—China. | Philosophy, Chinese.
Classification: LCC RA790.7.C2 M45 2021 (print) | LCC RA790.7.C2 (ebook) |
DDC 362.20951—dc23
LC record available at https://lccn.loc.gov/2021008094
LC ebook record available at https://lccn.loc.gov/2021008095

DOI: 10.1093/oso/9780197505915.001.0001

1 3 5 7 9 8 6 4 2

Printed by Integrated Books International, United States of America

This book is dedicated to my advisor and mentor, Joel J. Kupperman (1936–2020), a true junzi, who always made me want to be better.

德不孤，必有鄰。

Contents

Introduction

In the Shadows of the Chinese Tradition

In his famous exploration of madness and civilization, Michel Foucault claims, "The Reason-Madness nexus constitutes for Western culture one of the dimensions of its originality."[1] This claim, like many claims about the distinctiveness of Western culture, philosophy, and tradition by scholars over the years, is demonstrably false. Part of my aim in this book is to offer such a demonstration. It is nearly impossible to encounter non-Western traditions in any kind of depth and fail to recognize a distinction made between reason and madness, between the cultivated and the wild, between sanity and insanity. Indeed, this distinction seems a hallmark of human society, and perhaps it is even necessary to form the boundaries of a society. In this sense, at least, Foucault is on to something. Human societies are defined not only by characteristic actions and cultural norms but also by what is deemed as *outside* of these boundaries, transgressive of the norms. Madness is indeed a necessary category for the creation and maintenance of a society and social norms.

If this is the case, then claims like the one from Foucault entail that non-Western cultures were not and are not capable of societies at all, as long as they do not contain this essentially Western idea of the reason-madness dichotomy. This is so bold and astonishing a claim as to be truly absurd, especially when not a shred of support is supplied for such a claim. If one is going to make such a sweeping claim, one had better have a mountain of evidence to back it up. One can be forgiven for claiming that the moon is made of rock without providing evidence, but when one claims that the moon is made of cheese supplied by Wisconsin farmers as part of a CIA conspiracy, one places a heavy burden of proof on oneself. And Foucault's claim is more extreme than the claim about the cheesiness of the moon. Could one really believe that non-Western people have been incapable of the most basic distinctions

[1] *Madness and Civilization*, xi.

The Dao of Madness. Alexus McLeod, Oxford University Press. © Oxford University Press 2021.
DOI: 10.1093/oso/9780197505915.003.0001

underpinning developed society, and that insofar as any non-Western people today have such society, it is only through their adoption of Western categories? This position is so absurd as to be a *reductio* of itself. Nonetheless, people did, and many still do, believe it.

In this book, I offer a picture of madness as a category and a tool in the early Chinese tradition, offering an account of how early Chinese thinkers developed a conception of mental illness connected to both medicine and ethics (which were never seen as wholly separable, although they become more clearly distinct during the Han Dynasty). Specifically, I am concerned with the connections between madness, mental illness in general, and philosophical positions on personhood, moral agency, responsibility, and social identity. Madness, I argue, is a near universal category in human thought. In early China, madness (*kuang* 狂) has particular unique forms, shaped through consideration of the features of mind and body, cultural norms, and illness and health. While madness and other forms of mental illness were taken as either foils or ideals by different thinkers in early China, they were nearly always contrasted with operability, proper communal development, and progress on a specifically moral path.

***

A personal note here can help explain the genesis of this project, as well as how I hope it will contribute to the historical discourse on mental illness. Two major topics in my own life are unified in this book: early Chinese philosophy and mental illness. I have struggled with a severe mental illness (known clinically as bipolar I disorder) since I was young (though I have not always known what it was—this lack of awareness by mentally ill characters is a theme that will recur throughout this book in the various early Chinese figures we will meet). Sometimes it has been managed well, and sometimes it has been debilitating. I have studied, taught, and written about Chinese philosophy for close to twenty years now, and throughout that time I have been in and out of institutions and dealt with all manner of psychiatrists and mental health experts. With my difficulties, getting through undergraduate and graduate schools intact, and then landing and keeping a job as a philosophy professor was even more difficult than this track usually is. Learning Chinese, first Mandarin and then Classical Chinese, and learning the rich and enormous tradition of early Chinese philosophy—these tasks were made far more difficult than they otherwise might have been due to mental illness.

Mental illness has often made it difficult, if not impossible, for me to function in even the most basic of ways.

I have always thus had a special fascination with the depiction of mental illness in ancient texts, and with mentally ill characters in philosophy, literature, and history. One of my favorite works of fiction is the second part of *Don Quixote*, the madman's reflections on death and meaning. In the early Chinese tradition, it was Jieyu, the infamous "Madman of Chu" (楚狂), who first caught my attention. The cryptic stories from the *Analects* and the *Zhuangzi* concerning the Madman piqued my interest—especially the seemingly positive evaluation of the Madman in the *Zhuangzi* version. I continued to work on early Chinese philosophy without thinking much about the Madman of Chu or other similar characters. Though the Madman himself made it into some of my work looking at personhood and agency,[2] I hadn't thought of the Madman as a key character in early Chinese philosophy. This changed when I recently, when going through a number of early Chinese texts mentioning madmen and other plausibly mentally ill persons. I recognized that mental illness arose as a theme in early Chinese texts an unusually large number of times. I wondered what role mental illness played in these texts. This issue became even more interesting to me when I reflected on the self-cultivation in early Chinese texts and related this to my own difficult experiences both developing a career and growing as a person throughout my life. The instructions for moral development in ancient texts such as the *Analects*, *Mengzi*, and even *Zhuangzi* seemed to presume a roughly general agentive self, and one without compromised features. What, I wondered, could a person with mental illness hope to achieve in following such systems? Did these ancient philosophers think it was possible for a mentally ill person to engage successfully in moral self-cultivation? Or did they think their processes of reasoning, choice, action direction, and motivation were too badly compromised by their illness? As I looked to the ancient texts to try to discern answers to these questions, I discovered that there seemed to be a variety of different views on offer. And not only this, but almost *none* of this had been discussed in previous scholarship on early Chinese thought. Indeed, most scholars who discussed mental illness in China at all seemed to think that the concept of mental illness in China began only in the modern period, with Western influence. This series of puzzles concerning madness

[2] In particular, my 2012 paper "In the World of Persons: The Personhood Debate in the *Analects* and *Zhuangzi*."

(*kuang* 狂), agency, and moral self-cultivation had gone almost completely unrecognized. Why, I wondered, was this the case? A large part of the reason I noticed this problem and the host of different answers to it in early Chinese texts, I concluded, was my own sensitivity to the issue as someone for whom mental illness has always been a key obstacle to activity, tied into the issue of agency. I resolved to reveal this issue in early Chinese texts—and this became the origin of the project that forms the basis of this book.

Meeting with madmen, the excited and manic, as well as the immobile anxious, the catatonic, and the depressed—I recognized at least some of what I saw in the stories of these figures. I was also intrigued that they always seemed to be part of the story, part of the *lesson* of the texts I was reading. This lesson was not always (or even often) a positive one, but the fact that madness had been made part of the issue at hand struck me as interesting and unique. Especially given that the issue at hand always seemed to have to do with self-cultivation and success in action. I noticed that hardly any scholarly work that touched on passages or texts in which madness, mad characters, or mental illness played a role actually discussed these aspects of the texts in question. I had always experienced mental illness as an obstacle to activity—social as well as intellectual. As I read these accounts of mental illness and surrounding issues in early China, I came to think that my experiences with mental illness and my intellectual life, much of which surrounded Chinese philosophy, could not be as easily kept separate as I had believed. Reading and reflecting on the accounts of *Zhuangzi* and *Huainanzi*, I came to realize that perhaps my old belief that I had succeeded in becoming a scholar and a philosopher *despite* my mental illness was, if not wrong, not the whole story. Some of the accounts of madness I encountered in early Chinese literature (in particular that of the Zhuangists) suggested that it is at least sometimes the divergent mental states and worldviews of the mad and otherwise mentally ill that allow them to see possibilities that others miss.

I began to recognize that the various accounts and discussions of mental illness, particularly "madness," playing out across Chinese texts in Warring States and Han periods represented this very same tension writ large. Is mental disorder (in its various forms, which the early Chinese certainly understood differently than most contemporary people) a problem, a failure, or even an illness—or is it instead a boon, an assistant to freedom and creativity? I found these questions and others surrounding mental illness and moral self-cultivation in early Chinese philosophical and medical texts. Indeed, what I initially thought was a modest amount of discussion I came to find was truly enormous, and the project I originally envisioned as an article (perhaps even a short one) on mental illness and issues in ethics in the Chinese tradition turned into this book. At each stage, I became more convinced that there was something crucially important here, something that was being missed in other studies of early Chinese thought. Important not only for developing our understanding of self-cultivation and surrounding issues in early Chinese philosophy but also for aiding our understanding of mental illness itself and the role of mental illness in moral development and agency.

Thus, this book has both philosophical and personal significance for me, and I hope for others interested in Chinese philosophy, ethics, and the possibilities for those with mental illness and other forms of illness of living meaningful lives. As with much of early Chinese philosophy, the ultimate aim is to help us to live better lives. Though I cannot claim to have mastered their ways, in encountering these early Chinese texts, I learned new ways I might be in the world with mental illness, learned new strategies to try to cope with or see meaning in the endless struggles I endure. I hope this book serves not only to illuminate views and answer problems in philosophy but also to help other people struggling with mental illness of whatever kind to better understand themselves, their role in the world, how to cope with their illness, and ultimately how to achieve a thriving life.

I present in this book, as is apparent in the title, the idea of madness as a *dao* (way of being). This book is about the ways of being and conceiving of the *kuang* person, from the perspective of a number of traditions—evaluations of them, in terms of their value, and the connection of the *kuang* to personhood and self-cultivation. A *dao* is not always a good thing. And here it is ambiguous, too. Sometimes a path is a dangerous or misguided one. The *kuang ren*'s *dao*, insofar as it is a characteristic way of the *kuang* person as *kuang*, is a disorder and a failure according to the "traditional" view, while it represents a higher form of knowledge or ability according to the Zhuangist view. This book is not only an attempt to investigate the different conceptions of the *dao* of the *kuang* person but also to understand the true *dao* of the *kuang* person. This book is an attempt to understand different conceptions of, as well as to find, the *dao* of madness.

The various characters and the discussions of the mentally ill and mental illness I cover in this book are, all parties would agree, at the periphery, in the shadows of the early Chinese tradition. This is the reason such people are ultimately rejected by people such as Confucians, while praised and idealized by Zhuangists, who take the peripheral, unusual, or socially unacceptable as representative of a deeper wisdom. It is my attempt here to take these figures from the shadows and bring them into the light—to offer a coherent account of views of and about these people and of mental illness in early China, and to understand how we might incorporate the best of these views into our own accounts today.

Another peculiar thing about this issue is the distance between a number of views of mental illness in early China and those of later times closer to our own. The concept of mental illness as it is understood in the West is relatively new to China (although there is an important analog in early China), and understandings of mental illness are undergoing radical changes in Chinese society today, as rates of mental illness rise precipitously in the nation.[3] According to a 2009 article from the medical journal *Lancet*, 17.5 percent of China's population has some form of mental illness.[4] While this number is smaller than the 26.4 percent of the US population diagnosed with mental illness, it also means there are far more mentally ill people in China than in the United States—the mentally ill population of China alone is equal in number to about 75 percent of the entire US population. The reasons for this rise in mental illness are unclear. There have been many explanations offered for it, attributing causes to everything from increasing industrialization and "modernization" to better diagnostic techniques that reveal mental illness that simply would not have been attended to as such in earlier years. And there is also the possibility that the rise in mental illness (in China as well as the West) is due to the outsized influence of pharmaceutical companies and others, who have effectively *created* mental illness as a widespread phenomenon.[5]

All of this is particularly interesting in the face of early Chinese thought, in which we see a number of views of mental illness very close to or consistent with modern conceptions. That modern understandings of mental illness in China represent such an abrupt and dramatic shift from ones of previous years, one of the large questions we must grapple with is, What happened? How did things change in the years from the early Han to the end of the Qing period in the twentieth century, to move the dominant view of mental illness away from approaches like those of modern medicine, and toward the kind of "cultivational" views dominant in early Confucian texts?

[3] Cyranoski 2010.
[4] Phillips et al. 2009.
[5] As I discuss later, this is a common criticism of the "anti-psychiatry" movement.

While I do not fully answer this question in the book, I do offer an account of early Confucian texts that explains their views on mental illness. The story of how the Confucian views became the dominant and entrenched position in Chinese society until the modern day is a major story, told by numerous scholars, and far bigger than the subject of this book.

Understanding the role of madmen, the catatonic, and other mentally ill people in ancient China also, and perhaps most importantly, has implications for views of personhood, agency, and self-cultivation in the tradition. The various philosophers and others who dealt with the issue of mental illness almost always recognized its connection to moral self-cultivation, either as a problem for theories of cultivation or as a result or example of proper cultivation. We see a variety of radically different views on the status and value of madness and mental illness in general, as well as what exactly it is. Not everyone in the early Chinese tradition would agree that mental illness is illness at all. We find a variety of attitudes about what we might call mental or behavioral "dysfunction" in early China even broader than what we find in the modern world. Today, there is widespread agreement about the nature of mental illness, its causes, manifestations, categories, and even its implications for law, ethics, and personhood more generally. Despite some resistance to modern medical or scientific ways of thinking about mental illness (represented by figures like Thomas Szasz and the "anti-psychiatry" movement, which we will encounter in Chapters 2 and 4, the contemporary world has largely accepted a particular understanding of mental illness—and this despite the fact that psychiatry has perhaps the most problematic track record of the sciences, with the level of uncertainty about even its most basic concepts and premises demonstrated by the fact that foundational texts like the American Psychiatric Association's *Diagnostic and Statistical Manual of Mental Disorders* radically changes with every edition. The history of psychiatry is one of radical revisions and rethinking, rather than progressive construction. None of this is to say that modern psychiatry has not helped many people and overall been a positive development. Rather, it is curious that such acceptance and certainty have been achieved in our society in the case of the most provisional and incompletely understood of areas in medicine and the science of the self.

Of course, it would be unfair to conclude that psychiatry is uniquely unscientific because it has been provisional and often revised. *Every* scientific field has undergone radical revision through its existence, particularly in its early stages, and even major shifts in its foundations. When Newtonian mechanics gave way to the theories of relativity, no one questioned the objectivity or truth of physics. Contemporary physics is still unable to give us certainty or explanation of many topics and outstanding questions, yet it does not arouse the same suspicion and rejection as psychiatry often does. Nonpsychiatric medicine constantly changes, revises, and updates, yet we generally do not question its objective nature. Medicine as a whole is highly provisional and revisionary. We do not understand what causes most cancers, for example, or ultimately how to treat them successfully. There are a host of physical conditions about which medicine provides little if any understanding. Indeed, there are conditions on which experts have disagreed that they *are* conditions, and which are continually being reformulated. Examples of this include irritable bowel syndrome, which has not been linked definitively with a single cause. The condition is thus diagnosed through symptoms, and similar presentations may have different causes in different individuals. In many ways, "irritable bowel syndrome" is a catch-all term for a host of functionally related conditions. To require some specific single biological etiology for the reality of a medical condition would mean that irritable bowel syndrome could not exist as a condition. Nonpsychiatric medicine is also continually in flux concerning causal claims about connections between particular activities, substances, and disorders. Knowledge about what patterns or levels of consumption of things such as alcohol, sugar, or caffeine (for example) lead to or whether they leave one at greater risk for particular illnesses is continually changing, which leads to continual changing in the recommendations for consumption given by health institutions such as the US Centers for Disease Control and Prevention (CDC).[6]

Part of the reason that psychiatry receives skepticism that the rest of medicine, which can be shown equally as volatile and frequently revised, does not, is that many are skeptical of the very existence of mind as such (as the continued influence of some eliminativist theories of mind in the philosophy of mind demonstrates).[7] Many people, adopting universal physicalist views, take seriously the idea that mind either does not exist or must be somehow reducible to physical stuff. I suspect that this suspicion of mind, and the scientific respectability of the category of mind, is behind much of

[6] A recent example of this is the revision of the Dietary Guidelines for Americans recommendation by the US Department of Health and Human Services for the maximum healthy amount of alcohol consumption for men from 2 drinks per day (where 1 drink = 12 oz of 5% ABV) to 1 per day. https://thehill.com/opinion/healthcare/503508-theres-now-progress-on-alcohol-in-the-dietary-guidelines

[7] Churchland 1981; Rey 1983.

the suspicion of psychiatry and the "anti-psychiatry" movement. It is difficult to take seriously a science based on a category of thing that one will not allow into their basic ontology. Though there are surely many physicalists among psychiatrists and those who take psychiatry seriously, no one can give an adequate account of just *how* mind reduces to the physical, and without such an account, physicalistically-minded skeptics will continue to have something to sink their teeth into (just as the skeptic in epistemology depends on our inability to demonstrate the inerrancy of any justification). In addition, some of the central arguments of anti-psychiatry skeptics (including Szasz himself) are inadequate to demonstrate that mental illness is a particularly problematic natural kind. As I argue in Chapter 2, demonstrating that social and cultural factors are relevant to what constitutes mental illness does not show that mental illness does not exist as a natural kind or is simply a social construct, any more than the fact that there are social and cultural factors that determine what constitutes illness of *any* kind undermines the reality of physical illnesses. Szasz's criticisms simply do not hit the mark—he cannot show that mental illness has any particular conceptual difficulties that physical illness does not have, yet he is not prepared to jettison the concept of physical illness as a natural kind—indeed, he explicitly claims that all illness should be understood in terms of physical illness. This is simply a misguided commitment to physicalism, and it masks the fact that the reality of physical things is often no less culturally determined than the reality of mental states (and illness). Indeed, this is one of the driving insights behind conventionalism about objects in metaphysics, both in its early Chinese and contemporary Western guises.[8] Rudolf Carnap expressed this in his conventionalist view of the connection between language and reality:

> "Are our experiences such that the use of the linguistic forms in question will be expedient and fruitful?" This is a theoretical question of a factual, empirical nature. But it concerns a matter of degree; therefore a formulation in the form "real or not" would be inadequate.[9]

My usage of the phrase "mental illness" here and throughout the book could be taken as anachronistic in the case of early China, especially if one

[8] The *Zhuangzi* can be read as endorsing a kind of conventionalism about language and kinds, in which things (*wu* 物) are constructed via conceptualization, rather than by the world itself independently of humans. See Coutinho 2014, 161.

[9] Carnap 1956, 213.

is inclined to skepticism about psychiatry and its basic concepts. I use the phrase for a few reasons. First—I am assuming the category of mental states, behavioral dysfunctions, and phenomena that *we* in 2017 refer to as "mental illness," which surely also existed in fourth century BCE China, even if they were thought of very differently. That is, psychiatry is a legitimate science (just as are nonpsychiatric medicine, meteorology, geology, and physics) and deals with natural kinds. While this must remain here largely an assumption (as it would take another entire other book on its own to argue for this, as many have), it is not a problematic assumption in our modern-day context. Many people in the scientific and medical communities take psychiatry seriously and view mental illnesses as real illnesses, real disorders that obtain in humans. Much, if not all, of the modern apparatus of our society takes for granted that mental illness is a real and natural phenomenon, even if we have not fully integrated appreciation of this into all of our institutions. The Americans with Disabilities Act of 1990 distinguishes between physical and mental disability, including in its very first line: "physical or mental disabilities in no way diminish a person's right to fully participate in all aspects of society."[10] The text goes on to discuss "mental disabilities" and "mental impairment" as distinct from physical disability and impairment throughout. Given this widespread acceptance of the reality of mental illness in our society, the burden is on the skeptic to demonstrate that we are mistaken in our acceptance of this category, and its defense is a task I leave to others.

Assuming that mental illness is a natural kind, we can refer to mental illness in early China, even if they did not have such a concept (although as I argue here, they did), in much the same way we can refer to *molecules* or *economies* in early China, even though people in early China did not think of these things in the same ways as we do, or even differentiate them as particular concepts. Early Chinese people *did* interact with and use molecules, even if they did not think of them as such. They also did have economies, even if there was no theoretical structure through which they thought of them as such. The same can be said of mental illness. If mental illness is a real thing, including conditions and dysfunctions human beings can have, independently of their cultural context, then mental illness existed in early China as much as it exists in the twenty-first century United States. It will, of course, be more difficult for us to identify cases of mental illness, because the

[10] *Americans with Disabilities Act of 1990*, Title 42, Ch. 126, Section 12101. https://www.ada.gov/pubs/adastatute08.htm

descriptions and classifications people in early China used to discuss it were different than those we use in the modern world. But there is also a great deal of overlap in the ways mental illness is conceptualized in early China and in our modern context, as I show in Chapter 2. This is perhaps surprising, given the vast differences between early Chinese society and our own modern societies (whether this is contemporary China, the contemporary West, or elsewhere). As I show, however, early Chinese thought about mental illness was much closer to current ways of thinking about these issues than the thought of much of the West for the entirety of its history, as well as other areas of the world during this time and later. Part of demonstrating this is to show that in early medical and other texts, there is a distinction drawn between mind and body, and a particular conception of illness (*bing* 病) as applicable to mind as a distinct kind of illness or disorder, though treated through similar methods as other kinds of illness.

The proximity of early Chinese thought about mental illness and its implications for philosophy make it possible for us to consider how these issues might be integrated into the ways we think about these issues within ethics and metaphysics. One of the key features of mentally ill figures discussed in early Chinese texts is that they are almost always mysterious, outside of society, ineffable, wandering in the shadows. Most of the time, such characters are peripheral to the main interests and themes of the situations, discussions, and stories in which they appear, and it is likely for this reason that their importance is often overlooked. But they appear so frequently as a trope in early Chinese philosophy, and are connected with such a variety of different positions, lessons, and assumptions, that there is much we can learn through them about early Chinese conceptions of the person, self-cultivation, and agency, in addition to their views about mental illness and the distinction between normal and abnormal or dysfunctional behavior and mental processes. There is much to be gained from hunting around in the shadows of the early Chinese tradition to draw out these hermits, madmen, shell-shocked ministers, and various other mentally ill persons. Just as in any society, including our own, we can learn much about a people from investigating the "dysfunctional," including the concept of (in this case mental) dysfunction, people who are so dysfunctional, and the ways these people are conceived of in the society.

The particular states I will consider in this book, such as "madness" (*kuang* 狂), anxiety (*chu* 怵), depression (*dian* 癲), and a number of emotional excesses deemed as *bing* 病 (illness), have a very different history and construction in the early Chinese context than they do in contemporary or modern Western thought. We see a narrative surrounding these states as limiting or creating obstacles. Mental disorder or illness is thought of as something that makes it impossible to live in the world with others in the expected ways. It is causative and constitutive of unusual ways of thinking and behaving, ways that fall outside of both the normal activity of people in society and norms concerning what acts *should* be performed in society. As we will see, the conception of mental illness in early China, as in the contemporary world, is descriptive as well as normative.

Although there are a number of concepts in early Chinese texts that suggest mental disorder, distress, or difficulty, the central focus of this book is on the particular concept of *kuang* 狂 (madness). The reason for this is that *kuang* appears in a number of texts as a particularly potent image, and it is used as a tool in arguments for particular conceptions of personhood, agency, and value. While I look at a few of these concepts through the book, the central focus remains on *kuang* as a frame for a particular debate between three strains of thought in early China concerning madness and personhood (that do not easily align with "schools"). This debate is directly relevant to the numerous early Chinese understandings of *kuang*, which range from the more traditional and "mainstream" views of *kuang* as a disorder or illness to alternative views of *kuang* persons as wise, guides, or extranaturally knowledgeable. This range of meanings of *kuang* does not represent independent innovation or differences, but rather emerged out of a sustained debate surrounding personhood, social norms, and community that raged among early Chinese thinkers, who often responded to one another in their texts, sometimes explicitly and sometimes less so. *Kuang* thus serves as a particularly powerful concept through which to focus the multifaceted debates surrounding personhood, agency, moral and social norms, and physical and mental illness in early China. Interestingly enough, many of the same debates going on today concerning personhood, character, and mental illness (some of which are discussed in Chapter 2) can be found in early Chinese texts. The topic is clearly one that taxes people in the contemporary West no less than it did people in ancient China.

As I explain in the chapters that follow, part of the reason that *kuang* plays such a central role in this debate tying mental illness to personhood and norms is that *kuang* is the mental state most closely tied to the "uncultivated" and wild, the ignoring or flouting of social norms. The broad range of what we might call mental disorder ranges from pure ignorance and incorrect or improper synthesis of the senses to pathological states like anxiety, depression (*dian* 癲), and *kuang*. Only *kuang*, as associated with openly and loudly flouting norms and living outside of respectable social boundaries, became a symbol for the rejection of dominant and traditional social norms and conceptions of personhood. The symptoms of *kuang* documented in texts such as the *Huangdi Neijing* show that such a state is inconsistent with the ritual activity deemed proper in early Confucian, Mohist, and other texts. The *kuang* person is not only mentally disordered, but this disorder manifests itself through socially problematic behavior. The *kuang* person is one whose activity disrupts and throws into disorder the harmonious working of society, and thus presents a danger to this society. In this way, the *kuang* person is associated also with the wilds, uncultivated, and unshaped, which is unsuitable for human life and must be formed and reshaped in order to be habitable for humans (as I discuss in Chapter 4). Most parties seem to agree that there is a connection between the mad, the wild, and the uncontrolled. And this shows that the activity of the mad person is somehow connected to human nature and does not arise from outside of it. A key difference between the *kuang* person and the sane, civilized person, however, is that the latter has, through proper socialization, controlled and subordinated the "natural" responses to put them in their proper places and allow their manifestations to be expressed properly and curbed through social norms. This is also why the wild and the mad are connected to the concept of barbarity. The barbarians are those without civilization, those without proper norms, and thus those always in some state similar to *kuang*. If we think about symptoms of *kuang* (which seem to mirror symptoms of our concept of *mania*), we cannot say these are "unnatural" in the sense of activities that cut against normal human tendencies. Rather, *kuang* actions are done without the restraints or modifications of social norms, as if the subconscious of the individual has been given free rein as in individual imagination without the constraints of social demands. The pure individual demand for gratification, excitement, and immediate expression of emotion is unfiltered through the social demand on shaping or constraints on such expression. So anger immediately results in bursts of shouting and abuse, feelings of joy result in spontaneous outbursts of singing or dancing, and sexual arousal results in immediate satisfaction, even in public. Madness thus has a special place in consideration of the issues of personhood and self-cultivation. Michel Foucault, like the Zhuangists, recognized this uniquely transgressive quality of madness and its link to social norms and personhood. He discusses the link between madness and "animality" in the West (mirroring the Chinese link between madness and the wilds and uncultivated).[11] Foucault wrote:

> We see why the scandal of madness could be exalted, while that of the other forms of unreason was concealed with so much care. The scandal of unreason produced only the contagious example of transgression and immorality; the scandal of madness showed men how closely to animality their Fall could bring them; and at the same time how far divine mercy could extend when it consented to save man.[12]

We see much the same in early China, with ritual (*li* 禮) and social norms more generally playing the role of Foucault's "divine mercy" in its transformative power, shaping the raw, "animal" stuff of human nature to the uniquely and properly human, in its constrained and socially contextualized full formulation. Thus we can see why madness would become a central fulcrum for a debate between cultivationists like Confucians and Mohists and advocates of a less constrained and more "natural" expression of human activity, such as the Daoists and Zhuangists.[13]

This book is organized into six chapters. The first lays out the dominant views of self, agency, and moral responsibility in early Chinese philosophy. The reason for this is that these views inform the ways early Chinese thinkers approach mental illness, as well as the role they see it playing in self-cultivation as a whole (whether they view it as problematic or beneficial, for example). In this chapter I offer a view of a number of dominant conceptions of mind, body, and agency in early Chinese thought, through a number of philosophical and medical texts.[14]

[11] Foucault 1988, 78.

[12] Foucault 1988, 81.

[13] I discuss later the extent to which these can be taken as distinct but related groups, or even as coherent groups at all.

[14] The distinction between "philosophy" and "medicine" is somewhat artificial when applied to early Chinese texts. While I separate the two here for purposes of bringing focus to medical texts that have not commonly been considered part of the early Chinese philosophical tradition, there is a great deal of philosophy done in "medical" texts in early China. One of the things I hope to show in this book is that philosophers and others interested in philosophy in the early Chinese context cannot afford to ignore medical literature and other relevant literature. Zhou Guidian put this well in his book *Qin Han Zhexue* 秦漢哲學, writing: "Chinese philosophy and science have a considerable amount of connection. Philosophy speaks about 'the oneness of Heaven and persons' [天人合一 *tian ren he yi*], and this is closely connected to astronomy and medicine. Since we are discussing Qin and Han philosophy, one also needs to investigate traditional Chinese sciences, and this requires investigation of the systems of astronomy and medicine." Zhou 2006, 190.

In Chapter 2, I consider the question of "mental illness" more specifically, looking to both modern accounts and early Chinese accounts mind and body, of what illness is in a broader medical sense, and mental illness in particular as a form of illness. I offer a view of illness in general in early China, linking it to development of the person, and consider mental illness in terms of *qi* 氣 (vital essence), mind, and community based on the conception of person of the first chapter. I consider here also how illness affects agency—both physical and mental.

In Chapters 3 and 4, I look at two distinct reactions to madness and mental disorder broadly seen running throughout early Chinese philosophy, the "feigning" and "celebratory" accounts. While there is temptation to connect these to Confucianism and Zhuangism, respectively, I show that the positions are intertwined in a number of texts and cannot be associated with particular schools. The celebratory approach focuses on the ways in which the mad and "disordered" are rendered valueless based on certain social choices. The Zhuangist, among others, focuses on the way we can understand there being an inherent value in these states depending on how we conceive of situations in given perspectives, and that we have reason to resist understanding particular people as mad or disordered objectively. The idea here is to include any mental state that is regularly seen as problematic or getting in the way of efficient or proper human functioning. Certain texts, I argue, have as a goal getting rid of these states, as do the Buddhist and Hellenistic texts. One thing numerous scholars have missed, because of comparisons with these texts, is that a host of other early Chinese texts reject the view that we should aim to get rid of problematic mental states such as *kuang* or *chu*. Texts such as *Zhuangzi* and *Huainanzi* argue that we need to understand how to use these states to see their value. In this chapter I also discuss a host of mad or mentally disordered individuals found in early Chinese texts, with the aim of understanding how they fit into the structure built thus far, and how various appearances of these characters (such as the "Madman of Chu") in different texts will often serve to illustrate the divergent messages about mental disorder we find in these texts.

In Chapter 5, I discuss what I call the *syncretic* view of madness and mental illness in early Chinese texts. This view, I argue, is the most plausible account of mental illness and self-cultivation of those on offer in early Chinese philosophy. This view is mainly associated with the syncretistic texts of the early Han Dynasty, such as *Huainanzi* and *Chunqiu Fanlu*, though the seeds of this view can be found earlier in Warring States material. The syncretists reject both the negative and positive views, arguing that a complex of nature, circumstances, and individual activity is responsible for most mental illness, and that the key to avoiding or eliminating mental illness is the undermining of conceptualization and elimination of desires. The syncretic view of mental illness and cultivation creates the groundwork for the development of naturalistic medical texts such as the *Huangdi Neijing*, constructed during the Han. The conception of "controlled madness" based on the synthesis of views found in texts such as *Huainanzi* suggests that a view like this not only had some influence in later Chinese philosophy, but that it can also help us better understand the connections between illness and agency. The problem is recognized and worked out with an eye to avoid what we might see as the shortcomings of the two approaches discussed in Chapter 3. I consider also whether the syncretist approach solves the problems with the other two without creating difficult problems of its own. Finally, I tie the developments of the early Han syncretic movement to the "medicalization" of mental illness in the *Huangdi Neijing* and later medical texts.

In the conclusion, I consider some of the implications of early Chinese views of mental illness and self-cultivation for contemporary thought concerning mental illness. I argue that some of the views of early Chinese thinkers can be adapted using contemporary conceptions of mental illness, and that difficulties for certain kinds of character, virtue, and role ethics that arise surrounding issues of mental illness might be solved by adapting these views to contemporary contexts.

Note on Primary Sources

I would like to make a final note concerning citations of early Chinese texts. My citation practice in this book is to use the chapter and line numbering of the Chinese Text Project (ctext.org) website. Many scholars of early China today are using such online sources, most of which (like ctext) contain notes linking to print versions for those who would like to consult these versions. Given that our practice of using digital sources has become standard, it seems to me appropriate to cite the digital sources, especially when one's preferred print version can be easily located by consulting the digital source (the

Chinese Text Project site contains links to numerous print editions, while locating a passage in one print edition from another is more difficult to do).[15] Thus, for all early Chinese texts (with the exception of some not included on the site, flagged in the text that follows), citations follow Chinese Text Project numbering.

[15] It is true, of course, as a reviewer points out, that the digital version on ctext.org sometimes contains mistakes. This, of course, can happen in print versions as well. For any early text, readers are encouraged to consult multiple sources.

1
Self, Mind and Body, Agency

Traditional Views of Personhood and Agency

Perhaps the most traditional view of the person in early Chinese thought is the one I associate here with the Confucians. While we can refer to this as the Confucian view of personhood, it was shared (roughly) with other thinkers, such as Mohists and Legalists, and was only in its key aspects challenged by Daoists and Zhuangists, both extending criticisms originally made by Yangists. Although this conception of personhood was not solely the purview of the *Ru* (Confucians), and it had much wider influence, it is most famously associated with them, because of the way various early Confucians put forward and developed such a view, far beyond what we find in other sources.

There have been a number of contrasting interpretations of Confucians and other early Chinese thinkers on the self or person. These interpretations differ so radically that one suspects that the scholars putting forward these views do not have the same thing in mind when they purport to outline early Chinese views of the self, person, or individual. One thing that makes this task difficult is the fact that the English language and Western philosophical concepts often have only a loose connection to similar Chinese terms and concepts. Sometimes, there are no equivalents at all in Western languages and traditions to early Chinese terms and concepts. While this does not mean that we are unable to make sense of Chinese philosophical concepts,[1] it does greatly complicate the task of locating the concept in mind.

A number of scholars understand the self as the focus or center of a complex of roles and relationships. Roger Ames's "role ethics" interpretation of

[1] Alasdair MacIntyre infamously argues for the "incommensurability" of philosophical systems in MacIntyre 1981, 8 and MacIntyre 1988, 380. Relatively recent philosophical work, such as Van Norden 2007 and Stalnaker 2009, argue against this view and, convincingly, that we can isolate certain concepts and thoughts in early Chinese thought even if there was no specific term corresponding to such concepts.

The Dao of Madness. Alexus McLeod, Oxford University Press. © Oxford University Press 2021.
DOI: 10.1093/oso/9780197505915.003.0002

Confucianism reads the tradition along these lines. Tu Weiming explains well much of what is going on here. He writes:

> the Confucian idea of the self as a center of relationships is an open system. It is only through the continuous opening up of the self to others that the self can maintain a wholesome personal identity. The person who is not sensitive or responsive to the others around him is self-centered; self-centeredness easily leads to a closed world . . . to a state of paralysis.[2]

I think we can go even further than this, to say that for the Confucian, no person outside of communal integration and concern is possible. It is the human way that guides our actions and our understanding of the world. Even in trying to escape society or ignore it, the variety of ways we understand our own experience is due to community and its traditions, as is every aspect of our physical selves. There was certainly recognition of inherited features from ancestors and parents, and this is part of the reason the Confucian view took filiality as an ineliminable responsibility of the child to the parent. Filiality was central to self-cultivation, because what our parents are is intrinsically also what we are. The physical features, the mental traits, and the characteristic ways of action of the individual are in each case due to the actions and traits of their parents and wider community. Thus, the individual is not, at most basic, an autonomous self, but rather a collection of elements of ancestors, community, and tradition.[3]

Wen Haiming argues for what he calls a "co-creative" conception of the development of the self (person) in Confucian ethics.[4] On this picture, the person is created through self–other exchanges and relationships.[5] Much of this in consideration of Confucian conceptions of the self is grounded in the Confucian ethical system. In particular, many contemporary scholars are interested in the question of whether Confucians can accept a concept

[2] Tu 1985a, 114.

[3] Sungmoon Kim criticizes this "social self" view that he sees underlying modern Confucian communitarianism as an extreme version of a view of the self that can recognize the centrality of community in human life. Kim 2014, 34. The more autonomous "liberal self" Kim discusses can also make sense of the Confucian communal point. This is presumably close to what Tu Weiming has in mind as well (see previous note). While I agree with them on these points, I disagree with this as a reading of the early Confucians, who for the most part seem to have actually held the "extreme" view. I am also not convinced that the extreme view is not better than its liberal opponents.

[4] Using a term from Tu Weiming. Wen 2012.

[5] There must be a self prior to the person construction through self–other interaction, or we have no way to make sense of this as interaction at all, unless the conception of self develops from this activity in which there come to be drawn self–other distinctions. But how does this happen?

such as rights. Communitarian interpretations, like those offered by Henry Rosemont,[6] seem to have little room for such a conception. This is part of the reason for the move toward more liberal (in the sense of traditional Western liberal democratic) conceptions of the person, with some seeing modest versions of such a view in early Confucian texts.

A general trend in recent scholarship is to understand early Confucian texts advancing a view of the person as relational, while still maintaining the possibility of the discrete individual morally appraised on its own.[7] While there are many passages in early Confucian literature that seem to refer to persons as individuals, this alone is unhelpful in determining whether a kind of "extreme" relational view is the right one or whether the person on a dominant Confucian view is a relation-dependent individual. Indeed, it is not clear that for the earliest Confucians, there would even be a meaningful distinction between these two views, as their theories focused on the ethical and political implications of certain evaluations rather than the metaphysics of self and person, and it seems that *either* of these conceptions of the self and person might have the same ethical and political implications. The key here is that relationality, and the roles this relationality entails, are seen as a central to what a person is.

Likewise, it is unclear to me that which of these views of the person one adopts will even turn out to be relevant to the issue of *rights*. While in the Western tradition, rights are generally conceived of as belonging to autonomous individuals, there is nothing about the concept of rights that *requires* this sort of rights bearer. A locus of roles or confluence of communal elements could also be understood as the kind of thing that could bear rights.[8]

All of these interpretations of the person in Confucianism share the view that the person is fundamentally communal for the Confucians. Whether we understand this in the radical sense of my own interpretation, in which the individual is nothing more than the confluence of particular communal elements and that agency is understood primarily in a communal sense (Ames's position comes closest to this), or instead adopt a more modest view

[6] His final and developed statement of this can be found in Rosemont 2015.

[7] Chenyang Li and Peimin Ni attribute such a position to Joel Kupperman. They write: "Although [Kupperman] often references and seems to appreciate the relational nature of the Confucian person, he is still consistent in maintaining that an individual can be accurately described, analyzed, and evaluated independently of other human beings." Li and Ni 2014, 25.

[8] I also, however, share with Henry Rosemont and others the suspicion that a concept of rights may be unnecessary or even problematic in Confucian theory. And that this may show more of a problem with the concept of rights than with Confucian theory. Rosemont 2004.

in which the community is necessary for self-development, expression, or maintenance of the ideal, proper integration into the community in terms of obtaining of roles and then proper performance of roles is central to the Confucian conception of personhood. All of this has implications for their views concerning abnormal or dysfunctional mental and behavioral states, their cause, and their implications for self-cultivation.

There are a number of interpretations on offer of the Confucian conception of personhood underlying their conception of self-development.[9] While my own view shares some elements with each of these interpretations, I offer here a modest account, pulling back somewhat from the more complete account I offer in other work.[10] My reason for this is not that I no longer accept this view, but rather that here I want to offer a general enough account of Confucianism on the self to capture the plausible aspects of a variety of positions, as well as to show the fundamental features of this conception of the self that are relevant to helping us understand Confucian views concerning madness and its connection to self-cultivation.

While my own interpretation offers a (perhaps radically) communalistic version of Confucianism, additional support for it comes from the fact that it adequately explains the Confucian views concerning madness and mental illness more generally, including Confucian ambivalence about the causes and the results of mental illness. I do not make a *strong* connection between my views of agency in Confucianism and the Confucian views of mental illness and self-cultivation I discuss in later chapters, because my interpretation of their views on mental illness and its roles stands independently of their view of the person. If one accepts the interpretation I offer of personhood in Confucian sources, however, the views of the Confucians concerning mental illness and self-cultivation become far more explicable. Thus we can see these interpretations mutually supporting one another.

I have to make one note on my categorization of these views by school, such as Confucian, Daoist, Zhuangist, Mohist, and so on. School (*jia* 家) affiliation is in many ways an anachronistic way to classify these positions. Thinkers like Mengzi, Xunzi, and Dong Zhongshu certainly saw themselves as

[9] My own views are outlined in McLeod 2013, 2012a, 2012, and 2009. Joel Kupperman offered a similar view in Kupperman 2004. Roger Ames discusses what he calls the "focus-field" self in numerous works, including Ames and Hall 1998, ch. 2, and most of Ames 2011, 60–61, 66–69, while Erica Brindley considers individual agency more specifically as part of the Confucian conception of personhood in Brindley 2010, 128–130. Brindley uses different categories than "Confucian," "Daoist," and so on, which are in some ways more proper and applicable to the Pre-Han period.

[10] See, for example, McLeod 2011 and McLeod 2012.

inhabiting a larger tradition that we can associate with the *ru* 儒, but this certainly never amounted to anything like a "school" with coherent doctrines or teachings, let alone other scholarly traditions like the amorphous "Daoism," which contains myriad tendencies, viewpoints, and teachings which are often in tension.[11] Among the *ru* as well, we see key disagreements between the adherents of Mengzi and Xunzi, among others. The separation of texts in the Han and Pre-Han periods into different school categories is itself a later phenomenon, started by the Han historian Sima Tan. Sima Tan invented the names for Daoism (*Daojia* 道家), Legalism (*fajia* 法家), and the School of Names (*mingjia* 名家), and applied the other already existing categories, *Ru*, Mohist, and *Yinyang* thought, in new ways.[12] Given that these categories were not in use before his time, the thought of texts in those times does not perfectly correspond to coherent schools of thought with shared doctrine, arguments, or positions. Though Sima Tan's categories are philosophically very useful, in part because they do show us relative similarity in strains of thought, there are vast divergences within these so-called schools. Perhaps a better way to render *jia* 家 then is "tradition," not in the sense of individuals and groups who shared a set of shared texts, teachings, or revered figures (although sometimes they did), but in the broader sense of the term used in the phrase "Chinese philosophical tradition," of a grouping of thinkers with certain important shared features, explained by shared influences, goals, and motivations of their unique time and place, recognized or not.[13]

The question naturally arises, of course, why use *any* affiliation term, rather than simply referring to the views found within a particular text or passage as the views of the author of that text or passage? The answer is that I think Sima Tan was onto *something* when he categorized texts into his *jia* classification.

[11] See Zufferey 2003, 149–150.

[12] Smith 2003, 129.

[13] Part of the difficulty here is that this term is standardly used to translate *zhuan* 傳, referring to the commentarial texts on important early documents such as the *Chunqiu*, or the *Liji*, associated with schools, which is a far more coherent and specific sense of "tradition" than intended here. Ironically, *zhuan* had more connection with actual schools, in terms of groups of people with shared doctrines, commentarial views, and transmission, than did the very loosely defined *jia*. I will render *jia* as "tradition" throughout the book, and it will be clear when I use the term to refer to something other than *jia*. Paul Goldin (Goldin 2011, 90) renders Sima Tan's *jia* as "house of thought," which is in the ballpark of what I intend here with "tradition," though I think Goldin's terminology suggests more coherence than *jia* often had. It is a tricky term to translate, given the connotations of any English word or phrase we might choose (and adding to the mix the fact that Sima Tan's conception of these groupings was itself problematic). I agree with Goldin's general position that Sima Tan "referred to philosophies that does not correspond to any organized school of thought" and grouped them according to ideological similarity. The situation is similar to labels used to describe philosophical views in contemporary philosophy: "realist," "naturalist," and so on. On "naturalism" as a particularly broad (and often problematic) moniker, see Brown and McLeod 2020, ch. 1.

And these shared features of texts and thinkers are relevant for my purposes here specifically because one of the fault lines along which thinkers of the relevant intellectual tendencies diverged was that of personhood—particularly concerning social norms, proper action, and mental state. The terms "Confucian," "Daoist," "Zhuangist," and so on do not work for every issue. These categories would not be particularly useful for helping make sense of the variety of early Chinese views of action (*xing* 行), ritual (*li* 禮), or even *dao* 道. They are indeed relevant on the issues of personhood and its attendant states, however, as this seems to be one of the main lines of disagreement between those categorized as Confucian, Daoist, and Zhuangist. The distinctions I make in this book between "traditions," however, do not completely match those of Sima Tan in his categorization of *jia*. While I follow Sima Tan's categorization of Confucianism and Mohism (which are the easiest, as these are the most coherent "school-like" traditions), I distinguish "Daoists," "Yangists," "Zhuangists," and "Syncretists" in a different way than Sima Tan did.[14] Perhaps the greatest divergence from his categories is in my use of "Zhuangist" and "Syncretist." The former is a category not included by Sima Tan at all, and the latter is a category understood very differently by Sima Tan. My justification for distinguishing "Zhuangist" from "Daoist" views likewise has to do with this particular issue of personhood and mental state. The view on personhood and states such as madness in the *Zhuangzi* goes far beyond what we find in texts such as *Daodejing*. The celebration of *kuang* and the elevation of the *kuang* person is a particular feature of the *Zhuangzi*, found throughout this text, but not in other texts known as "Daoist." Thus, the use of "Zhuangist" in this book flags a particular view of personhood found primarily in the *Zhuangzi*, although one that occasionally surfaces in other texts, as discussed in Chapter 4.

Given that there is such diversity within these traditions, due to the post-facto creation from independent sources, we should not expect to find coherent positions that we can call the "Confucian" position or the "Daoist" position. I want to concede this right up front. When I discuss the Confucian view of personhood, I am drawing a very broad picture of one dominant conception of persons found within many of the texts of the Confucian tradition in the Han and Pre-Han periods. Though I make the case for this view on the

[14] One complication is that it is not altogether clear exactly who Sima Tan considered representative of these *jia*. Some hold that his categorization of "Daoism," for example, referred primarily to Huang-Lao thought. See Song 2016.

basis of a number of positions put forward in early Confucian texts, this view of personhood cannot be said to be a strictly "Confucian" view, and to use this terminology is shorthand for this. The same can be said when I use "Daoist" and "Zhuangist" later. More than any of these, "Daoist" is vague, referring to the myriad method-based views found in texts such as the *Daodejing* or the *Liezi*.[15] I also refer to "Zhuangist" views rather than the views of Zhuangzi or the views of the *Zhuangzi*, mainly because the composite text *Zhuangzi* is so varied that many different views can be found within.[16]

The "Confucian" view of the person I outline here is a dominant view of personhood in the pre-Buddhist early Chinese tradition,[17] and it is challenged most seriously by the Zhuangists. In the Pre-Han philosophical milieu, the Confucian and Zhuangist conceptions of persons were the primary options, even though we find some other conceptions, all of which are variations on these larger themes.

The Confucian view of personhood, as I have argued in previous work, is that the person is primarily a communal entity.[18] The elements of the individual self, most notably roles, relationships, characteristic mental and physical features, and positions, come from other individuals to whom we are related, either biologically or communally. Certain physical and character traits may be attributable to my father, and through him my paternal grandparents, great-grandparents, and so on, while others may be attributable to my mother and her ancestors. The language I speak and the accent with which I speak it are attributable to my community—this is why I speak English as a first language, with a "General American" dialect and accent, as I grew up in urban and suburban areas on the East Coast of the United States, in a middle-class family. Had I grown up in Alabama, I would likely have a southern accent, and had I grown up in Beijing, Mandarin would likely be my first language, and I would speak it with a northern accent.

We can understand the elements of the individual self as resulting from a nexus of properties and elements from other sources.[19] Sometimes these are adopted by choice, as in the case of my selection of a school, which thereby creates in me certain attitudes and characteristics. Others are completely independent of our choice, such as the mental and physical features we inherit

[15] See Barnwell 2011.
[16] Liu 1994, 14–15; Ziporyn 2009, ix–x.
[17] Things change dramatically with the rise of Buddhism in China. See Berger 2016, 151–177.
[18] A view somewhat close to this can also be found in Kupperman 2004.
[19] This shares some similarity with the "role" self that Roger Ames discusses in Ames 2011.

from our parents, who themselves inherited them from their parents, and so on. Joel Kupperman points out that these features of the individual self, as themselves features of the community, commit the individual to respect for communal and traditional elements, according to the Confucians.[20] My own view follows this, arguing that for the Confucians the person is primarily a communal entity—this is much of the reason for the Confucian rejection of "primitivist" or anti-society approaches to self-cultivation and thriving, such as those they see as being offered by Daoists and Zhuangists.[21] We will see in Chapter 3 how this position underlies the Confucian negative portrayal of madness and mental illness, as well as their suspicion of the legitimacy of madness.

The *Analects* and *Xunzi* are perhaps the best early Confucian texts to consult for a picture of the Confucian view of the self. While the *Mengzi* is, of course, important, the shift toward *xin* 心 (mind) as a central aspect of the person shares much in common with Daoist/Zhuangist positions, and the *Mengzi* offers us a kind of hybrid Confucian-Daoist view. In the focus of the *Mengzi* on the development of aspects of the *xin*, we find a new position in Confucianism that has implications for their views of mental illness.

The key to the Confucian conception of personhood is its *communal* and social nature. A number of interpreters have commented on this aspect of Confucianism, which grounds the general Confucian commitment to society and the development of and maintenance of social order.[22] In numerous Confucian texts, we find explanations of the Confucian moral and political project—the attempt to bring about social harmony (*he* 和) through the construction of humanity (*ren* 仁) in terms of features of the human being. For the Confucians, the political project and the moral project of self-development go hand in hand, as the person is fundamentally political, fundamentally communal.

We find arguments throughout the early Confucian texts appealing to aspects of human nature or identity to establish moral or political norms. In the "Discussion of Ritual" chapter in the *Xunzi*, for example, the funerary rites are linked with care and concern for parents. Similarly, in *Analects* 17.21, Confucius chides his student Zaiwo for suggesting that the standard three-year ritual mourning period for a parent might be reduced to one year. After

[20] Kupperman 2004.
[21] McLeod 2012.
[22] Tu 1986; Tu 1985b; Yao 2006, ch. 6; Li 2014b, xii; among many others.

asking if Zai Wo would feel comfortable acting without grief for parents after only a year, the passage continues:

> 女安則為之！夫君子之居喪，食旨不甘，聞樂不樂，居處不安，故不為也。今女安，則為之！」宰我出。子曰：「予之不仁也！子生三年，然後免於父母之懷。夫三年之喪，天下之通喪也。予也，有三年之愛於其父母乎？(Confucius said): "If you are at peace with this, then do it. A morally exemplary person, however, throughout the period of mourning—even though he eats excellent food it is without taste, even though he listens to music he cannot enjoy it. If he remains in place, he does not feel at peace. Thus he does not (cut the mourning period short). But if you are at peace with it, then go ahead and do it." When Zai Wo left, Confucius said, "Yu [Zai Wo][23] is not humane. Not until a child reaches three years old does it leave the arms of its parents. The three years of mourning for one's parents is a common practice throughout the world. Didn't Yu receive three years of care from his parents?"

While Confucius's criticism of Zaiwo may appear to be primarily based on consideration of reciprocity, there is more than this going on. Zaiwo fails to be a *junzi* because he does not have the proper feelings simply on the basis of a consideration of who he is and who his parents are. For the morally exemplary person, this is enough. Moreover, Zaiwo fails even on a lesser standard of virtue. Even if one does not rise to the level of the truly filial son, one should *at least* be able to appreciate the need for reciprocity for care of one's parents, and Zaiwo fails even on this level. One's parents spend three years caring for and maintaining an individual when one is a baby, too young to fend for oneself. This care and concern creates a reciprocal obligation on the part of the child to observe ritual norms as they concern the parent. Still, the fundamental consideration should not be for repayment of benefits accrued, but a care for one's parent grounded in one's sense of shared identity.

The binding nature of rituals has to do with the person's identity as part of a particular community.[24] Confucius suggests in *Analects* 18.6 that the

[23] Yu 予 was Zai Wo's given name (Zai Yu 宰予). It is unclear how he got the courtesy name Wo 我, which ironically is a term for "self," and could be meant to express the inherent selfishness of Zai Wo, demonstrated in passages such as this one. I am indebted to a reviewer for raising this possibility.

[24] Mark Berkson, discussing Xunzi on ritual, writes: "individuals and communities have been shaped by rituals, meaning that their very identities might be, to a degree, constituted by the rituals that give their lives meaning. An emphasis on innovation and getting rid of old rituals risks divorcing people from their pasts and from the traditions and practices that have given their lives meaning." Berkson 2016, 262.

reason morality itself (including the rituals) is binding on the individual is due to one's identity as a person. To be a person is to be committed to the *dao* of the person—the moral way, which includes work on behalf of the community. Criticizing a number of hermits we might, following Chad Hansen, refer to as "proto-Daoists," Confucius says:

> 鳥獸不可與同群，吾非斯人之徒與而誰與？We cannot group together with the birds and beasts. If I do not follow the path of the human, then what can I follow?

If we understand *roles* created by a particular positioning within a community as part of one's identity and what creates obligation, we can make some sense of this communal conception. Roger Ames has developed what he calls "role ethics" as a way of understanding Confucianism. The idea behind this is that for the Confucians, roles are part of the self, defining it within the community, and that for the Confucian there can thus be no selves independent of a communal network of roles.[25] The reason particular norms are binding on an individual is because of the roles those responsibilities attach to. These include natural and selected roles. If one is a son, for example, the responsibility of filiality attaches to the individual, as this role requires filiality as part of its proper performance. Roles are fundamentally things that are *performed*, rather than static states or substances, and performance of role is understood in terms of the norms that guide this performance. To be a teacher, for example, is to act in certain ways, instructing and guiding students. To fail to instruct and guide students is not to be a teacher badly, but is to fail to be a teacher, as this particular kind of action defines the role of teacher.

This is part of what is behind the early Confucian focus on *zhengming* 正名 (rectification of names).[26] We can understand it as an attempt to define the particular kinds of action that constitute a role. Roles, as considered by the early Confucians, are not states that individuals have, but communal relations and norms connected to these, in part determined by standards for success discovered and constructed though successive generations. The *Xunzi* discusses this basis for norms, in looking closely at the funerary norms in the chapter *Lilun* 理論 ("On Ritual").

[25] See Ames 2011 and Mattice 2019.
[26] Mattice 2019 discusses this naming aspect of role ethics.

The funerary rituals, according to Xunzi, are part of the expression of grief for a parent who has died, and the performance of this grief is properly (and only) manifest in such rituals because what it means to be a son is determined by the construction of these ritual actions. That is, the role of son is defined by a certain range of activities, which are specified by history and culture (although the extent to which they are thus conventional rather than found in human nature or the world is a matter of debate).[27]

The source of *agency* for the person, according to the Confucians, is role and communal context. Individual choice and will are operative in that they allow one to perform a particular role, but there is a sense in which one does not act in capacity as a person until one acts in ways that are contextualized by one's roles, which are determined by various positions in community. The person, for the Confucians, is a primarily communal entity, determined and defined by roles based on communal position and communal features.

Given that the individuating features of the individual are features belonging to the community in some sense, either in a shared genetic sense or in the sense of shared cultural features or knowledge, an individual is always and only a combination of elements of a community or communities. This is true even if the individual rejects community and runs off to be a hermit in the fields or mountains like the proto-Daoists of *Analects* 18. One's mental and physical features are due to (and part of) one's parents, grandparents, and so on. One's speech is a feature of the community in which one learned to speak—and so on.[28] To reject the community and the social project is to fundamentally reject what one is, something from which one can never escape, no matter how much one may want to. If my communal roles and obligations obtain on the basis of my identity as *this* individual, with *these* parents, those roles and obligations do not change as long as I exist. To attempt to remove myself from this social context is like taking a car and putting it in the water to sail.

Not all human beings, on the traditional Confucian view, are persons. This is because persons have to be constructed, given their ineliminable social nature. There are necessary conditions for personhood that are not met by possessing all of the necessary and sufficient conditions for being a human

[27] I myself have come down on the strongly realist side of this debate (McLeod 2018b), following Goldin 1999, 73–75. Kurtis Hagen reads Xunzi as offering a conventionalist view on this. See Hagen 2003.

[28] This view is reminiscent of a traditional view among the Classic Maya of Central America, who extended this even to identity, in the view I call "embedded identity." I make this comparison in more detail in McLeod 2018c, 82–89.

being. This is not only the case for early Chinese views—the Kantian conception of agency holds autonomy and rationality as necessary features, and one might be a human being without full rationality or autonomy, even though these exemplify the nature of the person. The insufficiently rational individual does not qualify as a full person, and thus does not have the same rights and privileges as full persons. This is enshrined in the laws of a number of governments as well. Prior to the "age of reason" (however this is defined), individuals are not allowed participation in certain institutions or legal standing on certain decision, and so on.

On the Confucian view, a certain communal contextualization is necessary for personhood. This minimal threshold can be met in a number of ways, and self-cultivation continually happens beyond this to perfect oneself as a person. Given that certain key relationships between an individual self and others in a community are constitutive of personhood, one must actually be within a communal context to be a person. Individuals without communal context have no roles to exemplify, as they have turned their backs on this central constituent of their selves. While Confucius in *Analects* 18.6 suggests that such people do not reach minimal personhood because they lack communal context, it is unclear what they would say about the fact that, as Confucians in other places often admit, even those who completely reject the community still have a communal context in that they are children of particular parents, whether these parents are living or dead, whether they know them or not. As much as any individual might desire to decontextualize oneself from community, this is ultimately impossible to do for such reasons. One simply *is* the collection of states inherited from one's parents. The duties incumbent upon one as bearer of these roles, such as filiality, are generated not on the basis of choice, identity construction, or acceptance, but rather on the basis of unchangeable and unavoidable facts about who one is, about who one's parents are. You can't fail to have parents, and you can't change who your parents are. This is one of the most necessary truths about the individual. One could not have different parents than one has and yet still be oneself. That an individual has the two particular parents one has is a necessary feature of that individual. There are other central and determinative relationships, but this is the most basic, and the one that makes the best case for the Confucian position. This is perhaps one of the reasons the parent–child relationship (from the standpoint of the child) is one of the most discussed of the relationships in the Confucian tradition.

This communal conception of personhood is taken for granted for the most part in early Chinese texts, with the exception of a group of texts that resist the idea of communal personhood, instead locating the core of the person in conformity with natural patterns. Many of these texts are compiled in the *Zhuangzi*, with some found in other sources such as the *Daodejing*, and *Guanzi*. We find a direct attack on the communal conception of personhood in chapter 4 of the *Zhuangzi*, titled *Renjianshi* 人間世 (In the World of Persons). I argue in previous work that this title is a play on the Confucian conception of personhood—to be in the midst of persons is, according to the Zhuangist author(s), to fail to recognize the source of effective action. The chapter goes on, however, to engage in a subtle shift. While the Zhuangists may appear to be rejecting the concept of personhood, and arguing that rather than engaging in person-making-and-perfecting projects we should aim to deconstruct or eliminate the person, they actually argue for a very different conception of personhood. Personhood as properly understood, according to the Zhuangist view, is something we should aim for. The Confucian conception of personhood, however, makes it impossible to achieve true personhood, to become *true persons* (*zhen ren* 真人).

The Zhuangist conception of the *zhen ren* was a person who acted completely in accord with the natural patterns inherent in the *dao*, which for the Zhuangist required the undermining of particularizing commitments based in *shi-fei* (this–not this) conceptualization. This kind of conceptualization is what grounds critical kinds of distinction making, including right-wrong, true-false, and other fundamental distinctions without which we cannot make sense of a Confucian conception of personhood. While we see a variety of criticisms of personhood built on *shi-fei* conceptualization in the *Zhuangzi* as a whole, there are also a number of places in which there appear to be claims made about the essence of personhood that are inconsistent with this picture.[29] Part of the reason for this, I contend, is that there is no consistent position on this issue across the entirety of the *Zhuangzi* text. The *Zhuangzi* is a composite text, drawn from a number of roughly related sources that we might call a Zhuangist school, with "school" here used in the weakest of senses similar to the way we speak of a "postmodernist school"—that is, as referring to ideology, strain of thought, or philosophical family resemblance.[30] While there are a number of views developed throughout the text,

[29] Zhuangzi's discussion with Hui Shi about the essence (情*qing*) of humans and 是非 *shi-fei* conceptualization of chapter 5, for example.

[30] Liu 1994.

some to a greater degree than others, the most well-developed and supported view of personhood in the *Zhuangzi* is that developed in *Renjianshi* (although, as we will see in Chapter 4, this view is echoed elsewhere in the text).

A number of scholars have investigated the connection between Zhuangist views of self and person and those of Buddhism, which appears to have close connection with Zhuangist positions.[31] These scholars argue that in the *Zhuangzi* we find a deconstructive view of personhood and self we might understand as a "no-self" view.[32] The similarity in phrasing to the Buddhist *anatman* (no self) doctrine is not coincidental, as these views hold that the Zhuangists advocate something in important ways similar to the Buddhist doctrine, in which practitioners are encouraged to reject the view that selves exist (in terms of enduring and eternal bases of subjectivity, the *atman*). While the Zhuangist position is clearly not a rejection of anything like the *atman* of the Brahmanist Indian tradition, it does vehemently reject some conceptions of person construction, including that of the Confucians.

Part of the difficulty here is with the ambiguous use of the terms "self" and "person." Chris Jochim argues that the *Zhuangzi* does not offer a "no-self" view in anything like the Buddhist sense,[33] and this is certainly correct. There were no *atman*-like views being advanced in the time of the *Zhuangzi* for these thinkers to object to. In order to reject such a concept, they would have to be the ones to propose it—and why would they do this, if it were not already the kind of thing people were inclined to accept? There is some sense in which the Zhuangists can be said to have a "no-self" view, on a particular conception of "self."[34] But I think the use of the term "self" here is problematic, for a few reasons. The *ren* (human, person) the Zhuangists reject in *Renjianshi* is far from the kind of metaphysical entity most have in mind when they discuss the concept of self, as subject of experience. The reason we can accurately translate the Brahmanist concept of *atman* as "self" is that the eternal and changeless ground of personal identity in this tradition was *also* the subject of experience. Part of what was at

[31] Certainly early Chinese Buddhists thought so, leading to the loaning of Daoist terms to render Buddhist ideas originally discussed in Sanskrit and Pali, and leading to the development of the Chan (Zen) tradition, clearly involving heavy elements of Daoism. See Chen 2008.

[32] Berkson 2005; Graham 2001; Mair 2000.

[33] Jochim 1998.

[34] Something Mark Berkson points out in Berkson 2005, 294: "The meaning of 'no-self' in the context of any thinker or tradition will depend, of course, on the notion of a 'self' against which he or she is reacting. Two thinkers can both hold a position that can be accurately defined within their specific dialectical contexts as 'no-self' but hold very different positions from each other because the self each denies is different."

issue in the Buddhist rejection of the *atman* was whether we could make sense of the idea of a subject of experience without something like the eternal and changeless ground of personal identity. Numerous Buddhist philosophers argued that we can, and that we can thus reject the latter without losing the former.[35]

On the contrary, the Zhuangist rejection of the Confucian conception of *ren* was the rejection of certain ways of understanding the development of the self and the purposive behavior of the individual as tied to the community. The Zhuangists had little to say about either the issue of personal identity or the issue of the self as subject of experience. Their view is best understood, like that of the Confucians, in terms of the concept of the *person* rather than that of the self. I take here as a key component of the term "person" as used in English its reference to what John Locke called a "forensic notion" tied to agency and moral responsibility primarily. It is persons, rather than selves, who have roles, responsibilities, and even rights. Thus the Zhuangist view might be understood as a "no-person" view, but even this does not quite capture what they are after. The Zhuangists are careful, after all, to avoid doing the very thing they criticize others such as the Confucians for—devaluing certain things (whether valuations, discriminations, mental states, persons, or objects) in preference for others. Also, while they seemingly reject a Confucian conception of persons, they develop an alternative to this that allows them to explicitly endorse the idea of properly becoming a *ren* 人 (person), such that we might perfect ourselves and ultimately become "true persons." This perfection of personhood, though, takes place through undermining commitment to and habitual performance of *shi-fei* 是非 discrimination and performance of intentional agentive activity, and instead following the natural patterns (*tian li* 天理).

Notice that the difference here between the Confucian and Zhuangist is *not* that one requires conformity while the other values the development of autonomy. Both the Confucian and the Zhuangist are committed to a kind of robust conformity. This is certainly out of step with a common understanding of the Zhuangists as promoting individualism in opposition to Confucian communalism. The conformity called for by the Zhuangist (and similar thinkers) is complete, and perhaps beyond that called for by the Confucians.

[35] Discussion of a number of these philosophers can be found in MacKenzie 2008 and MacKenzie 2007.

The source is the key difference. Conformity to the natural patterns, for the Zhuangist, requires undermining *shi-fei* discrimination, which also thereby undermines desire, individual will, and choice. It is for this reason that the "true person" (*zhen ren* 真人) has the ability to act spontaneously (*ziran* 自然) in a manner others cannot. We will see in Chapter 4 that this has important implications for the Zhuangist view of madness.

The true person can act in this way because such a person follows along with the natural patterns, subsuming one's own agency in that of the patterns themselves. A number of passages across a range of early discuss this following of natural patterns. A passage from the *Chunqiu Fanlu* associates following *tian* with *dao* itself:

> 循天之道，以養其身，謂之道也。Following the way of *tian*, and using this to nourish oneself—this can be called *dao*.[36]

In chapters 24 and 15 of the *Zhuangzi*, following along (with the natural patterns, or with the world) is said to be the key to being a true person. The key passage from chapter 24 reads:

> 以順天下，此謂真人。And when one follows the world, they can be called a true person.[37]

The *Heshanggong* commentary to *Daodejing* 65 explains the *da xun* 大循 (great following) of the *Daodejing* passage:

> 玄德與萬物反異，故能至大順。順天理也。Mysterious potency and the myriad things are inverted, and thus one is able to arrive at the great following. Following the natural patterns.

For the Zhuangist (and later *Huainanzi*), conformity to the basic patterns of nature perfects the person, who is defined by a certain set of patterns. This presents an interesting difficulty for the Zhuangist view of madness and mental disorder. There is a tension at the heart of the Zhuangist view that is never completely resolved in any of their texts, and it suggests that perhaps the Zhuangists intended it to be left unresolved. Namely, they make the

[36] *Chunqiu Fanlu*, 77.1.
[37] *Zhuangzi* 24.13. Chapter 15 discusses 循天之理 (following the natural patterns).

distinction between perfected ways of following the natural patterns and nonideal ways, but at the same time hold that the myriad ways of human activity can all be held to have their own intrinsic value. This is not only a tension found across Zhuangist texts, but even within them—thus, it cannot be written off simply as a conflict between the views of different Zhuangist thinkers. It is structurally similar to the problem often leveled at the Academic Skeptics—if humans cannot have knowledge, how can we know *that*? There are a number of ways we might look to solve the Zhuangist problem, and it may be that the distinctions Zhuangists draw between things like "greater knowledge" (*da zhi* 大知) and "lesser knowledge" (*xiao zhi* 小知) are meant to solve this problem. Given their view of the person as based on pattern and their privileging of certain patterns as the natural patterns, it is hard to see how they can avoid the problem.

The Mind–Body Distinction

Numerous scholars in the West have advanced the view that there is no mind–body distinction in early Chinese thought. This claim is generally connected to the view that Chinese thought also had no room for distinction between human activity and agency and the operation of the natural world.[38] These views generally appeal to the organic metaphors and the discussion of whole entities such as persons or nature rather than body and mind or human and nature. It is not the case, however, that early Chinese texts *never* speak in terms of mind and body, or humanity and nature. Vivien Ng makes this claim as well in her book on madness in late imperial China.[39] She writes:

> Chinese physicians universally understood the many forms of madness to be organic disorders, and the language used to explain the pathology of *dian* and *kuang* was not at all different from that used to explain other illnesses. The notion that madness could be a *mental* illness was never advanced, not even by those who saw a distinct relationship between emotions and madness. The holistic approach of classical Chinese medicine has made the distinction between "physical" and "mental" alien to the Chinese

[38] A number of scholars have made such claims through the years. Some prominent examples include Ames and Hall 1998, 39; Hansen 1983, 178n18; and Hansen 2000, 17–18.
[39] Ng 1990, 50.

experience . . . behavioral disorders were certainly recognized—for example, the classic symptoms of *kuang* madness—but only as manifestations of physiological dysfunctions.[40]

There are a number of problems with this view.[41] While early Chinese thinkers likely did not conceive of the mind and the body in a Platonic or Cartesian sense, they certainly did posit a mind–body distinction, which can be found throughout early Chinese works. In this section, I offer some argument for the view that we should understand early Chinese thinkers as recognizing a mind–body distinction, one that becomes important in their thinking about behavior, illness, and the implications of both for self-cultivation. Indeed, disorders such as *kuang* 狂 (madness) could only have presented the kind of difficulty and opportunity for these thinkers that they did if there was a robust understanding of such a distinction.

While early Chinese thinkers did maintain a mind–body distinction, their conceptions of the distinction do not map neatly onto familiar historical Western ways of making the distinction. We find nothing like the kind of substance dualism offered by Descartes in early Chinese texts, in which mind and body form two separate and incompatible categories of basic "stuff" in the world. If we confine our conception of a mind–body distinction to substance dualism, however, we are likely to come away with the impression that early Chinese thinkers, and indeed anyone who lacked a Cartesian substance dualist conception of mind and body, made no distinction between mind and body. And this is simply false. Cartesian substance dualism is not the only way to distinguish between mind and body.[42]

The term most often associated with the body, and translated in English as such, is *shen* 身. Erica Brindley, following to some extent an "organicist" approach, claims that *shen* refers to "psychophysical aspects of the self," as

[40] Ng 1990, 50.

[41] Edward Slingerland argues against the view of mind–body holism in early China in Slingerland 2016, and most recently in Slingerland 2019. See also Slingerland and Chudek 2011. Martha Li Chiu also challenges this view in Chiu 1986. Paul Goldin argues for the mind–body distinction in early China as well as the separability of soul (through views of continuity of soul after death) in Goldin 2015.

[42] Zhang Zailin argues an integrative mind–body position such as that of Merleau-Ponty may be closer to that of early Chinese thinkers (Zhang 2011), though Zhang makes the common mistake of reading Descartes's view of mind and body in humans as nonintegrative. There are a variety of kinds of dualism, including property dualism, predicate dualism, and even views of mind that do not generally go by the moniker "dualist," but take mind as a different category of entity than the physical, such as emergentism, functionalism, and other theories that render mind as distinct from physical stuff, if not a distinct type of stuff.

distinct from *ji* 己, which is simply a reflexive term to refer to the self.[43] She understands *xin* 心 as an aspect of this *shen*, which she translates as "psychology," and associates it with *qing* 情. A particular reading of Western "dualism" may be behind the curtain here. Brindley presents the Western tradition, exemplified by Descartes, as associating the self with a disembodied mind, "disassociated from its psycho-physiological aspects by positing a sharp dichotomy between the mind and body."[44] This reading of Descartes is associated with the Western tradition by a number of other scholars as well.[45] There are some problems with this view. First, these positions tend to misconstrue the dominant Western conceptions as well as Cartesian substance dualism. Brindley writes:

> The self was conceptualized in terms of essences or essential characteristic—like that of the "ghost in the machine"—rather than embodied experiences. [. . .] Such an idea is also expressed very prominently in famous proclamations such as Descartes' "I think, therefore I am," which strips the self down to its most mental, essential, and disembodied nature.[46]

This interpretation of Descartes is problematic, as is this view of the mind–body distinction, which is certainly a radical thesis not widely held, if held at all. Descartes himself recognized the implausibility of the "ghost in the machine" view, as seen in the Sixth Meditation in his *Meditations on First Philosophy*, in which he describes the self as a mind–body unity, suggesting either a third substance, or something in nature distinct from either pure mental or physical substance. In his correspondence with Elizabeth of Bohemia, he insists on this, as a response to Elizabeth's objection concerning the seeming impossibility of mental causation on the dualist account Descartes appears to offer in the *Meditations*.[47] While he may be shifting his view to some extent in his response to Elizabeth, the mind–body union does feature prominently in the Sixth Meditation. It seems that Descartes may have at least had some hesitation concerning the dualist position outlined earlier in the *Meditations*. Part of Descartes's own explanation to those who challenged him concerning these points underscored an important feature

43 Brindley 2010, xxviii. While *shen* is also used in this reflexive way, *ji* is much more limited in its use, though it occasionally refers to something more substantive as well.

44 Brindley 2010, xxix.

45 See Zheng 2008, 397.

46 Brindley 2010, xxix.

47 Letter to Princess Elizabeth, May 21, 1643, in Cottingham et al. 1991, 217.

of the *Meditations* that is still often missed by scholars. Namely, that all of the claims Descartes makes prior to the Sixth Meditation are provisional steps that are superseded later in the text. For example, the *cogito* (purely thinking thing) envisioned in the Second Meditation is what Descartes uses to gain certainty of his existence, but it is *not* his settled view on the nature of the self. Descartes needs only the fact that he is *at least* a thinking thing to establish his own existence. And the *cogito* is all he can demonstrate in the face of radical skepticism. This does not, however, entail that the *cogito* is all he takes himself to be or is the fundamental constituent of the self. If this were the case, Descartes could have stopped with the Second Meditation. While he does speak in terms of *having* a body, we equally speak of *having* a mind—it is not clear that an identity is made between the self and either of these. What he fundamentally is, according to the final view of the *Meditations*, is a mind–body unity. While mind and body are understood as distinct substances, it is incorrect to say that Descartes understood the self to be a mind inhabiting a body—rather, Descartes understood the self as a mind–body unity.

Thus, to hold that early Chinese thought does not recognize a clear mind–body distinction on the basis of its failure to identify the self with purely mental function is problematic. Descartes, at least in some parts of his work, also does not identify the self with purely mental function, yet he is seen as the archetype of a thinker who drew a clear distinction between mind and body (Plato aside). Indeed, Plato and Descartes are often linked in consideration of this view, but it is Plato rather than Descartes who had something much closer to a "ghost in the machine" type view. Even in the case of Plato, however, this is not quite right. We cannot properly call the self a soul enmeshed in a body, because the body ultimately has a lower level of reality than the soul, as the body is a changing, noneternal thing. It is not that the soul and body are two distinct substances that interact, but rather are distinct kinds of thing altogether. Clearly, a mind–body distinction can be drawn without commitment to the kind of disembodied conception of the self often associated with the Western tradition. And the fact that Chinese texts often stress the physical embodiment of mental effects does not in itself show that they made no hard distinction between mind and body, *xin* and *shen*.

We can look to the terms and concepts employed in early Chinese texts to draw out a fuller picture of mind–body distinction in these texts. The term *shen* refers to the body of the individual, but it sometimes also refers to the self in a reflexive way similar to *ji*. The two can be interchangeable, and we see them as such in numerous early texts. As reflexive, *shen* could refer to the body specifically, or the entire person, and thus we have to take care with a reading of this concept. The term *ti* 體, which is also used to refer to the body, is much more specific and narrower in scope, lacking the kind of reflexive self-referential use of *shen* or *ji*. We also find use of the term *xing* 形, which, like *ti*, is not used reflexively, and can also refer to other physical forms, but also in some cases refers to the *person* more generally, and many cases the body more specifically.

We see a number of places in early Chinese texts in which distinctions are drawn between the mind and body, and states of body contrast with and can be cultivated separately of mental states. A key test of whether a thinker posits a distinction between mind and body is that of causal independence. Descartes, for example, held that different mental states are possible even given exactly duplicate physical states. The physical states involved do not have a causal effect on the independent mental states, or the mental states retain independence of these states.

While early Confucian texts often suggest that mental and physical states are dependent on one another (in terms of motivations and behaviors), there are also numerous places within early texts, including Confucian texts, where different views are suggested. In the final passage of the last chapter of the *Xunzi*, for example,[48] the author claims the possibility of putting on a visage (*se* 色) of madness while retaining the mind of a sage.[49] While it is unclear exactly what is entailed by having the appearance of a madman, the text seems clear that it is consistent with retaining a sage's mind, such that the behavior alone does not affect the mental state. The *Zhuangzi* also suggests the possibility of retaining certain mental states while altering our behavior and physical states. In Yan Hui's discussion with Zhuangzi's version of Confucius in *Renjianshi*, he offers as a possible solution to the problem of remonstration that internally (*nei* 內) he retains his uprightness while externally (*wai* 外) conforming.

> 則我內直而外曲，成而上比。內直者，與天為徒
>
> Thus I will internally remain straight and externally bent (to circumstances), completing my task by conforming to the superior. Those who remain internally straight are the followers of heaven.[50]

[48] A passage we return to in Chapter 3, as it bears on Confucian views on madness.
[49] *Xunzi* 32.7.
[50] *Zhuangzi* 4.1.

This internal/external distinction here plausibly equates to the mental state/behavior distinction, where behavior is seen in terms of what is accessible by other people, which is physically manifested. Others can see one's physical behaviors, but cannot see one's mental states, at least directly. Even though Confucius criticizes this approach of Yan Hui, the fact that the possibility is raised here shows that the author is aware of a mind/body distinction, and that such a distinction would also have been accepted by contemporaries.

Edward Slingerland argues for a distinction between mind and body in early Chinese thought along similar lines, in his book *Mind and Body in Early China*. After criticizing "monistic" readings of mind and body in scholarship on early China using methodology similar to my own here, Slingerland applies what he calls a "digital humanities" approach to the material, demonstrating that terms for mind and body are contrasted and used in ways that show that various kinds of mind–body dualism can be found in early China well before the advent of Buddhism. Arguing against what he calls the "myth of holism" in early China, Slingerland shows that *xin* is understood as a distinct kind of entity from physical organs, organizing and in charge of these organs. He argues for the intrinsic "otherness" of the mind in early Chinese texts,[51] as discussions associated with *xin* are fundamentally different from those involving physical organs and states. In addition to the concept of mind (*xin*), Slingerland discusses various conceptions of soul and locates a variety of passages in early Chinese texts that take *xin* as immaterial, in control of the self, and the source of free will and moral responsibility. In one of these passages from chapter 21 of the *Xunzi*, we find a particularly compelling dualist view of *xin* as "ruler" or "lord" (*jun* 君) of the body, which suggests not only a mind/body distinction, but importantly for our purposes, a sense that behavior is explained ultimately by features of the *xin*. Such a view makes it a natural move to propose that disordered conduct is caused by disordered mind. The passage from *Xunzi* reads:

> 心者，形之君也，而神明之主也，出令而無所受令。自禁也，自使也，自奪也，自取也，自行也，自止也。故口可劫而使墨云，形可劫而使詘申，心不可劫而使易意，是之則受，非之則辭。

The *xin* is the lord of the body, and master of its spiritual intelligence. It issues orders and takes orders from no one. It restricts itself, manages itself, struggles

[51] Slingerland 2019, 111.

with itself, takes hold of itself, allows itself to proceed, forces itself to stop. Therefore, while the mouth can be forced to remain silent or speak, and the body can be forced to bend or straighten, the *xin* cannot be forced to change its mind. What it considers right is accepted, what it considers wrong is rejected.[52]

When we look to early medical literature, such as the *Huangdi Neijing* 黃帝內經 texts and the *Nan Jing* 難經, we find additional information on early conceptions of the body and its connection to mind. The conception of body and mind in early medical texts is particularly important for this project, as it informs the way mental illness was conceived in early China. The *Huangdi Neijing* texts remind us that while we can certainly make sense of a mind/body distinction in these texts, nothing like substance dualism can be found in them. To the extent that there are differences between them, mind and body are different formations of *qi* 氣, but ultimately they are both caused by and constituted by (the formulation depends on which text we look at) *qi*.

The *Huangdi Neijing* discusses physical attributes in distinction with others in a number of places. In the first chapter of *Suwen*, three aspects of the individual are related to *qi*:

是以志閑而少欲，心安而不懼，形勞而不倦，氣從以順，各從其欲，皆得所願。

This is why when the *will* (zhi) is relaxed there are few desires, when the *mind* (xin) is at peace one is without fear, and when the *appearance* (xing) is toiling one is not worn out. The *qi* follows its course, each thing follows its desires, and all obtain their ends.[53]

Here, will and mind are distinguished from appearance, that which is accessed externally, but which here seems to refer to the entire body. It is not simply that one *seems* to be toiling, but that one is actually toiling, without being worn out. Appearance in the sense of "seeming" is generally indicated by *se* (色), as in the case of the *Xunzi* passage earlier. The *Huangdi Neijing* attributes the particular state of physical and mental entities to *qi*. *Qi* is stored in the five *zang* 藏 (organs, storehouses) of humans. The quality and quantity of *qi* in these organs as well as their transformations—the way the *qi* moves

[52] *Xunzi* 21.9. Hutton 2016, 229.
[53] *Huangdi Neijing Suwen* 1.2.

and interacts with other organs as well as the outside world—determines one's physical and mental state. Various kinds of illness, physical and mental, are caused by particular quantities and movements of *qi* in the organs. It is not only disorder that is thus caused by *qi*, however. Strength, health, and the proper functioning of the entire human organism (body and mind) are likewise due to *qi*. Whether or not it turns out that all physical and mental phenomena reduce to *qi*, it is clear that *qi* is at least causally responsible for all of our mental and physical states.

According to the *Huangdi Neijing* and other texts such as *Neiye* and Zhuangist texts, the key to cultivation of health is ultimately the same as that of cultivating normatively proper action. Following the *dao* (or natural patterns, *tian li* 天理) is this key. This may seem vague, as the Confucians, Mohists, and other thinkers would all agree that there is a particular *dao* we should follow.[54] The issue here is just what this *dao* amounts to—is it the ritual and social *dao* of the Confucians, or the *dao* of following "natural patterns" of the Zhuangist? Texts such as the *Huainanzi* envision the possibility of unifying these various *dao* in a single *dao*. The natural patterns for the social human, we might say, comprise the human *dao* the Confucians discuss. The natural patterns applied to statecraft, perhaps, entail the *dao* of Han Feizi. The *dao* the *Huangdi Neijing* seems to have in mind is that of following the natural patterns for the proper transformation of *qi*, the increase and decrease of *qi* in the organs, in concert with the transformations of *qi* external to the body, connected to aspects of the world such as the seasons, climate, time of day, and other regularities of nature. The key to ideal functioning of the entire human organism (body and mind) is the retention and skillful transmission of *jingshen* 精神 or *jing qi* 精氣 (essential spirit), which is the definitive *qi* of human life. The cultivation of this kind of *qi*, according to *Huangdi Neijing*, has not only physical effects but effects on the functioning of the entire human organism. Ethical considerations cannot be taken as separate from medical considerations. A passage from *Suwen*, chapter 1, describes the state of those who follow the *dao*, and its physical, mental, and moral effects:

> 余聞上古有真人者，提挈天地，把握陰陽，呼吸精氣，獨立守神，肌肉若一，故能壽敝天地，无有終時，此其道生。中古之時，有至人者，淳德全道，和於陰陽，調於四時，去世離俗，積精全神，游行天地之間，視聽八達之外，此蓋益其壽命而強者也，亦歸於真人。

[54] *Analects* 18.6.

> In high antiquity there were true men (*zhen ren*). They upheld the patterns of heaven and earth and they grasped the regularity of yin and yang. They exhaled and inhaled essence qi. They stood for themselves and guarded their spirit. Muscles and flesh were like one. Hence, they were able to achieve longevity, in correspondence with heaven and earth. There was no point in time when their life could have come to an end. Such was their life in the Way. At the time of middle antiquity, there were the accomplished men. They were of pure virtue and they were entirely in accord with the Way. They adapted themselves to the regularity of yin and yang and they lived in harmony with the four seasons. They left the world and they departed from the common. They accumulated essence and preserved their spirit. They roamed between heaven and earth and their vision as well as their hearing went beyond the eight reaches. This way, they added to their lifespan and were strong. They, too, may be counted among the true men.[55]

Notice here the connection of these sages of the past who acted in accord with *dao* and the "true person" (*zhen ren* 真人). This is the same terminology used in Zhuangist texts to describe the ideal person who follows the natural patterns rather than cutting against them by engaging in *shi-fei* conceptualization. The suggestion here is that the following of the natural patterns is to preserve one's essential *qi* through mental and physical cultivation that amounts to *qi* retaining and transforming processes. The chapter goes on to discuss two different kinds of person, the sage (*sheng ren* 聖人) and the worthy (*xian* 賢), which are presented as less than the other two but still skillful. The main focus of this ranking of persons for the *Suwen* is to describe the actions of these persons and how these actions issued in a certain length of life. The *zhen ren* seems to be connected to immortality,[56] while the other categories of person attain long lives.

Texts involving related concepts of the person, such as the *Zhuangzi*, *Huainanzi*, and *Huangdi Neijing*, see self-cultivation as involving mental, physical, and moral elements.[57] Moral and other normative elements are ineliminable parts of how we determine both illness and health, and proper functioning of the human organism. The physical effects of certain states of *qi* are

[55] *Huangdi Neijing Suwen* 1.4; Unschuld and Tessenow 2011, 42–43.

[56] The later Daoist concept of the 仙 *xian* (immortal) develops from this. Note that the idea of reclusion in the mountains (the person of the mountains) is inherent in this term—an image also connected with madness, as I discuss in Chapter 4.

[57] This can even be found in texts such as the *Mengzi*. Recall Mengzi's discussion of his 浩然之氣 (flood-like *qi*) and its effects in *Mengzi* 2A2.

paralleled by mental and moral effects, and likewise one cannot cultivate the body to attain health and long life without developing and guarding the very thing that also leads to mental and moral well-being, namely the essential *qi*. While mental and physical features were taken as substantially similar parts of a single organism, both explained by *qi*, early Chinese thinkers did recognize a difference between the two and would focus on one or the other depending on the primary aim of the text. Thus, in *Huangdi Neijing* we find a greater focus on the body and on aspects of the mind closely related to physical health. In the *Huainanzi*, we find greater focus on morality and knowledge.

Mind in Early Chinese Texts

We don't find much explicit discussion of the *xin* 心 ("heart-mind" or "mind") in Confucianism until the *Mengzi*, which develops a view concerning *xin* as central to the person unlike anything else in early Confucian thought. The Mengzian view is likely influenced by Daoist/Zhuangist sources.[58] While we certainly do find discussion of mental illness in early Confucian texts outside the *Mengzi*, it is never discussed in terms of the disorder of one's *xin*. We will see that this is an important distinction in early Confucianism and Chinese philosophy in general. In general, thinkers will attribute as much to the mind in the case of behavioral disorder or "mental illness" as they do with normal or ideal human behavior. Thus, when communal patterns or situational features are most operative in causing behavior on a particular view, disorder will be a function primarily of dysfunctional communal patterns and situational features. Part of the reason we find an underdeveloped view of mental illness in much of early Confucianism is the early Confucian suspicion of individual agency and the decentered nature of their theories of mind. Mengzi, of all the early Confucians, was best placed to offer an account of mental illness, but there is oddly a silence on this topic in the *Mengzi* when compared with other early Confucian texts like the *Analects* and *Xunzi*.

In the *Analects*, we find *xin* as the locus of desires (*yu* 欲), which can guide actions of the individual (*Analects* 2.4), and reflect on or otherwise contain *ren* 仁 (*Analects* 6.7). In the *Mengzi* we hear much more about *xin*, possibly as a response to concerns with the *xin* in competing texts such as the *Laozi*,

[58] Lee 2005, 13.

Zhuangzi, and *Guanzi*. These latter texts, which I look at later, flesh out a clear view of the *xin* that distinguishes it from other aspects of the person.

In the *Mengzi*, the *xin* plays the role of the ground of the sprouts (*duan* 端) of virtue contained in our nature. In 1A7, Mengzi in his discussion with King Hui of Liang claims that the king's compassionate response to an ox and his trading it for a sheep shows that King Hui possesses a *xin* sufficient to be a king. Mengzi makes clear that what he refers to is not the act of swapping the ox for a sheep, but rather the king's inability to bear the suffering of the ox (*bu ren* 不忍). He also there sees the *xin* as something that contains states such as compassion and joy. Mengzi elaborates on this in 2A6, explaining that all persons have minds that cannot bear the suffering of others (*bu ren ren zhi xin* 不忍人之心). Late in 1A7, Mengzi refers to the "constant mind" (*heng xin* 恆心). Mengzi claims here that certain states are necessary conditions for having a constant mind:

> 無恆產而有恆心者，惟士為能。若民，則無恆產，因無恆心。苟無恆心，放辟，邪侈，無不為已。
>
> Those who are without a constant livelihood yet can maintain a constant mind—only true scholars are capable of this. As far as the people in general, if they lack constant livelihood, they will not maintain constant minds. If they lack constant minds, they will break laws, indulge in vice and excess, and there is nothing they will not do.[59]

Mengzi also speaks about a similar concept, the "unmoved mind" (*bu dong xin* 不動心) in 2A2, which appears related to the unperturbed mind of 1A7. Notice that this claim in 1A7 is only for necessary conditions. It is not a claim that states of character constitute *xin*, rather that the *xin* can only be constant when one possesses these traits, which then leads to vicious action similar to that of the madman. Thus in the *Mengzi* we see the beginnings of a natural association with madness and abandon, with lack of the kind of constraints and cultivation that the civilized and socialized person is expected to have. The disordered *xin* will make it possible for a person to act without restraint, in the ways associated with the madman (*kuang ren* 狂人), whom we encounter in Chapter 2.

In 2A2, Mengzi gives us a more robust account of the *xin*, in discussing the unmoved mind, that begins to clarify its connection with conceptions

[59] *Mengzi* 1A7.

of the body and vital spirit. Discussing Gaozi's views of the mind, Mengzi says:

> 告子曰：『不得於言，勿求於心；不得於心，勿求於氣。』不得於心，勿求於氣，可；不得於言，勿求於心，不可。夫志，氣之帥也；氣，體之充也。夫志至焉，氣次焉。故曰：『持其志，無暴其氣。』
>
> Gaozi says: "what you do not find in words, do not search for in the mind, and what you do not find in the mind, do not search for in the vital energy (*qi*)." Now, the claim that what you do not find in the mind, do not search for in the vital energy—this is acceptable. The claim that what you do not find in words, do not search for in the mind—this is unacceptable. The will (*zhi*) controls the vital energy, and vital energy is what suffuses the body. Will is completed first, and the vital energy follows. This is why I say: "cultivate your will, do not brutalize your will."[60]

The *xin* clearly has a major regulative role to play for Mengzi, and one connected to elements of the person any Western philosopher would recognize as primarily or even wholly mental. In the earlier passage from 2A2, we find *xin* at least distinguished from the body. The term *ti* 體 here refers to the body, and the body is suffused or flooded (*chong* 充) with *qi*. But the text says here that the will, which is connected here with the mind, is distinct from, and controls, the *qi*. Thus, there is already a distinction made here between the *xin* and other aspects of the person, including the vital energy and the body. It seems too much to think of Mengzi's *xin* as "psychophysical" other than in the sense that the mind *controls* the physical and the psychophysical. If there is anything in this picture that should be seen as continuous with mind and body, it is *qi*.

As shown in the *Mengzi* passage earlier, the mind (or the will as contained in the mind) plays a coordinating role for *qi*. But notice that this does not show that Mengzi does not accept a clear distinction between the mind and body. Any conception of mind will have to have an account of mental causation, as one of the most basic facts of life we first notice is that we seem to have control over (many of) our bodily actions on the basis of thoughts, intentions, and aspects of what we call mind. Even Descartes and other

[60] *Mengzi* 2A2.

Cartesians, who many take as the arch dualist, had an account of mental causation. Descartes's own answer to the seeming problem with mental causation that his substance dualism created was to insist on the person as a third type of substance, a "mind–body unity."[61]

The mind has the role of controlling and guiding *qi*, which is directly responsible for motion of the body as well as thoughts. *Qi* is perhaps the most unique category of the person in early China as compared with much of Western thought. While it is not the same as the physical body, it animates the body and also has a vital and animate quality, unlike the mind. "Psychophysical stuff" has been proposed as a translation for *qi*,[62] as it has elements of both mind and body. It serves in some sense as an intermediary between the two, as we see in the *Mengzi* passages. As Bryan Van Norden writes, of Mengzi's conception of *qi*: "*qi* . . . straddles the dualism between mind and body that has become a fixture of post-Cartesian philosophy in the West: *qi* is embodied emotion."[63]

In other texts of the period, we find similar conceptions of *xin*. In the *Mozi*, the *xin* is presented as something that can investigate,[64] reflect,[65] discriminate,[66] and in which things such as care (愛 *ai*) can be collected.[67]

In *Neiye*, the *xin* is the source of emotions and has a natural state that can be lost through dissipative actions and attitudes (this will become central in consideration of the medical context). The mind in the context of *Neiye* is important for our purposes, as it is in this text that we see one of the strongest connections drawn between the natural patterns or the *dao* and particular states of mind. This is something we find in Daoist, Zhuangist, and Han correlative texts as well, but the *Neiye*'s formulation is one of the clearest.

In the *Zhuangzi*, the mind is taken as the source of most of the problems of humanity. Having a settled or "completed" mind (*cheng xin* 成心) is to be stuck within a particular perspective, and this makes it impossible to follow the natural propensities.[68] It is just this that the *Zhuangzi* recommends we rid ourselves of by engaging in the "fasting of the mind" (*xin zhai* 心齋) discussed in

[61] Descartes, *Meditations on First Philosophy*, Sixth Meditation. There has been debate among scholars concerning whether Descartes's mind–body unity was a third substance alongside mind and body, and whether Descartes should thus properly be considered a substance *trialist* rather than a dualist. See Nolan 2015.

[62] Also mentioned in Van Norden 2011, 97.

[63] Van Norden 2011, 98.

[64] *Mozi* 9.5; 40.91.

[65] *Mozi* 5.4.

[66] *Mozi* 40.93.

[67] *Mozi* 2.3; 40.98.

[68] *Zhuangzi* 2.4.

Chapter 4. Here, the mind is contrasted again with *qi*, with the suggestion that the mind includes our various conceptualizations, plans, will, and deliberation, while *qi* is something more instinctual, that can operate on its own without the higher-level deliberations of the *xin*, and which on its own can more effectively follow the natural propensities. In its imagined exchange between a Zhuangist version of Confucius and his student Yan Hui, Confucius says:

无聽之以耳而聽之以心，无聽之以心而聽之以氣。聽止於耳，心止於符。氣也者，虛而待物者也。唯道集虛。虛者，心齋也。

> Do not listen with the ears, but listen with the mind. Do not listen with the mind, but listen with *qi*. Listening stops at the ears, and the mind stops with signs. As for *qi*, it is empty and waits for things. The *dao* collects emptiness. And in emptiness is the fasting of the mind.[69]

The fasting of the mind Confucius enjoins here is a move away from dependence on the mind to a dependence on the (spontaneous) movement of *qi*. This suggests that the mind is the source of deliberation, planning, willful action, choice, conceptualization, and everything else that characterizes the human being. It is this conceptualization, *shi-fei* 是非, according to the Zhuangists, that is both the essence and nature of humans,[70] a view the Zhuangists seem to share with Mengzi.

In the *Zhuangzi*, the lesson seems to be that any conceptualization on the part of the mind is ultimately undermining. This position has deep implications for the way Zhuangists ultimately conceive of madness, disorder, and norm-divergent behavior of all kinds.

In Han texts, we begin to see focus on different aspects of the person. The concept of *jingshen* 精神, while we see it discussed in Pre-Han texts, comes to form the basis for thinking about the animation and abilities of the human person in the Han. In the *Huainanzi*, *jingshen* is understood as a uniquely human form of *qi*, perhaps connected with the abilities of the mind, distinct from forms of *qi* which lack these features.[71] The *Taiping jing* also discusses *jingshen*, offering the view that this complex (*jing* and *shen* as two forms of *qi*[72]) animates the body. Hubert Seiwert explains: "a body without *jing* and

[69] *Zhuangzi* 4.2.
[70] See *Zhuangzi* 5.6, Zhuangzi's discussion with Hui Shi on the human *qing* 情 (essence).
[71] See introduction to *Jingshen* chapter in Major et al. 2010.
[72] Seiwert calls them "the more subtle forms of *qi*" in Seiwert 2018, 270.

shen is just a corpse. The body is like a city, while *jing* and *shen* are like the senior officials. The officials control the fate of the people in the city."[73]

The Han period text *Huangdi Neijing* is the main source of medical understandings of physical and mental disorder in early China, and an additional place to look for understandings of mind and body and their relationship. In the *Huangdi Neijing*, mental phenomena are more commonly referred to in terms of *jingshen* or *jing qi*, referring to the kind of *qi* unique to humans, associated with sentience and mentality. When there is a dualistic distinction drawn in terms of internal/external, we see that it is not the mind (*xin*) distinguished from the body, but *qi*. Chapter 6 of the *Huangdi Neijing Suwen* reads:

> 陰陽𩾺𩾺，積傳為一周，氣裏形表而為相成也。
>
> Yin and yang move endlessly. Repeated transmission constitutes one cycle. The qi inside and the physical appearance outside, they complete each other.[74]

While the *qi* is put into this direct dualistic relationship with the body, or "physical appearance" (*xing* 形), it is the mind that controls the *qi*, according to *Suwen*, chapter 9, and forms the "root" of life. ("The mind is the basis/root of life; it is responsible for the changes of the spirit."[75]) This confuses things to some extent—there are numerous passages throughout the *Huangdi Neijing* and other early texts that claim both that *qi* is fundamental and that mind is fundamental. The same passage from *Suwen*, chapter 9 that claims the mind as the root of life also claims that the lung is the root of *qi*.[76] The opening passage of the *Neiye* claims that the *jing* 精 (essence) of all things is what gives them life. This *jing* seems to refer to the *jingshen* or *jing qi* discussed in *Huangdi Neijing* and *Huainanzi*.

> 凡物之精，此則為生下生五穀，上為列星。
>
> The *jing* of each thing is that in which it has life. Below, the five grains are generated, and above, the orders of stars are made.[77]

[73] Seiwert 2018, 271.
[74] *Huangdi Neijing Suwen* 6.3; Unschuld and Tessenow 2011, 135.
[75] *Huangdi Neijing Suwen* 9.7; Unschuld and Tessenow 2011, 178.
[76] The etymology of the term reflects this as well, with *qi* originally referring to the breath, with the view that the breath is what animates living beings. *Qi* retains this meaning of vapor, steam, breath. See Kuriyama 1999, 236.
[77] *Guanzi* 49.1.

We see the development of a particular conception of mind in the *Neiye* that suggests many of the features of the Zhuangist and later Huang-Lao accounts, and it can help us understand some of what is going on concerning the stark differences in attitudes concerning madness and similar states in early texts.

It is clear in the *Neiye* that *qi* is fundamental and the basis of life—in agreement with parts of the *Chunqiu Fanlu*, *Huangdi Neijing*, and a number of other texts. It is *jing* (essential *qi*), according to the first line of the text, from which things are born.[78] The text goes on to describe in a number of passages the particular features of the mind and its role in regulating states of the body:

> 我心治，官乃治。我心安，官乃安。治之者心也，安之者心也
>
> When our minds are regulated, the senses are regulated as well. When our minds are at rest, the senses are at rest as well. What regulates the senses is the mind; what places the senses at rest is the mind.[79]
>
> 人能正靜，皮膚裕寬，耳目聰明，筋信而骨強，乃能戴大圜，而履大方。鑒於大清，視於大明。敬慎無忒，日新其德；徧知天下，窮於四極；敬發其充，是謂內得。然而不反，此生之忒。
>
> When a man is able to attain balanced tranquility, his skin is sleek, his flesh full, his eyes sharp, his ears keen, his muscles taut, his bones sturdy. And so he is able to carry the great circle of heaven on his head and tread upon the great square of earth. He finds his reflection in the great purity and sees by the great light. Attentive and cautious, he never errs, and every day renews the force of his virtue. Knowing everything in the world and exhausting the four poles of the earth, he attentively nurtures his plentitude: this is called: grasping within. To be so and never to revert is life without error.[80]
>
> 全心在中，不可蔽匿。和於形容，見於膚色。
>
> When the mind completed lies within, it cannot be concealed. It may be known through the form and countenance, seen through the skin and expression.[81]

78 凡物之精，此則為生.
79 *Guanzi* 49.5, Eno trans., p. 8, adapted.
80 *Guanzi* 49.5, Eno trans., p. 9, adapted.
81 *Guanzi* 49.6, Eno trans., adapted.

This final passage suggests a deep connection between mind and body. While this is true in the case of *Neiye* and most other early Chinese texts, it does not show that the two are indistinct. In fact, in drawing this connection, it further demonstrates that there is recognition of the distinction of mind and body. The regulated mind has a certain causal effect on behavioral states, such that it becomes impossible to make one's physical states such that they do not manifest this regulated mind. Thus, one can use the body as a means for knowing the mind. Notice that this conflicts with the final chapter of the *Xunzi*, which claims that Xunzi was able to retain his sagely mind while appearing visibly as a madman. We might explain this by positing a kind of subtle distinction in appearance or visage (*se* 色) between the sage feigning madness and the true madman that a discerning person would recognize, but this does not seem like the kind of claim the *Neiye* passage wants to make. It is not that the regulated mind cannot be concealed from other sages or those who have a fine level of discernment, but that it cannot be concealed from *anyone*. Otherwise, the point of the passage is undermined. The implication of the inability to conceal the mind of this passage is that the regulated mind is manifest to everyone around the sage, such that it leads to *their* ordering as well.

> 氣意得而天下服。心意定而天下聽。
>
> But when the intent of the *qi* is in one's grasp, the world will submit. When the intent of the heart is fixed, the world will listen.[82]

A major part of the intended lesson of the *Neiye* in general is that control of the *qi* through developing aspects of the mind leads to thriving, in terms of physical, mental, and moral health. This is similar to what we find in the *Huangdi Neijing* medical texts, with the main difference in focus on the particular effects of cultivation. The general view that cultivating certain states of *qi* through operation on the mind has myriad effects on the various aspects of the human organism is common to early Chinese texts. We find something like it across the spectrum of schools and philosophical tendencies in early texts. The mind/body connection in early texts such as *Guanzi* is primarily understood in terms of cause and effect for particular mental and physical states relevant to thriving. The primary purpose of the mind,

[82] *Guanzi* 49.6. Eno trans., adapted.

according to *Neiye* and other texts, is to regulate the *qi* and thus understand *dao*, which then allows one to follow the natural patterns of *dao*, and thus generate an inexhaustible potency.

Neiye says of the relationship between mind and *dao*:

> 凡道無所，善心安愛，心靜氣理，道乃可止。
>
> The *dao* has no fixed place; it dwells at peace in a good heart. When the mind is tranquil and the *qi* aligned, the *dao* may be made to stay.[83]

Recognition of *dao* is attained through silencing or stilling the mind, according to the tradition in which *Neiye* falls. *Zhuangzi*, *Huainanzi*, and other Daoist texts follow this view. While the traditional Confucian view of the mind is somewhat different, we find significant overlap between it and this view as well, especially in texts such as the *Mengzi*. The *Huangdi Neijing* texts also discuss the role of the mind as restraining and modifying or otherwise operating on *qi*:

> 心者，君主之官也，神明出焉。
>
> The mind is the official functioning as ruler. Spirit illumination originates in it.[84]
>
> 心者，生之本，神之變也，其華在面，其充在血脈
>
> The mind is the basis of life; it is responsible for changes of the spirit. Its effulgence is in the face. Its fullness manifests itself in the blood vessels.[85]

83 *Guanzi* 49.2. Eno trans., adapted.

84 *Huangdi Neijing Suwen* 8.1; Unschuld and Tessenow 2011, 156. A number of different meanings of *shenming* have been proposed (see Small 2018), and its meaning differs with use as well. It is translated in this passage as "spirit illumination" and differently elsewhere as a result of this different use. Donald Harper writes: "whereas the philosophical texts use ideas of spirit and spirit illumination to speculate on the nature of mental faculties, in macrobiotic hygiene spirit illumination is a kind of mana which those who practice cultivation can concentrate in their body" (Harper 1998, 120). The *Huangdi Neijing* usage here seems to have both connotations.

85 *Huangdi Neijing Suwen* 9.7; Unschuld and Tessenow 2011, 178. Part of the reason we see ambiguity concerning *xin* between what we would consider mental functions and those of an organ is that early Chinese thinkers associated the mind with the heart, rather than the brain. This is why the various vessels are associated with it, as well as the myriad mental states.

The first chapter of the *Huainanzi* further stresses this centrality of the mind in controlling *qi* and creating mental and physical thriving:

> 是故以中制外，百事不廢；中能得之，則外能收之。中之得則五藏甯，思慮平，筋力勁強，耳目聰明
>
> if you use the internal to govern the external, then your various endeavors will not fail. If you are able to realize internally, then the external can be attended to. If you realize it internally, then your five organs (*wu zang*) will be in repose; worries and anxieties will be at peace. Your sinews will be powerful, and your muscles will be strong; your ears and eyes will be acute and clear.[86]

The mind is also discussed in this chapter in ways reminiscent of the *Huangdi Neijing*:

> 夫心者，五藏之主也，所以制使四支，流行血氣，馳騁於是非之境，而出入於百事之門戶者也。
>
> The mind is the master of the five organs. It regulates and directs the four limbs and circulates the blood and vital energy, gallops through the realms of accepting and rejecting, and enters and exits through the gateways and doorways of the hundreds of endeavors.[87]

The nature of the mind itself is discussed in these texts, as we see from the passages listed here, in terms of its effects on the human organism as a whole, rather than in terms of its substance, what it is made of, or explanation of how it is that the mind does its work. It may be in part for these reasons that some scholars (as seen earlier) have denied a mind/body distinction in early Chinese texts. But we can see from this it is difficult to maintain this view in the face of the textual evidence. What we *do* see evidence for is that early Chinese thinkers tended not to have the same kinds of concern with mind that Western thinkers have since at least the early modern period—that is, concern with mind as substance, the accuracy of the ideas of the mind as representations, and the particular problem of consciousness in a physical

[86] *Huainanzi* 1.16; Major et al. 2010, 67.
[87] *Huainanzi* 1.18; Major et al. 2010, 71.

world. It is not that early Chinese thinkers were not sophisticated enough to understand these problems; rather, it is that the dominant view of the world in early China, holding nature as including both the descriptive and normative, both fact and value, did not see these issues as problematic. They simply never presented themselves as difficulties to be worked out as they did in other traditions. This unique feature of mind and the mind–body relationship is of central importance in understanding the various responses to madness and mental disorder we see in early Chinese texts.

While some scholars may admit that there is discussion of "mind" as such in early texts, they take *xin* to be a particular organ alongside others such as the liver, spleen, and so on, and not as distinct in kind from the other organs.[88] Slingerland argues convincingly that mind cannot be seen as an organ in the sense of the physical organs discussed in numerous early Chinese texts, as it has a different function and is *contrasted* with physical terminology and concepts rather than combined with them.[89]

Personhood and Deconceptualization in *Huangdi Neijing* and Zhuangist Texts

There has been a great deal of scholarly discussion of the issue of self and personhood in the *Zhuangzi*. The attention to this issue is rivaled only by the issues of skepticism and relativism among contemporary scholars in the West. In the *Zhuangzi*, we find the development of an alternative conception of personhood that challenges the accounts we find in other texts such as the early Confucian and Mohist texts. The Zhuangist account is suggested in texts such as the *Analects*[90] and *Daodejing*, but it is in chapters of the *Zhuangzi* such as *Renjianshi* (most prominently) that we find a fuller development of the Zhuangist account of personhood going beyond the mainly negative claims made elsewhere.

The Zhuangist account of personhood presents itself as primarily a challenge to accepted conceptions of self-cultivation in many Yangist and Daoist-inspired texts. The conceptions of personhood the Zhuangists find throughout society come in for ridicule and rejection in numerous places in

88 See Slingerland 2019, 39–45 for a discussion of these views.
89 Slingerland 2019, 106–111.
90 *Analects* 18.5–7. See also McLeod 2011 and Chong 2016, ch. 5.

the *Zhuangzi*. The Zhuangists have a host of problems with received notions of the person, rather than a single overarching problem. These are outlined in various ways throughout the text, but the issues we see most prominently in the *Zhuangzi* are the following: (1) personhood relies on and bolsters *shi-fei* 是非 distinction making, (2) communal features contributing to *shi-fei* distinction making and thus the construction of persons are often problematic, and (3) the possibility of the development of a different kind of personhood without reliance on *shi-fei* distinction making.

Much of the difficulty of understanding Zhuangist views on personhood is that person-talk is criticized while at the same time modified. In deconstructing the received conception of the person, the *Zhuangzi* offers new ways of conceiving of the person, often phrased on nonpersonalist language. This tactic was well known from texts such as *Daodejing* and *Neiye*.

In the *Huangdi Neijing Suwen*, though we do find the terms *shen* 身and *xin* 心, the more common distinction is that between *jing qi* 精氣 (spirit) and *xing* 形(form). The various mental illnesses are not distinguished as occupying a different category of illness from ailments like malaria or other physical illnesses. It is ultimately the same kind of process, which has to do with *yin* and *yang*, the five *zang* 藏 (organs), the movement of *yin* and *yang* between these organs, and the amount of *qi* contained in them. Where mental effects of disease are mentioned, they are often mentioned alongside of physical effects of a particular disorder. The *Huangdi Neijing* texts operate with a clear conception of distinction between physical and mental features, and terms referring to body and mind and their aspects are explicitly utilized in the texts in the same way we find in other texts recognizing mind–body distinction.

As discussed above, part of the reason scholars resist mind–body dualism in early Chinese thought is based in something that is certainly true about the tradition. We do not clearly find a mind–body polarity in early texts. The reason for this, however, is not because the early Chinese thinkers do not posit these categories, but rather because they are not opposed to one another in a dualistic system as we see in early modern Western texts, for example. Rather than mind–body polarity, mind and body should be seen as two elements in an organic conception of the human including also *qi* and *jing* (or *jingshen*).

Qi is generated by *tian* and transformed via *yin-yang* in the body through the *wu zang* 五藏 (five organs), according to the *Huangdi Neijing* texts.[91]

[91] Most list the *zang* as lung, liver, gallbladder, heart, and kidneys.

Suwen, chapter 5, explains how the transformation of *qi* in the organs creates a number of effects of the mind or spirit:

> 人有五藏，化五氣，以生喜怒悲憂恐。故喜怒傷氣. . . 暴怒傷陰，暴喜傷陽。

> Man has the five organs; they transform the five *qi*, thereby generating joy, anger, sadness, anxiety, and fear. Joy and anger harm the *qi* . . . violent anger harms the *yin*; violent joy harms the *yang*.[92]

The five *qi* discussed here are the kinds of *qi* originating in each of the five *zang*, which the text connects to the "five phases" (*wu xing* 五行) of correlative cosmology.

The ways mind and body are conceived in much of Western philosophy created the particular problematics surrounding the ways mental disorder is conceived in contemporary Western medicine and philosophy. One of the most controversial issues surrounding psychology and the philosophy of psychology is the issue of physical reductionism (also a hot issue in the philosophy of mind). Given a fundamentally physicalist worldview, in which physical things and their interaction are the sole constituents of the world, any mental phenomenon ultimately has to be explained in terms of physical processes. Whether mental events are identical to physical events, are instantiated by physical events, supervene on physical events, are a function of physical events, or are in some other relationship, for physicalists there must be a physical basis, cause, or ground for mental events.[93] Because of this, mental disorder or illness must be a different category of disorder or illness than the kinds of physical illness represented by physical disease. Mental illness, according to contemporary psychiatric understanding, is not identical to brain illness, even though brain states may be (perhaps necessarily) involved in mental illness.[94] When we look at contemporary accounts of mental illness, they generally focus on behaviors but also reference mental causes of these behaviors—disordered patterns of thought, reasoning, or emotion that are not amenable to immediate control of the individual.

92 *Huangdi Neijing Suwen* 5.6 (Unschuld and Tessenow 2011, 103).
93 See Stoljar 2010, ch. 1.
94 Graham 2013, 29–30.

This is a different conception of mental disorder than what we find in the *Huangdi Neijing* and early Chinese texts in general. But it would be the wrong to conclude on this basis that there was no conception of mental illness in early China. Rather, early Chinese texts show no tendency to think of mental disorder and symptoms as different in kind from physical disorder and symptoms. The *cause* of such disorder does not need to be grounded in or instantiated by physical phenomena. In the early Chinese case, it is *qi* that forms the ground of medical explanation, of human activity, both mental and physical.

There have been numerous arguments made concerning basic ontology in early Chinese texts. A common interpretation, one that certainly finds support in many early texts, including *Chunqiu Fanlu*, is that *qi*, rather than mental or physical features or substance, is the "basic stuff" of early Chinese metaphysics.[95] Both mental and physical phenomena then are constructed by, reducible to, or ultimately grounded in *qi*. While there is evidence suggesting something like *qi* reductionism in early texts, we also find alternative views that seem to cut against this. The difficulty is that both of these positions can be found even within single texts, with *Chunqiu Fanlu* as a good example of this. Of course, much of what we refer to as single texts, such as the *Huangdi Neijing*, *Chunqiu Fanlu*, or *Huainanzi*, are actually compilations of works by a number of authors, and the ideas within represent a range of different viewpoints. In the *Chunqiu Fanlu* in particular we can see the seams of multiple authorship. As Xu Fuguan, and more recently Sarah Queen, John Major, and others have argued, the *Chunqiu Fanlu* is much more accurately understood as a compilation of *Gongyang* thought, rather than the work of any single individual, let alone Dong Zhongshu.[96]

Whatever the right view concerning reductionism, what is most important for our purposes is that in the *Huangdi Neijing* tradition, and in early China more generally, disease or biological disorder is fundamentally due to states of *qi*. That is, *qi* and its movements do the explanatory work, rather than either physical or mental phenomena. When discussing the etiology of the variety of disorders, the primary explanation is understood in terms of *qi*, of which both physical and mental symptoms are symptoms. While we refer to different etiological bases of mental and physical diseases in contemporary medicine, some of which overlap, in the *Huangdi Neijing* tradition all disease is understood in terms of *qi*. Thus, there is no need to distinguish mental and physical disorder as different categories of illness in need of differential

[95] Tiwald and Van Norden 2014, 27; Liu 2014a; Hansen 2000, 156.

[96] Queen and Major 2015, 16–17; Xu 1976, 309–311; Loewe 2011, 225–226.

explanation. Certainly there still are mental disorders, such as *kuang*, but these mental disorders are *qi* disorders no less than malaria or the myriad other illnesses discussed in the medical texts.

Numerous passages in the *Huangdi Neijing* illustrate the centrality of *qi* in the etiology of disease, physical as well as mental. The presence, absence, or transfer of *qi* in certain parts of the body manifests itself as physical or mental disorder of certain kinds. Physical or mental disorder is always a *symptom* of some underlying imbalance or disorder of *qi*. This may be part of the reason that chapters 66–68 of the *Suwen* focus specifically on the generation and transformation of *qi*, rather than specific medical applications. These texts are much different than the surrounding chapters, seeming much more at home in a compilation such as *Huainanzi* or early Daoist work, perhaps even the *Guanzi*.

As seen earlier, in the *Neiye* chapter of *Guanzi*, it is the *jing* 精 of things that leads to their creation. *Jing* in this sense is a kind of *qi*, a purified *qi* linked to the *jingshen* or *jingqi* discussed in *Huainanzi* and *Huangdi Neijing*. This "essential *qi*" is linked in humans with the tranquil mind—the mind unencumbered by the mental states that arise as a result of disordered *qi* (as explained in *Huangdi Neijing*). According to the *Neiye*, the natural state of the mind (that according to the natural patterns) is without the mental states caused by disordered *qi*.[97]

The Connection of Mind–Body and Agency

The final piece of the puzzle in this discussion of personhood in early Chinese texts is *agency*, the most important aspect of which for our purposes is moral responsibility. On what grounds are actions said to be actions of a particular person in early Chinese texts, such that the person takes moral responsibility for these actions?

If we measure agency by claims of responsibility made by early Chinese thinkers, we have a complex picture, on which agency seems to be far broader than it is in the context of much of Western philosophical thought. One of the primary differences between the traditions here is that autonomy, in anything like a Kantian sense, is not seen as necessary for agency. It is less clear what early Chinese traditions will say about rationality—this is a large part of the payoff of looking at the issues of madness and mental disorder as I do in the chapters

[97] *Guanzi* 49.1.

to come. For some traditions, such as the Confucian and Mohist, some amount of rationality and behavioral conformity is necessary for the perfection of the person, but agency in itself is not reliant on such rationality. For the Zhuangist and other traditions, rationality not only fails to be a necessary condition for perfection of the person, but it actively gets in the way of our ability to become perfected persons. They propose a very different conception of "rationality," as they do with the case of persons and other key concepts.

In many ways the hallmark of Western thought on personhood and agency, at least since Kant, the idea of autonomy is seen as grounding agency, as it makes the key difference between what is caused by the world and what is caused by the person. In some sense, we can see this as akin to the *tian-ren* 天人(nature/humanity) distinction in early Chinese texts. The nature/humanity distinction in modern Western texts is far more rigid than in early Chinese texts—so much so that it causes indissoluble problems for the metaphysics behind these ethical systems.

The concept of autonomy depends crucially on a distinction between person and world, such that a person can be caused to act by internal considerations independently of the world—that is, by reasons, emotions, or other considerations that do not originate in the world, but from the self.[98]

The language of autonomy is ubiquitous in contemporary philosophical work in the West, with most taking it to be central to ethical theory. Contemporary ethics is thus largely the legacy of Kant. Even virtue theorists have managed to take the concept of autonomy on board.[99] Much of the idea behind this is that autonomy is necessary to make sense of moral, legal, and other kinds of responsibility (that an individual bears responsibility for an action rather than others or the world),[100] and that without autonomy, control and (negative) paternalism results.[101] This latter claim is a particularly relevant one for consideration of early Chinese thought, as one of the perpetual criticisms of traditions like Confucianism in the West is that it engenders a kind of corrosive paternalism.[102]

While Kant's formulation of autonomy is the most well-known and historically grounded, it is perhaps not the strongest formulation.[103] And

[98] Christman 2020.
[99] Winter 2012, 160–162.
[100] Ripstein 1999.
[101] Feinberg 1986.
[102] Kim 2016, 64–65; Hu 2000, 31; O'Dwyer 2015, 33–54.
[103] For Kant and later Kantians, autonomy is the single central concept grounding all of morality. Freydberg 2005, 65: "autonomy of the will is called both the positive sense of freedom and the principle of all moral laws."

contemporary Western (analytic) philosophy is not known for its devotion to history, despite its unacknowledged dependence on it. The basic features of the view remain the same from Kant's version onward, however. While there is an enormous literature on autonomy, a helpful categorization of the necessary features is offered by Richard Arneson. He argues that to be autonomous, one must form a plan of life via critical reflection and re-reflection or review.[104] This follows the basic Kantian formation: that one acts on a moral law on the basis of rational consideration and acceptance of that law independently of coercion.

For Kant's formulation, there are numerous objections. One might argue that being responsive to reasons itself is a kind of external influence. Why can't we say that reasons compel one in such a way that they undermine one's autonomy? We might also object to the idea of independent rationality itself that the concept of autonomy seems to rely on. Given that one critically reflects and reviews one's choices, how is this enough to ensure autonomy if one's very system of reasoning is dependent on or otherwise part of extenuating conditions of the world that lead to one's decisions? We can understand this through something like genetics—the ways an individual thinks and reasons are understood as related to the ways one's genetic ancestors thought and reasoned, and when one engages in this activity of critically reflecting and reviewing, one is doing something already nonautonomous. What then makes this nonindependent, nonautonomous act into a condition for autonomy, beyond simply a stipulation?

John Christman summarizes a number of views characterizing what he calls a "self-rule" condition of autonomy in a way that attempts to bypass this problem. He writes:

> The idea of self-rule contains two components: the independence of one's deliberation and choice from manipulation by others, and the capacity to rule oneself. [. . .] it can be claimed that to govern oneself one must be in a position to act competently based on desires (values, conditions, etc.) that are in some sense one's own. This picks out the two families of conditions often proffered in conceptions of autonomy: competency conditions and authenticity conditions. Competency includes various capacities for rational thought, self-control, and freedom from debilitating pathologies, systematic self-deception, and so on.[105]

104 Arneson 1994.
105 Christman 2020.

Notice that on this account, deliberation and choice can be independent, in the sense of being "unmanipulated" by others. But can we truly make sense of this? Deliberation and choice in much of the Western tradition (as in the Indian tradition) are seen as being in the realm of the uncaused and independent—dependent on free will rather than the activities of the community and nature. Most of the early Chinese tradition would reject this, had someone explicitly formulated it. Not that there is no conception of free will in early China (there is), but it is both taken as a divergence from the normal operation of things and as a *problem*. Agency does not require autonomy in anything like a Kantian sense, in part because most early Chinese thinkers would have taken this kind of autonomy to be a metaphysical impossibility. Where such independence of the causal interference of the world does arise, it does so as a divergence from normative natural patterns.

Part of what explains this is a dominant view of normativity in early Chinese philosophy that takes it as part of the natural patterns, rather than as specifically connected to human construction. Of course, that which is created by humans is also part of the natural pattern (when consistent with nature), but normativity outstrips human concern and valuation. Normative features are part of nature itself—things to be discovered rather than invented, and to be followed rather than created, like rules of a game.

We can look at the two components of the conception of "self-rule" necessary to autonomy as described earlier in light of early Chinese texts. On the issue of the independence of deliberation and choice from the manipulation of others, it turns out the tradition has much to say. It is indeed just the *opposite* of this for most early texts that discuss agency. On the Confucian conception of the person, as seen earlier, deliberation and choice are only perfected or morally acceptable insofar as they are informed and shaped by the norms governing the roles one inhabits. These roles themselves are not chosen, but are accorded to the individual on the basis of where one stands in the community (as a child, parent, citizen, etc.)

In much recent literature on the question of autonomy in Confucianism, scholars have attempted to find space for the concept in early Confucian texts, mainly to ground something like a concept of rights, which is seen as dependent on autonomy.[106] This leads some to locate a particular kind of concept of moral autonomy in Confucian texts that nonetheless differs from that of Kant and the

[106] See Chan 2002, 281.

later Kantian tradition.[107] Doing this, however, papers over the extent to which the early Confucian tradition and other early Chinese traditions were largely concerned with undermining autonomy as the key to agency.

There were various ways of conceiving of the individual in early Chinese thought. In most of these conceptions, individual agency comes mainly into play in consideration of how the individual integrates into society, or with the natural patterns, in a sufficient way to make the individual either a fully developed person or a sage, a *zhen ren*. Some of these claims, in texts such as *Daodejing*, even link the ideal state with a kind of conformity so complete that it can be associated with total ignorance. For example, *Daodejing* 48:

為學日益，為道日損。損之又損，以至於無為。無為而無不為。

> Committed to learning, one increases daily. Committed to the *dao*, one decreases daily. One decreases and decreases further, until finally arriving at non-action (*wu wei*). Non-active, yet there is nothing that is not done.

The various appeals to keep without knowledge in Daoist texts[108] should thus not necessarily be seen as (only) authoritarian power moves or attempts to suppress the rights of individuals. Rather, in undermining the reasons people have to act in alternate ways to those dictated by the natural patterns helps ensure that they follow those very patterns. The sage, for the Daoist and Zhuangist, is not a person with supreme autonomy who makes reasoned choices on the basis of a law—but one who follows this "law" without the need for such autonomous choice. This is part of the point of the paradoxical sounding claims throughout the *Daodejing* such as "the highest virtue is not virtuous"[109] or "the *dao* that can be a *dao* is not the constant *dao*."[110] What we can take from such claims in understanding autonomy and choice is that the perfectly virtuous person is one who simply follows the natural pattern and exemplifies action on the basis of these patterns—such a person has no use for or necessarily even understanding of the concept of a *virtue*. Where there is no possibility for vice, there is no virtue. When one follows the natural

[107] Chan voices the motivation for this move particularly well: "the inclusion of personal autonomy would strengthen the contemporary appeal of Confucianism. Such an inclusion need not imply abandoning Confucian ethics for something else. Instead, it can be seen as an internal revision in response to new social circumstances." Chan 2002, 282.

[108] For example, *Daodejing* 3.

[109] *Daodejing* 38.

[110] *Daodejing* 1.

patterns, one exemplifies everything signified by those patterns, which as we have seen is normative as well as descriptive.

Kant himself is not completely unaware of the possibility of a person similar to the Daoist *zhen ren*. In the *Critique of Practical Reason*, Kant discusses what he calls the "holy will"—imagining a being of perfect intelligence that could act such that their will and the maxims acted on by their will could never come into conflict with the moral law. Such a being could thus never act in an immoral way. For Kant, this requires a kind of infinite rationality, since rationality is the basis for such moral action. For such a being, however, there could be no obligations in the sense there are obligations for imperfect beings like ourselves, as only the possibility of divergence between the maxims we will and the moral law makes obligation necessary and binding.[111]

Kant claims that the existence of a being with the holy will is a thought experiment introduced as a guide to determining the categorical imperative. Thus he says: "act that the maxim of your will could always hold at the same time as a principle establishing universal law."[112] While positing a holy will can serve as a guide to the structuring of maxims through the categorical imperative, Kant also does not suggest that we should try to imitate a possible being with the holy will—possibly because he thinks that such a being is impossible. There is some inconsistency on this notion of the holy will as a model, however. Bernard Freydberg explains:

> in the former *Critique*, Kant is careful to say that this notion is presented for purposes of illustration only, namely the illustration of our own finite intellect as requiring "thought, which always involves limitations" (B71). There is no exhortation . . . that we ought to strive to imitate such a being. Here, however [CPR V, 32], the holy will is called a "necessary *Urbilde*" (V, 32), usually translated as archetype or model, but literally connotes an *originary* or *primal image*.[113]

Kant's hesitancy about this idea seems to be based in the fact that he believes such a being to be impossible, and the realm of fiction. God could have no such will, as God would not be subject to the constraints of moral law in the same way as created beings are. And no finite being could have such a holy will—thus it looks as if the idea of a holy will can serve as a guide insofar as we can imagine what it would be like for one's will never to diverge from the moral law.

[111] *Critique of Practical Reason* V, 32.
[112] *Critique of Practical Reason* V, 30.
[113] Freydberg 2005, 64.

For early Chinese thinkers, not only is this seen as not impossible, but something for which we should strive. Replace correspondence between will and moral law with that between action and natural patterns, and we have a decent structural similarity between the views. Why do early Chinese thinkers see it as a real possibility to adhere perfectly to the natural patterns?

Well, there is some question as to whether they *do*. Perfect adherence, being a *zhen ren* (for the Daoists and Zhuangists) or a sage (for the Confucians and Mohists) is a goal toward which we work. But in texts across the schools and traditions, we find a great deal of evidence that achievement of these states is extremely difficult, if not impossible. This is certainly the case for the *Huainanzi*, which explains in its opening chapters just why it is impossible for modern humans (of the Han) to achieve the kind of perfection humans were capable of in the period of "grand purity" (*taiqing* 太清). Perfect adherence to the natural patterns is understood in the *Benjing* chapter of *Huainanzi* as premoral and prereflective. The only way to understand and follow these natural patterns is to undermine the tendencies we have to form desires incompatible with them. The opening section of *Benjing* reads:

> 太清之始也，和順以寂漠，質真而素樸，閒靜而不躁，推移而無故，在內而合乎道，出外而調於義
>
> The reign of Grand Purity was harmonious and thus silent and indifferent; substantial and true and thus plain and simple; contained and tranquil, it was not intemperate; exerting and shifting, it followed no precedents. Internally it accorded with *dao*, externally it conformed to righteousness.[114]

It further explains that the decline from this period of grand purity resulted in the development of morality, ritual, and government, which only have meaning in the divergence from natural patterns.

> 是故德衰然後仁生，行沮然後義立，和失然後聲調，禮淫然後容飾。
>
> when potency declines, humaneness is born; when conduct fails, rightness is established. When harmony is lost, there are sounds and ditties; when rituals are decayed, comportment is gaudy.[115]

[114] *Huainanzi* 8.1; Major et al. 2010, 267 (adapted).
[115] *Huainanzi* 8.3; Major et al. 2010, 273.

Insofar as it is difficult or impossible to become a *zhen ren* or a sage, it is not, as in the case of Kant, that our rationality is limited or imperfect, but rather that our ability to *conform* to the natural patterns is limited and imperfect. It is in particular our *desire*, *shi-fei* discrimination (which can be seen as the basis of rationality), and our ability to deliberate and choose that is the problem. While there are different claims and different focuses in each of the texts and schools, this seems to be a general feature of early Chinese texts. In Confucian texts, it is generally *desire* that stands in the way of our ability to perfectly follow *dao* or natural patterns. This explains the "overcoming the self and returning to ritual is *ren*" (克己復禮為仁) of *Analects* 12.1. Adhering to ritual, which is not a matter of deliberation, choice, or rationality (primarily at least) is the key to achieving ideal personhood—in this case, attainment of the elusive property of *ren*.

The *Mengzi* in particular has much to say on this point. It is not ridding oneself of desire altogether that is the goal, according to the text, but rather making one's desires consistent with the way of morality—with the natural patterns grounding the human Way. The discussion of the *heng xin* 恆心 (constant mind) in *Mengzi* 1A7 (quoted earlier) expresses some of this.

Mengzi here makes a distinction between the learned person and the average people (*min* 民). What allows one to have the mind that does not alter in its movements is either instruction and learning such that one understands the natural patterns or the *dao* (in the case of the scholar), or that one has a livelihood (in the case of the people), which allows one to avoid the kinds of desires that lead to disordered action, to action opposed to the natural patterns of *dao*. Notice that what enables proper action here, the unmoved mind, is not independence, autonomy, or rationality. Indeed, it is only in the case of the learned person here that anything like rationality will come into play, or that the understanding at all comes into play. In the case of ordinary people, constant livelihood plays the key role because it is constant livelihood that averts the kinds of seeking desires that lead to diverging from the natural patterns. The idea seems to be that action consistent with the natural patterns is the base state for humans (and all other things), and that divergence from this state only happens with the kinds of instigating factors represented by desire, breakdown of order, or irregularity.

The idea that mirroring the patterns of nature makes one *zhen* (or a complete person) is something we first see in the *Zhuangzi*. Mirroring the patterns of nature has been understood through a number of different phrases: "following *tian*," "following *dao*," "adhering to the natural propensities," and other constructions. The general idea is that nature itself, or the ground of nature, has certain normative patterns such that when we align our conduct with these patterns (most often a matter of getting rid of our own biases, etc.), then we act effectively. According to the *Xunzi*, to follow the dao (*xun dao* 循道) rectifies our conduct (*zheng xing*).[116] In the outer chapters of the *Zhuangzi*, the idea is discussed in terms of "following the pattern of *tian*" (*xun tian zhi li* 循天之理) (chapter 15), and linking this to potency (*de* 德). The Heshanggong commentary to the *Daodejing* explains this following in terms of "following the natural patterns" (*shun tian li* 順天理). The *Jingfa* (one of the unearthed texts of the Mawangdui excavation in 1976) discusses "following patterns" (*xun li* 循理), following *dao* (*xun dao* 循道), and "following the regularities of nature" (*xun tian chang* 循天常).[117] We will see in the following chapters that much of the difference between schools and thinkers in early China, and the way they conceived of madness and mental illness in general, turned on just what they took the natural patterns or propensities to be.

[116] *Xunzi* 32.7
[117] *Jingfa* 5.3, 9.2.

2
Illness, Disorder, and Madness

The Role of Community in Behavior

In Chapter 1, I laid out the position that early Chinese texts generally view the person in terms of both body and mind, related to (or reducible to) *qi*. Construction of personhood and operation of human agency are understood as related to the subordination of one's autonomy, will, or desire and the use of the mind to align with natural patterns (or the moral *dao*). Another part of the picture as it pertains to madness and mental illness is the way that the mind and body are constrained or caused to act by parts of the world. One's acts are constrained (to various degrees) by one's *ming* 命 (allotment). Another part of the picture is human nature or inborn characteristics (*xing* 性), broadly understood as the features one naturally has simply on account of being human. The final major part of the explanation here that leads us more fully to consideration of madness and other forms of mental illness is community. Many early Chinese texts discuss the role of community in the formation of mental states and determination of behavior. The *Analects*, *Daodejing*, and the "Legalist" texts are particularly interested in the subject, though assumptions concerning it can be found across a wide range of early texts.

The community is important in two ways insofar as it concerns ordered and disordered behavior. First, as suggested in Chapter 1, many early Chinese thinkers held that the community played both an individuating and identifying role (one cannot possess a role without a community). Second, the norms of a particular community play a role in the determination of which kinds of behavior are ordered and which kinds are disordered. To determine this, we must refer to the natural patterns, but natural patterns might be differently manifest in particular communities.

Some scholars have stressed a seeming pluralist strain of thought in early Chinese texts.[1] While this view can be found in some early

[1] David Wong's own account of moral pluralism (or relativism) is inspired by his reading of early Chinese philosophers—see Wong 2009, xv, 37–41. A number of essays responding to and supporting Wong's position can be found in Xiao and Huang 2014.

The Dao of Madness. Alexus McLeod, Oxford University Press. © Oxford University Press 2021.
DOI: 10.1093/oso/9780197505915.003.0003

texts,[2] I do not think that this strain of thought is very prominent in early Chinese philosophy prior to the Han, despite the arguments of some contemporary scholars, who see a kind of moral pluralism in Pre-Han Chinese thought.[3] There are at least never explicit claims of such pluralism in the texts—most of the argument for this view comes from what seems entailed by some of the views presented in early texts. Almost every time there is direct discussion of the issue, however, most early thinkers insist that there is a uniquely correct *dao*. Even the Zhuangists, perhaps the best case for Pre-Han Chinese moral pluralists, hold such a view.[4] The way of Confucians, Mohists, and others, bound by and caught within a particular perspective, is ultimately a flawed way, because it is limited.[5] The way of true human thriving is to follow the way that is unbounded, that can shift and transform—that is, echoing the *Daodejing*, the *dao* that is not/cannot be *dao*ed.[6] Thus, the issue of the culture-boundedness of disorder and illness will only be problematic for a few of the early Chinese traditions. Confucians, as we will see, can easily sidestep the problem, as for the most part they accept a kind of cultural anti-relativism that holds behavioral standards as ordered or disordered on the basis of universal human features, rather than ones that change with culture. Order and disorder of behavior and mind can only be understood, according to such views, in terms of human nature (*xing* 性). If there are certain cultural norms that play a role in determining order and disorder, this can only be the case insofar as these cultural norms are based in or otherwise track human nature. For this to be so, there must be cultural norms that can so track, and others that do not. For the Confucians, it is clearly the cultural norms of the Zhou (at least in their morally relevant features).

Things are somewhat different for Zhuangists and the later synthetic thinkers of the Han, such as the authors of the *Huainanzi*. The *Zhuangzi* chapters take specific aim at the view that there is any one comprehensive and authoritative human nature or culture, the following of which will constitute order and lead to thriving. Such a view, contend the Zhuangists, is just the kind of thing that cuts against our thriving in general. There are cultural

[2] Though more often associated with metaphysical and linguistic types of pluralism than moral pluralism.

[3] Wong 2004, 32; Hagen 2003, 379–381.

[4] As we will see later, particularly in Chapter 5, pluralism of various kinds becomes popular in the Han Dynasty, developed in texts such as *Huainanzi* and *Chunqiu Fanlu*, among others.

[5] While the *Zhuangzi* is often read as advocating skepticism, relativism, or at least some kind of pluralism, some scholars disagree with this. See Ivanhoe 1993, 640.

[6] *Daodejing* 1.

determinations that lead to certain kinds of conceptualization, discrimination, and thus valuation—and insofar as this takes place, it is disordered or improper only insofar as it limits an individual from recognizing the contingent nature of this conceptualization or valuation. The influence of culture then tends to be toxic, as it lulls us into the sense that the valuations it sanctions are the natural and solely proper valuations. For the Zhuangists, then, the answer must be to *transcend* culture.[7] The *Huainanzi*, while it agrees somewhat with the Zhuangist picture, goes even further. The reason that no single culture or perspective can be the authoritative one is that each of them only represents a limited aspect of the expansive *dao* comprised of them all.[8] The key to order (and disorder) is understanding how cultural patterns can be manifestations of an underlying pattern of nature, without being necessary structures.

Communal norms, such as the Confucian *li* 禮 (ritual) or the *fa* 法 (standards) of Legalists and others, including the *su* 俗 (customs) of the *Huainanzi*, are central in the construction of personhood in much of early Chinese thought. Almost all the early schools and thinkers accept something like this, but the Zhuangists are the main opponents of this kind of view, and as we will see, their conception of madness and illness is also much different than ones commonly found in other schools and more conventional thinkers.

In their focus on character and virtue, early Confucians understood the critical position of *role*. A role can only be understood in terms of community, and it can only be carried out in terms of expected and publicly accessible behaviors within this community. That is, to perform a role properly, one must act in concert with norms governing the performance of the role, and in such a way that others in the community recognize one's performance and can respond to it, in ways dictated by their own role norms. Ethics, according to this view, can only be understood in terms of the community. The development of the individual must be seen as a social development. This view does not, of course, go unchallenged—we can see the Yangist, Daoist, and Zhuangist strains of thought each representing resistance to certain features of this view. But a particular conception of the person as requiring

[7] The *shi-fei* valuations discussed throughout the text suggest this, particularly in Zhuangzi's discussion with Hui Shi about *qing* 情 in *Zhuangzi* 5.6. The injunction to engage in "fasting of the mind" (*xin zhai* 心齋) in *Zhuangzi* 2.2 also suggests this.

[8] *Huainanzi* 2.7: 己自以為獨擅之，不通之於天地之情也. "Each thought he alone had a monopoly on true governing; he did not understand the genuine disposition of heaven and earth" (Major et al. 2010, 97).

communal integration via role and ritual norms connected with these roles is a basic feature of much of early Chinese thought, and it is relevant to the way these thinkers conceive of madness and illness.

In the *Analects*, we find numerous discussions of the place of the community in forming character of the individual, though these discussions are mainly suggestive. In *Analects* 4.1, Confucius says that the best state is to be in the vicinity of humaneness (*li ren wei mei* 里仁為美), while in 4.7, Confucius says that the faults or mistakes (*guo* 過) of a person are attributable to their kind or group (*dang* 黨). Numerous scholars have made sense of these passages by connecting the communal features of society to those of the individual. One way of understanding this is that individual character traits are shaped by the community in the sense that communal norms and shared knowledge set the parameters within which one constructs one's character.[9] The ways in which we express features of character are constrained by the meanings of actions supplied by the culture of our communities. Which actions constitute benevolence, disagreeableness, courage, or rebelliousness, for example, will be culturally contextual. In traditional societies like that of Han Dynasty China, individualism, resistance to authority, and skepticism about received doctrines would have constituted rebelliousness (as we see in the case of Wang Chong) and likely have led to one being rejected or ignored (as also in Wang's case). In the modern West, however (at least in my own cultural context in the United States), these same traits are normative and expected, such that one must at least appear to display them if one is to be taken seriously. In that context, commitment to a kind of traditional collectivism would itself be a form of rebelliousness.

If we consider the ways particular traits manifest themselves in behavior, the picture is complicated even further. One of the difficulties in talking about virtue and character is the extent to which these are culturally contextual. There has been discussion of the effect of culture on our consideration of what kinds of traits *are* virtues,[10] but the more relevant question here is to what extent culture plays a role in what kinds of traits constitute the relevant virtues in question. For example, we might determine that the virtue of *charity* plays a more central role in some cultures than others, or that all cultures seem to equally value *benevolence*. But this tells us relatively little.

[9] This is discussed in a different cultural context by Corey Barnes (2016), in the case of person construction in the Akan tradition of West Africa, building on the interpretation of Kwasi Wiredu.

[10] Van Oudenhoven et al. 2012.

It may turn out that what benevolence means in one cultural context is very different from what it means in another. That is, the traits—actions, attitudes, dispositions—that constitute benevolence in one cultural context may differ (and quite radically) from another.

Culture, Illness, and Rectification of Names

Given a complex of different actions and attitudes, which ones constitute virtue (or a particular virtue) or illness will differ between cultures. This is something critics of the idea of mental illness in the West[11] have remarked on—though there is some question as to how much we can conclude from these attacks. What is certainly the case is that aspects of culture are central to the construct of mental illness. Hans Agren considers this in his discussion of Chinese conceptions of mental illness, going so far as to challenge the objective basis of mental disorders:

> Medical diagnostics is learnt labeling. Disorders do not "exist" as entities that never change, but are invented as hypotheses about the proper grouping together of signs and symptoms that tend to be connected and change concurrently in time. [. . .] Which symptoms to take "seriously" is a personal choice highly influenced by social and cultural values.[12]

This holds for illness as much as character traits such as virtue. The characteristic actions and attitudes we associate with a particular virtue will be different based on culture. The question arises—given such variability, why should we think different cultures are dealing with the *same* virtues? That is, if different actions and attitudes are associated with a virtue in two different cultures, why should we conclude that these cultures have different conceptions of the same virtue rather than that they are simply talking about two *different* virtues, each of which has no counterpart in the other culture? There has been a great deal of discussion of similar issues concerning translation of not only virtues but general concepts between cultures.[13] While some,

[11] Such as Michel Foucault and Thomas Szasz, whose work I deal with more explicitly later.

[12] Agren 1982, 574.

[13] Aaron Stalnaker discusses what he calls "bridge concepts" in Stalnaker 2009, 17–19, while Bryan Van Norden relies on the thick-thin concept distinction in Van Norden 2007, 16–20. I discuss this issue in McLeod 2015, 33–34.

such as Alasdair MacIntyre, famously advance the view that there is incommensurability between such culturally contextualized concepts,[14] both the possibility of coming to understand different cultures as well as culture-independent facts about human makeup and ways of conceiving the world suggest that there must be some way of independently categorizing states and concepts.

Early Chinese thinkers for the most part seemed aware of the central role culture plays in virtue, illness, and other concepts connected to human activity and character. This is likely part of the reason for the focus in early Confucian texts on the "rectification of names" (*zhengming* 正名) as a major concern of the ruler as organizer of the community.[15] The issue seems to be that there must be regularity in the ways we conceive of virtues, illness, or any other concept, in order to have a shared understanding of what constitutes a given state. This is not a completely foreign concept to us today—in order to properly diagnose someone with a particular illness, we have to have a functional definition of what constitutes symptoms of this illness. Notice that this is distinct from an etiological definition (especially in the case of mental illness). A person is diagnosed with depression or schizophrenia, for example, not on the basis of certain brain states that might cause these conditions, but on the manifestation of certain activities characteristically associated with these conditions.[16]

While there are numerous suggestive claims about *zhengming* in early Confucian texts such as *Analects*,[17] the *Xunzi* is the most descriptive source for information on the idea in early Chinese philosophy, though the views of the *Xunzi* may be different from those of other Confucian texts on the issue. The *Zhengming* chapter explains that the reason for having correct names is communication and the ability to distinguish between things.[18]

[14] Which ultimately suggest the inability to translate concepts from one cultural context or language to another. See MacIntyre 1991 and MacIntyre 1981, 9.

[15] Rectification of names is generally associated with early Confucians, such as Xunzi, although it is a concern throughout early Chinese schools, discussed in Mohist and Legalist texts as well. Graham 1989, 283–284; Makeham 1994, 163–165.

[16] This fact leads some, such as Thomas Szasz, to reject the reality of mental illness as illness (although this is certainly a minority view in Western scholarship). Szasz's own view depends on the assumption that all illness should be understood in terms of specific physical causes. There are numerous problems with this, however. Among other problems, our conception of a physical disorder is, when pushed on, ultimately no clearer or culture-independent from our conception of a functional disorder. See Szasz 1974 (2003), 12–13.

[17] The term *zhengming* is used only a single time in the *Analects*, in *Analects* 13.3, but numerous scholars argue for the relevance of the concept to a number of other passages of the text. See Loy 2003.

[18] *Xunzi* 22.3.

It is primarily the sage who has responsibility for fixing names, but Xunzi suggests that since the sage kings are no longer to be found in his day, and no new sages are likely to arise, regular people can use their own minds to investigate the connections between names and things. Xunzi offers an account of the rectification of names that clearly ties it to self-cultivation, understanding of proper action, and *communication* of action and intent:

> 貴賤明，同異別，如是則志無不喻之患，事無困廢之禍，此所為有名也。
>
> When noble and base are clearly distinguished, and like and unlike are differentiated, then the problem of intentions not being understood will not happen, and the disaster of affairs being thereby impeded and abandoned will not occur. This is the reason for having names.[19]

This suggests that not only are the constructions of distinctions between virtue and vice, and illness and health, dependent on rectification of names, but the communication of these states to others is of central importance. The visible traits we can distinguish in the actions of others and how we categorize those with respect to our conceptions of virtue and vice or illness and health depends on having shared names, with names here being similar to the idea of definitions. We can make sense of early claims often connected with a *zhengming* doctrine in this way, such as *Analects* 12.11 (君君，臣臣，父父，子子. "Call the ruler a ruler, the servant a servant, the father a father, and the son a son.") While both Xunzi's claims and those of the *Analects* suggest that *zhengming* is an objective pursuit—that what counts as the proper actions of a father is not based on facts about a particular culture but facts about the nature of humanity, we do see here that how the virtues are understood, and what counts as health and illness as well, depends on how names have been constructed. A virtue is defined in a particular way, and the actions and traits that are relevant to the expression of that virtue are selected through this process of definition.

Part of the *Zhengming* chapter of the *Xunzi* that draws a great deal of scholarly attention is the claim by Xunzi that there are no patterns fixing names but that they are decided upon by people. This seems to be a bold claim of conventionalism about names or definitions—what we call *kuang* or other

[19] *Xunzi* 22.4, Hutton trans.

names is a matter of cultural or individual convention. The critical passage here reads:

> 名無固宜，約之以命，約定俗成謂之宜，異於約則謂之不宜。名無固實，約之以命實，約定俗成，謂之實名。
>
> Names have no unchanging appropriateness. Naming is based on agreement. Once agreement is established and the naming practice has become custom, they are called appropriate, and what differs from the agreed usage is called inappropriate. Names have no unchanging referent. Referents are picked out by names based on agreement. Once agreement is established and the naming practice has become custom, they are called the referents of those names.[20]

This seeming conventionalism can be explained in ways that ground the *Xunzi* in a broader realism concerning names, but there does seem to be here some sense in which there is a kind of cultural relativity concerning at least what features of activities and objects we take as relevant to point out and organize under certain headings. In the case of disorder—while there may be particular ways in which functional disorder like mental illness is caused and universal presentations in all humans, much of how these illnesses present will be dependent on the features of our norms and expectations that we have internalized through our culture.

Sarah Mattice draws out well what I think is behind much of the early Confucian conception of *zhengming*.[21] We can understand the process as connected to performance of roles and determination of the relevant actions of a role. A father might eat meat or be vegetarian, might wear silk or hemp, but what we are looking for in fixing names is to determine which of the actions of a father are normative—acts performed by a father *as* a father. It is these acts that are determinative of the role. The place of naming is to point out which acts we are concerned with, in offering an act-based definition of the role.

Culture plays a necessary role in the rectification of names, and this may have been the point Xunzi was trying to make in *Xunzi* 22.8 (cited earlier). As I argue later, culture, including understanding of how actions suggest or

[20] *Xunzi* 22.8.

[21] In Mattice 2019, 27–28. A number of other scholars offer different views of *zhengming* in the *Xunzi*; some outlined Hagen 2003, also Hagen 2007, ch. 3.

manifest certain kinds of identity, including disorder-based identity, will be relevant to the manifestation of madness and mental illness more generally in a given time and place. What constitutes mental disorder in some times and places will not in others, and vice-versa. We might see this as part of the Zhuangist point. It is less clear, however, to what extent the Zhuangists think of the norm dependence of disorder as relevant to its rejection or disvalue from within any given perspective. There is a perspective from which the state of the madman is not disorder at all, and rather everyone sane is disordered. What such a perspective might be (that of the madman?) the Zhuangists don't specify—but we are left to imagine a range of possible cases in which the madman or other "disordered" person has the better position, as in the numerous stories of the *Zhuangzi*.

Community norms can enter into behavior in other ways—our behavior is often guided by internalized expectations, connected to our roles, the character traits we believe we have, and even the disorders we believe we have. Confucians, as discussed earlier, famously recognized the place of community expectations in the behavior of individuals, going so far as to suggest that accepting and internalizing certain norms (rectification of names) and engaging with certain kinds of groups will have the critical effect on the formation of our behavior. As I discuss further later in considering mental illness in particular, numerous scholars have pointed out that a unique feature of mental disorder as opposed to physical illness is that it is susceptible to what some call a *looping effect*.[22] The idea is that knowledge of the particular features associated with a state will itself tend to play a role in production of those features in a person who believes that they have the state in question. Thus, for example, if one has been diagnosed with a particular mental illness and understands the symptomatic functional definition of it, this knowledge will have an effect on the way they act, and they will act in ways that conform to the disorder as it is defined.

And this makes perfect sense. We can understand why seemingly strange symptoms of madness (*kuang* 狂) mentioned by early Chinese texts, such as climbing high in trees and buildings, taking off one's clothes and running, and shouting abuse at people,[23] were so regularly associated with this disorder. This seems like a strange set of actions to coincide, and we might imagine that only a negligibly tiny percent of the population would

[22] Hacking 1995, in Graham 2013, 61; Sadler 2004, 359, in Graham 2013, 62.
[23] *Huangdi Neijing Ling Shu Jing* 10.9; Chiu 1986, 278.

exhibit them all or even multiple actions. Nonetheless, these actions seem to have been performed by single individuals in sufficient numbers for these definitions of *kuang* to widely be taken seriously. Likely there was something about knowing what the *kuang* person does that caused one expressing some feature of their psychology in *just these* ways rather than other ways. Just as there must be a similar explanation for why people deemed to have mental illnesses in the modern West have startlingly similar actions to one another. Mania, according to the American Psychiatric Association's *Diagnostic and Statistical Manual of Mental Disorders*, has seven characteristic symptoms. In the *DSM*, the "criteria for a manic episode," that is, a functional description of symptoms necessary for a diagnosis of manic episode, are the following (that must persist for at least a week):

> 1. Inflated self-esteem or grandiosity. 2. Decreased need for sleep (e.g. feels rested after only 3 hours of sleep). 3. More talkative than usual or pressure to keep talking. 4. Flight of ideas or subjective experience that thoughts are racing. 5. Distractibility (i.e., attention too easily drawn to unimportant or irrelevant external stimuli). 6. Increase in goal-directed activity (either socially, at work or school, or sexually) or psychomotor agitation. 7. Excessive involvement in pleasurable activities that have a high potential for painful consequences (e.g., engaging in unrestrained buying sprees, sexual indiscretions, or foolish business investments).[24]

Notice that the seven symptoms listed here are highly specific to the way we think about ourselves in modern Western culture. Our conception of goal-directed action, grandiosity, and so on—these are all things that will make sense only within a cultural context. Also compare this with other actions we might take a manic person to engage in that *do not* count as relevant symptoms according to the *DSM*, but are seen as relevant in other cultural contexts. I don't want to beg any questions just yet concerning how we should view *kuang*, but numerous scholars[25] have seen the symptoms of *kuang* as discussed in *Huangdi Neijing* and *Nan Jing* as similar to the contemporary conception of mania. Interestingly, though, while there may be overlap as far as the symptoms of the *kuang* person and the manic person, the criteria the two traditions focus on to establish the disorder are completely

[24] *DSM-5*, "Bipolar I Disorder: Manic Episode."
[25] Chiu 1986, 43.

different. While in the contemporary medical tradition, the earlier criteria from the *DSM* are used, the classic symptoms of *kuang* according to the early Chinese medical texts are lack of sleep, tendency to argue, climbing high into trees, and running with one's clothes off. While these symptoms may be present in the manic person, they are much less likely to specifically present themselves in this case. Part of the reason for this may go beyond simply what kinds of symptoms are noticed and taken as disease relevant. The way disorders present themselves may be guided in part by these cultural norms and expectations.

It is surely not due to its universality that we in fact find these symptoms coexisting in manic persons. Because if this is so, what explains why people in other times and places did not recognize such regularity of action among some part of the population? Was it that the early Chinese simply did not suffer from mental illness or things like mania? This seems incredibly implausible—what about *this* culture could make us more prone to mental illness than people in other times and places? It is much more likely that there is something about our *conception* of mental illness that makes the difference. Because the same could be said concerning *kuang* in early China. Is it just that there are no (or hardly any) *kuang* people in the modern West? What explains these differences? We should, I suggest, give up on the universality of behavior and mental disorder before we give up on the view that human biology and nature are the same everywhere. That there are certain features of particular cultures that tend to activate particular flaws in human organisms is an enormously problematic claim, and there are easier, clearer, and more compelling answers, that are informed by phenomena, such as the looping effect, that we already know are active in humans.

Illness and Health in Early Chinese Texts

The concept of illness in general (*bing* 病) is developed in a number of early Chinese texts. Medical texts such as *Huangdi Neijing* are the first to treat illness specifically in terms of a naturalistic approach to medicine. In many early texts, we find *bing* as indicating symptoms of illness or ill feeling, and in the late Warring States and early Han we begin to see movement toward consideration of *bing* in terms of underlying disease states and etiology. Paul Unschuld and Hermann Tessenow write of two senses of *bing* in the *Huangdi Neijing*:

Bing appears in contexts suggesting a meaning of being ill from the perspective of a patient, and it was used in other contexts to denote what medical theory believes to be the pathological change or dynamics in an organism underlying visible or otherwise noticeable signs.[26]

The conception of illness found in the *Huangdi Neijing* is understood as deviation from the healthy or "natural" state of humans, and it is tied to both energy and longevity. Chapter 1 of the *Suwen* of *Huangdi Neijing* explains that the divergence of the human organism from health has a natural progression with age, but that if one follows the *dao*, the natural degradation of the body will be slowed, if not altogether stopped, and one can live past one hundred years. At the limit, the perfect sage can live indefinitely, having the knowledge of how to guard *qi* from depletion and improper movement.[27]

It is *qi* that lies at the center of the consideration of health and illness in *Huangdi Neijing*. While the medical conception found in this text is certainly due to a naturalistic shift in the late Warring States and Early Han that made it possible to think of disorder in terms of qualities of *qi* and physical and mental functions, *qi* is far from naturalistic in the way current-day scholars (philosophers and otherwise) think of it. In the first chapter of *Huangdi Neijing Suwen*, *qi* is understood as retained through a skillful or agentless following of the natural patterns, here understood in terms of "following/regulating oneself with *yin* and *yang*" (*fa yu yin yang* 法於陰陽),[28] and depleted through divergence from these patterns. According to the text, it is the unhealthy activity of modern people, in terms of the overindulgence in desires, which takes them away from natural patterns, that is to blame for their illness and lack of energy and longevity in comparison with the ancients who understood the *dao*. Health, on this understanding, is closely tied to proper activity in a moral sense, particularly in a Daoist/Zhuangist sense. Insofar as the main aim and normative concern for the Daoists is to "follow the natural patterns," we find this echoed in the *Huangdi Neijing*. And in this sense, the medical cannot be seen as separable from the moral for these thinkers. The authors of the *Suwen* saw their medical considerations as tied directly to the overarching project of helping ensure proper human activity through following of natural patterns, with the aim of health, understood as proper

[26] Unschuld and Tessenow 2011, 20.
[27] *Huangdi Neijing Suwen* 1.2: "When essence and spirit are guarded internally, where could a disease come from?" (Unschuld and Tessenow 2011, 34).
[28] *Huangdi Neijing Suwen* 1.1 (Unschuld and Tessenow 2011, 30).

functioning of the human. This proper functioning can be understood as having implications for physical and mental energy and longevity (that is, medical implications) as well as for success of our goal-directed activities or attempts to understand the world (that is, political, ethical, and epistemological implications). The *Huangdi Neijing* provides us with an account of health that is already tied to key aspects of the view of the thriving and properly functioning human being that has become dominant in Chinese intellectual society by the Han Dynasty.

A key passage from the beginning of chapter 1 of the *Suwen* gives us a picture of the related concepts of health and illness in the *Huangdi Neijing*:

> 上古之人，春秋皆度百歲，而動作不衰；今時之人，年半百而動作皆衰者，時世異耶，人將失之耶？歧伯對曰：上古之人，其知道者，法於陰陽，和於術數，食飲有節，起居有常，不妄作勞，故能形與神俱，而盡終其天年，度百歲乃去。今時之人不然也，以酒為漿，以妄為常，醉以入房，以欲竭其精，以耗散其真，不知持滿，不時御神，務快其心，逆於生樂，起居無節，故半百而衰也。

> (Huang Di asked Qi Bo): "The people of highest antiquity all reached the age of 100 years without their energies or abilities weakening (in the least). The people of today reach the age of 50 years when their energies and abilities begin to weaken. What is the difference between these times and generations, such that people lose this capacity?" Qi Bo answered: "The people of highest antiquity understood the *dao*. They followed *yin* and *yang*, and were harmonized by the human arts and calculations. They were restrained in their eating and drinking, and regular in their rising and resting. They did not act or exert themselves foolishly, therefore they managed to keep their bodies and spirits together, and lived out their naturally allotted years, reaching 100 years old before dying. Now, the people of today are not like this. They drink wine like it's soup, and engage in foolish activity like it's regular. They drunkenly enter the bedroom, and through their lust they exhaust their essence.[29] Through overconsumption they dissipate their true natures. They do not understand how to keep hold of satiety, and do not continually maintain their spirits. In immediately attending to their desires,[30] they turn away from the true joys of life. Because they lack

[29] This may be connected to overemission of and thus perceived reduction of semen and seminal capacity, also associated with "essence" in this sense.
[30] Literally, their minds (*xin*), or what is in the mind, without consideration for proper action.

restraint in their rising and resting, they only reach 50 years old when they begin to weaken."[31]

This beginning of a consideration of medicine from the analysis of health is a unique aspect of early Chinese medical thought, and one that allows us a ready-made understanding of illness and disorder as divergence from the normal patterned functioning representing health. Once there are divergences from this pattern, generally through the excesses caused by following desires, human function begins to break down, whether in terms of loss of vital energy (*qi* 氣), reduction of longevity, or ineffective action. If we properly understand "potency" (*de* 得) as tied to the effectiveness of proper human activity, we can see how this concept bridges the moral, political, medical, and every other aspect of human activity. While the Confucian concept of *de* is often contrasted with that of the Daoists or other thinkers,[32] the concept is widely shared, even though the aspect of this general human potency of concern to particular schools is different. The effectiveness of proper human activity, when it comes to the moral, will involve communal expertise, understanding of and adherence to ritual, skilled interpersonal activity, and care and concern for community. Ni Peimin describes the Confucian conception of *de* as "a power or an art that enables a person to develop their human potential creatively."[33] This Confucian *de* need not be understood as opposed to that of the Daoists/Zhuangists. The key difference is that the Daoist/Zhuangist conception of *de* is tied to consideration of effectiveness *in general*, rather than specifically moral concern. The syncretistic thinkers of the early Han, such as the authors of the *Huainanzi*, and those of "Huang-Lao" persuasion, seem to have recognized the fundamental similarities and potential compatibility of these worldviews, and it is out of this syncretistic and increasingly naturalistic worldview that the medical thought represented by the *Huangdi Neijing* developed.

Health, according to the *Huangdi Neijing* view, is what is consistent with natural allotment—a normative conception of what a thing should be like given what it is supplied by nature (*tian*). This allotment from nature was often understood in terms of *ming* (allotment) in early texts. The Eastern Han philosopher Wang Chong understood this in terms of "natural allotment"

[31] *Huangdi Neijing Suwen* 1.1.
[32] Nivison 1996, 17–19.
[33] Ni 2013, 62. He adds: "Confucian *de* . . . centers on the affective aspect of caring and loving."

(*zheng ming* 正命), as opposed to "consequent allotment" (*sui ming* 隨命), connected to outcomes based on cultivation, and "incidental allotment" (*zao ming* 遭命), connected to outcomes based on accident.[34] The *Baihutong* makes a similar distinction, but it renders the first kind of *ming* as "fortunate ming" (*shou ming* 壽命).[35] While Wang's use of *zheng ming* seems to track the notion of its positive value, Wang leaves open space for the possibility that one's natural allotment may not lead to overall good outcomes, given that one may be supplied with a low quantity of *qi* by nature (*tian*), for example. This, of course, leads to an additional complication for medical thinkers and others associating health with the natural human state and retention of *qi*. Is the health of an individual here understood in terms of correspondence of the individual's patterns of action with a *general* human standard, or instead with an individualized standard relative to the natural allotment of the individual? Trying to make sense of natural allotment brings us squarely into this difficulty. One's allotted *qi* may be relatively little, and it may determine on its own that one has little strength, little moral and intellectual ability, or will live a relatively short life. Such allotment of *qi*, while perhaps divergent from the general allotment of humans *as such*, is perfectly in line with the allotment of the individual as such. That is, there is one way of understanding natural allotment as the maximization of individual *qi*, which is different from thinking of it in terms of the standard or average allotment of general human *qi*.

The primary cause of illness, according to the first chapter of *Suwen*, is failure of the individual (for whatever reason) to "internally guard the essential spirit" (*jingshen nei shou* 精神內守).[36] This is put in terms of lack of knowledge, as we see in the earlier passage. The dissolute activity of the people of the current day, according to the *Huangdi Neijing*, is attributable to lack of knowledge or skill, of "not understanding how to keep hold of satiety." The implications are, of course, that if people did have the knowledge of how to maintain health (and thus proper desire fulfilment for continual thriving), they would act in healthy ways. There is little motivation problem here, as we find in some moral theories, because we can all assume along that health is something all people naturally desire.

Of course, this assumption tells us more about the conception of health in *Huangdi Neijing*. In chapter 1, there is no single term used specifically to

[34] *Lunheng* 6.4. Also see McLeod 2018a, 229–231.
[35] *Baihutong* 31.1.
[36] *Huangdi Neijing Suwen* 1.2.

capture the concept of health, but the concept of health is discussed through a consideration of proper functioning and the divergence from proper functioning. For the motivational component, health is understood in terms of absence of illness. The person who operates properly, following the natural patterns (such that their *qi* moves as it ought to), illness has no way of arising. "When one internally guards the essential spirit, how can illness arise?" (精神內守，病安從來).[37]

Let us look to the rest of this passage, describing what the fully healthy person is like:

> 是以志閑而少欲，心安而不懼，形勞而不倦，氣從以順，各從其欲，皆得所願。故美其食，任其服，樂其俗，高下不相慕，其民故曰朴。是以嗜欲不能勞其目，淫邪不能惑其心，愚智賢不肖不懼於物，故合於道。所以能年皆度百歲，而動作不衰者，以其德全不危也。
>
> This is why (in such a person) the will is at ease and desires are few, the mind is calm and not afraid, the body toils but is not tired, the *qi* follows its proper pathways, each (part) follows what it desires, and all attain what they wish for. Thus one is able to enjoy whatever they eat, accept whatever they wear, and take joy in the commonplace. When the high and the lowly don't long for one another's places, the people can be called simple. This is why overreaching for desires could not tax their eyes, and wicked excesses could not confuse their minds. The stupid, the wise, the worthy and non-worthy are not afraid of things. Thus they are united in the *dao*. It was through maintaining their potency (*de*) that they were all able to attain 100 years of life, without their energies or abilities weakening (in the least), and avoid danger.[38]

Clearly, knowledge of the *dao* and ability to follow the natural patterns (somehow grounded in the *dao*) are fundamentally what allow for health and avoidance of disease. While this picture of health and illness sits well with some of the syncretistic approaches to mental illness we find in the early Han, it clashes in some key ways with both early Confucian and Daoist/Zhuangist ideas. For the Confucians (as I discuss in Chapter 3), particularly Xunzi, the unhewn and uncultivated individual, "natural" and "simple" in that sense,

[37] *Suwen* 1.2.
[38] *Suwen* 1.2.

cannot be taken as the moral standard or the image of thriving. (This will turn out to be the case for Mengzi as well.) The Daoists and Zhuangsts (with the Zhuangists taking the more radical stance), on the other hand, will reject the idea of illness (particularly *kuang*) as necessarily a divergence from the natural state. That being said, the *Huangdi Neijing*'s conceptions of health and illness are closer to those of the Daoists/Zhuangists than the Confucians. Like the Daoists/Zhuangists, the *Huangdi Neijing* takes following natural patterns and one's original and uncultivated nature to be the key to thriving (and health). This simplicity is associated with the absence of excessive desires (whether self or other directed) and the retention of *qi*—both ideas that can be found in Daoist/Zhuangist work. A key difference between what we see in the *Huangdi Neijing* and Zhuangist texts, of course, is that madness and other states of illness or disorder are taken not as divergent and unnatural, but as themselves potential expressions of understanding of the *dao*. One possibility, of course, is that the Zhuangists are playing on the conventional conception of madness, making the claim[39] that what we conventionally take to be madness is (often) not madness at all, but is instead wisdom. We do see, however, that Daoists/Zhuangists, for all the basic similarities between their worldview and that of the authors of *Huangdi Neijing*, seem to eschew the question of proper functioning of the human in terms of natural allotment (according to *Huangdi Neijing Suwen* 1, a mark of proper functioning is "living out one's naturally allotted years"). Instead, they focus on following the natural patterns as ensuring success and thriving, which might be (at least sometimes) at odds with the human allotment from *tian* or features of human nature.[40]

The General Concept of Disorder (*luan* 亂)

My interest here is with mental disorder and madness in particular, but a necessary preliminary to this is discussion of the concept of disorder in general, and how it is understood in early Chinese texts. Disorder (*luan* 亂) is infamously one of the things Confucius is said to have never spoken about

[39] There is precedent for this, on my reading, as Zhuangists make a similar move concerning the Confucian conception of "persons" in *Zhuangzi*, chapter 3. Zhuangists do not reject personhood per se, but rather a particular narrow Confucian conception of personhood. The case is much the same for their rejection of "knowledge"—that is, they reject pursuit "lesser knowledge" as the final goal, but accept the primacy of "greater knowledge."

[40] *Zhuangzi* 5.6.

(*Analects* 7.21), despite its being a subject of discussion numerous times throughout the text.[41] We can chalk this up, of course, to the fact that the *Analects* is a composite text, based on numerous sources not all of which agreed with one another on what the Master said and did. But clearly, for each of the strains of thought within the text, Confucius and other early Confucians cared deeply about order and disorder, and the nature of the two.

While there was a focus on a distinction between the mind and body, madness was primarily understood in terms of *behavior* (*xing* 行), rather than in terms of functioning of the *xin*. Mental causes of behavioral disorders and disorders of reasoning could be assumed, given the dominant views concerning the mind's role in controlling behavior, but the medical texts point to another source of madness—*yin* and *yang*, and imbalance of *qi*. A number of texts discuss the connection between disordered *qi* and mental states such as madness in particular. A passage from *Chunqiu Fanlu* reads:

> 公孫之養氣曰：「裹藏泰實則氣不通，泰虛則氣不足，熱勝則氣，寒勝則氣，泰勞則氣不入，泰佚則氣宛至，怒則氣高，喜則氣散，憂則氣狂，懼則氣懾。凡此十者，缺之害也，而皆生於不中和。…」
>
> The "Nourishing *Qi*" of Gongsun Nizi says: "when the organs are overly full, *qi* will not transmit, and when they are overly empty, *qi* will be insufficient in quantity. When heat is victorious, then *qi* [. . .]; when cold is victorious, then *qi* [. . .].[42] When overworked, *qi* will not enter; when overindulgent, *qi* will fail to be complete. When angry, *qi* will be heightened; when happy, *qi* will be scattered; when anxious, *qi* will be *kuang*; when afraid, *qi* will be terrified. In each of these ten cases, there is a deficiency that harms *qi*, and they each come to be when one is not centered and not harmonious.[43]

This passage not only draws an association between emotion, state of *qi*, and mental state, but suggests that *qi* itself can have characteristics such as *kuang*. The connection between *qi* and mental state here is so close that the two are essentially interchangeable—a connection further strengthened in the next line of the passage, connecting fear to terrified or afraid (*she* 懾) *qi*.

[41] *Ren* 仁 is similarly claimed to be something Confucius rarely spoke about, despite much evidence to the contrary in the *Analects*.

[42] The sections in the ellipses here are points in the text where the words are missing. Presumably heat and cold, like the remaining states discussed, also have some effect on *qi*.

[43] *Chunqiu Fanlu* 77.1.

Madness (*kuang* 狂) and related states have reference not just to the *xin*—indeed, not *primarily* to the *xin*. Rather, they refer to disorders or illnesses of the entire body, that result in behavioral dysfunctions. The connections between madness, other mental states, and *qi* demonstrates this. *Qi*, as animating force associated with both body and mind, plays a governing role here. Some have taken the ubiquity of *qi* in the human organism and its use as an explanation for both physical and mental activity to show that early Chinese thinkers were monistic and did not make a distinction between mind and body, or somehow reduced mind to body in a physicalistic reduction.[44] This view neglects the fact that *qi* cannot unproblematically be taken as a physical substance, and that any dualistic view of mind and body will have to have some explanation of how the two categories interact. Mental states, physical states, and behaviors are all linked to *qi* in early Chinese texts. The behaviors of madness are considered dysfunctional on the basis of two features—their divergence from normal behaviors and their negative effect on the individual and the community. Divergent behaviors alone cannot be the basis of illness—this would rule out the possibility of mere eccentricity. Although in early China as in the West and every other part of the world, there has always been a thin line between eccentricity and madness, there is a *clear* line, and a widespread desire not to run one into the other. Sometimes placement of an individual on one side of the divide rather than the other is a matter more of the community and its concerns than any property of the individual. The same individual may be deemed mad in one social context who is deemed merely eccentric in another. Indeed, as I discuss later, this is one of the reasons skeptics about mental illness such as the Zhuangists in early China and scholars like Michel Foucault and Thomas Szasz in the modern West reject the reality of mental illness as such.

There must be some objective determination distinguishing what is mental (or behavioral) illness from what is not. We can use, as the early Chinese did use, standards for illness more generally to do so. Certain eccentric or abnormal behavior is also harmful to the individual and/or society. But won't this, too, be constrained by cultural and communal consideration? What causes harm will be highly dependent on the particular cultural

[44] Jeeloo Liu, for example, writes: "In the Chinese worldview, mind and body are not separated, and all dimensions of existence are placed on a continuous spectrum of *qi*'s operations. Furthermore, the standard view held by *qi*-philosophers is that there are qualitative differences in *qi*. The purer forms of *qi* are directly responsible for mental capacities, and the mind is closely associated with the *qi* in the body." Liu 2015, 39.

norms of a community, and thus harmful abnormal behavior will be very differently interpreted by cultural context. Take, for example, a person with an illness we understand today as schizophrenia. In certain social contexts, the behavioral aspects of this disorder would have been taken as merely eccentric—perhaps far out of the norms of behavior, but nothing that could be taken as dangerous to society or the individual and as representing a uniquely problematic level of disorder. We can certainly make this distinction between harmful and unharmful norm infraction in our own societies today, and it most often has to do with whether we take a norm to be a *moral* norm (but not always).

A person whose mental/behavioral abnormalities lead them to regularly eat insects they find on the ground we might regard as perhaps in need of help, and possessive of an unfortunate eccentricity. Few would regard this as dangerous to either the individual or society. A person with the same mental illness who felt compelled to run naked through the streets, however (a noted symptom of *kuang*), more may regard as problematic, as they might take this to present a harm to society. I use this example purposefully—there are differences about the harms presented by public nudity in our own society. Some do not see it as a harm at all, and would view a person like this as no more harmful than the person who eats insects. Others, such as traditionalists and those of certain religious backgrounds, would likely take this public nudity to be a clear social harm. This will certainly have some effect on how we view the nature of the person's behavioral abnormality. The same divergence from the norm is understood by some as eccentricity and others as a sign of disorder.

An important and controversial area we find this at play in the contemporary world is (though far more in previous decades than today) is in the realm of sexuality. Homosexuality was listed as a mental illness in the diagnostic manual of the Chinese Psychiatric Association as recently at the early 2000s (being finally removed in 2001). Its counterpart in the United States, the American Psychiatric Association, removed the designation of homosexuality as mental illness in 1973. The idea behind this, in both cases, was that homosexuality did not, as previously thought, create dangers to the individual or society, and that it did not interfere with the ability of the individual to lead a "normal" life. The prevailing view prior to this was that homosexuality was an unnatural form of sexual behavior, with heterosexual penile-vaginal intercourse being the normal and natural form of sexual activity. This was, of course, on the basis of the idea that humans were constructed to have sex only in certain ways, following a kind of "natural law" picture constructed by such medieval Christian thinkers as Thomas Aquinas. This all had to be done on this basis, as no one had ever done surveys or undertaken attempts to collect empirical data to determine whether male-female vaginal penetrative sexual activity was the most *common* kind of sexual activity, so as to determine its "normality."[45]

Thus we see that the idea of the *abnormality* of behavior is just as contentious and socially variable as that of the harms connected to such activity. We might be tempted to define abnormality in terms of divergence from common forms of behavior, but it turns out that all kinds of things we deem normal are uncommonly practiced or thought, and things we deem abnormal very commonly practiced and thought.

The role of *mind* in all of this is still very much in the background. Today, we understand mind, specifically the *brain*, as the entity responsible for behavioral characteristics, and in the absence of indirect causes of behavioral disorder dependent on illness that has an original source outside of the cognitive system, such as the speech problems that may result from certain nervous disorders (such as Tourette's syndrome, Parkinson's disease, etc.), we attribute behavioral disorder to illness affecting the cognitive systems—that is, mental illness. Early Chinese thinkers, particularly the Confucians, understood behavior as determined not primarily by the heart-mind (心 *xin*) but also by the community, the organization of the community, communal norms, roles, leadership, and other communal factors. The early Confucians in this way bore a strong similarity to psychological situationists in contemporary philosophy and psychology. Situationists will argue that behavior is explained by situational features, such as role, communal context, and expectation, rather than by what we might call *character*, which is formed by individual states of choice and disposition.[46]

The issue of *behavior* is also of key importance here. Disorders, for many early Chinese thinkers, involve aspects of the person manifest in unusual activities and functioning of the body. This could range from the pained

[45] Arguing against the normality view, figures such as Sigmund Freud and Havelock Ellis argued that homosexual desires were inborn in humans (rather than the result of cultural or environmental features) and widespread. Freud argued that initially bisexual desires of humans were shaped into socially acceptable heterosexual desires (Freud 1918; Ellis 1900). Alfred Kinsey argued for the inborn nature of homosexual desire in males in the 1948 classic *Sexual Behavior in the Human Male*. Psychologist Evelyn Hooker published a study in 1957 demonstrating no significant psychological differences in homosexual and heterosexual men. See Drescher 2015.

[46] Famous statements of this can be found in the work of philosopher John Doris (2002, 28) and psychologist Philip Zimbardo (2008, vii–viii).

groanings or regurgitation of someone with a stomach illness to the wild and uncontrolled dances of the *kuang ren*. What manifests disorder in all cases of illness (as I discuss in Chapters 3 and 4) is ultimately *behavior* or *conduct* (*xing* 行).

Disorder of the Mind (*xin* 心)

In a number of early texts, we see discussion of what it is for the mind (*xin* 心) specifically to be disordered. While there is little discussion in Confucian and Mohist texts about specifically mental disorder, Daoist texts have much to say about it. They seem to be in general agreement that mental disorder is associated with the obtaining of certain improper or problematic mental states—most often, desire (*yu* 欲). Desires, according to these texts, disorder the mind primarily because they get in the way of our ability to perceive the world as it is. Thus *Daodejing* 3 claims that the answer to mental disorder is to rid the mind of desire by making it empty (*xu* 虛). We can understand this in connection with *Daodejing* 12, which talks about the effect of particular kinds of desire associated with the mind, and why we should seek to undermine them:

> 五色令人目盲；五音令人耳聾；五味令人口爽；馳騁田獵，令人心發狂；難得之貨，令人行妨。是以聖人為腹不為目，故去彼取此。

> The five colors blind the eyes, the five sounds deafen the ears. The five flavors dull the tongue, galloping and hunting in the fields drives the mind to madness (*kuang*). Goods that are hard to obtain obstruct human behavior. This is why the sage attends to the stomach and not to the eyes—rejects "that" (*bi*) and takes up "this" (*ci*).[47]

Commentaries on the passage can help explain what is going on here (though we always have to take them with a grain of salt.)[48] Wang Bi reads this passage as making a point concerning the mind's following of its nature or inborn characteristics (*xing* 性). When we fail to follow the nature of the eyes, ears, tongue, and mind, we do harm to the spontaneity (*ziran* 自然)

[47] *Daodejing* 12.
[48] Much of this depends on what layer of the text or the historical context we're trying to get to.

of our actions, and the negative states described in *Daodejing* 12 result.[49] The *Heshanggong* commentary also explains this passage in terms of desire, seemingly the natural reading.

We see that in addition to addressing desire and disorder, our main theme of madness is also packed into this dense passage from the *Daodejing*. Strangely, we see here a claim that recreations such as horse riding and hunting can lead to madness. The *Heshanggong* commentary on the passage understands this in terms of the depletion of the *jingshen* 精神 (quintessential spirit/pure vitality), or uniquely human form of *qi*, which is commonly associated with the mind (and thus in this commentary madness). The relevant bit of commentary reads:

> 人精神好安靜，馳騁呼吸，精神散亡，故發狂也。
>
> The *jingshen* of humans is peaceful. When one gallops on horses, one breathes vigorously (from exercise?), and the *jingshen* is diminished and lost. This is why one becomes mad.[50]

Mental disorder thus appears to be caused by both the obtaining of negative emotions (particularly ones based in desire) and the depletion or elimination of *jingshen*, which is inconsistent with these emotions. As an explanation of the final part of *Daodejing* 12, the *Heshanggong* commentary goes further, instructing us to:

> 守五性，去六情，節志氣，養神明
>
> Guard the five inborn characteristics, reject the six (problematic) emotions, unite the will and vitality (*qi*), and nourish spiritual intelligence.[51]

To follow the inborn characteristics (in the *Heshanggong*'s terms) or the natural patterns (in the *Zhuangzi's* terms) requires elimination of problematic emotions, and in particular the desires connected to these emotions. Early Chinese medical texts such as *Huangdi Neijing* have much more to say about the connection between particular emotions and organic disorder, mental and physical.

[49] Wang Bi *Daodejing* 12 commentary.
[50] *Heshanggong, Daodejing* 12.
[51] *Heshanggong, Daodejing* 12.

Organic and Mental Illness in Early Medical Texts

Earlier, I discussed the issue of disorder in early Chinese texts, particularly mental disorder. But how does disorder link to the concept of illness (*bing, ji*) as we find it discussed in early texts? A key place to look for this link is in the so-called medical texts of the early Han (which include material dating back much earlier).

The term *bing* 病 does not neatly map onto the English word "illness." Though what English speakers would recognize as illness is part of the meaning of *bing*, *bing* seems to be a more general term than this, often allowing a sense fairly close to that of *luan*. In *Analects* 15.19, *bing* is used in the sense of "concern" or "worry."[52] Xunzi also refers to the world (*tianxia* 天下) as possibly becoming *bing* in some places.[53] In the *Zhengming* chapter, Xunzi writes that *bing* is what results from the harming of one's nature/inborn characteristics.[54]

A *bing* is clearly a kind of disordered state, more commonly of organic entities such as human beings, but also of communities and states. *Bing* does not seem to have as wide a scope as *luan*—as *luan* can attain to rules, activity, and other artifacts created by humans, while *bing* is limited to functional disorder. *Luan* can then be understood in terms of *structural* disorder. The failure of things to fit with natural patterns or of the parts of a thing not to fit with one another is *luan*. The *Zhengming* chapter of *Xunzi* describes the difference between *bing* and *ming* (allotment)—or the negative outcomes due to *ming*. When one's nature is harmed, this is a matter of *bing*, while when one meets with bad circumstances, this is a matter of *ming*. Thus, for example, one might die at thirty years old for different reasons. Having a congenital disease that leads to one's death is a matter of *bing*, a functional disorder of the body that causes death. Being killed in war or crushed in a collapsed house, however, is a matter of *ming* (allotment, sometimes translated "fate"). There is no organic disorder responsible for this; rather, it is based on external cause and situation.[55]

[52] *Analects* 15.19: "The exemplary person is concerned (*bing*) about being without ability—not concerned about being not well known among people."

[53] *Xunzi* 17.1.

[54] *Xunzi* 22.2. 性傷謂之病.

[55] The Eastern Han philosopher Wang Chong (27–100 CE) later attributes such differences to distinctions in type of *ming*—he distinguishes between three kinds, "natural" allotment, "consequent" allotment, and "incidental" allotment, to make this distinction. The first kind, *zhengming* 正命, is similar to the *Xunzi*'s appeal to *bing*. *Lunheng* 6.4; McLeod 2018, 228.

Brook Ziporyn's interpretation of *li* 理, which he translates as "coherence," is useful here.[56] Coherence emerges, according to Ziporyn, from an ordering or patterning of things with one another, which must involve the interests and creativity of humanity as well as the world. There are numerous (innumerable?) ways that things can fit together, and the construction of a well-formed coherence can be understood here as exemplifying *order* (*zhi* 治), with its lack as *luan*.[57] I disagree with Ziporyn that such coherence formation could always (or even often) be a matter of human convention—otherwise it would be impossible to make sense of *luan*. Certain patterns (and values) must be then privileged by the world, mind-independently, which form the basis of order and disorder.[58] The idea of coherences, however, can help us understand how disorder and illness might arise. Failing to cohere would be a kind of *luan*, and from this *luan* it is almost certain that *bing* would result—the functional effects of the failure of parts of a worldview, system, community, or organism to cohere. *Bing* can result from *luan*, just as functional disorder can result from structural disorder.

We can understand this, and early medical texts *do* understand this, in terms of the coherent activity of parts of the body and the human organism as a whole. In my view, not nearly enough philosophical attention has been paid to the early medical texts. In these texts, we see accounts of order, disorder, and illness developed in concert with a key case of the interaction of things—the various parts of the body. The most obvious purpose of texts such as *Huangdi Neijing* are medical—the diagnosis and treatment of illnesses of the human organism (physical and mental). But we also find

[56] Ziporyn 2013.
[57] Ziporyn 2013, 217–218.
[58] Ziporyn suggests a way out of this difficulty, by taking disorder to consist of the divergence from accepted and agreed-upon coherences, thus salvaging the conventionality of coherence. This seems to conflict with much of what is said in early texts regarding such things as the authoritativeness of ritual in Confucian texts or the centrality of impartial care in the *Mozi*. Appeals are made to the nature of humanity and the world—if this is simply a coherence based on one community's conventional conception of humanity and the world, then the appeal loses its force as based on a kind of natural law, and the appeal to humanity and nature turns out to be a red herring. But then why appeal to humanity and nature at all, rather than to purely communal norms, pointing out one's membership in the community? And in addition, how can there ever be meaningful debate outside of shared communal contexts (in which people structure coherences in the same way)? The discussion between Confucius and the "Proto-Daoist" hermits of *Analects* Book 18 and others like it become almost incoherent. Confucius appeals to the standard of humanity to people outside of civilization, but his appeal is baldly question-begging if the standard he has in mind is his own cultural construction of coherences. How can he hold those not in the community and with no desire to be in the community accountable to *those*? What ground does he appeal to in order to do that, if the communal formation of coherences is all he has? If that's all he has, then why shouldn't *he* form coherences like the Proto-Daoists do? What makes his way better? There should be nothing he can say. But he does!

detailed conceptions of natural patterns, order and disorder, correlative cosmology, and the link between various elements of the person and the world. In these texts, we thus also find much on self-cultivation in general.

The *medical* and the *moral* were not cleft from one another in these texts as we tend to see them in contemporary Western medicine and moral texts. We may see it as a central feature of the modern world that these two are delinked, but as I show later (and as many scholars have noted), mental illness in particular is the most difficult test case for the cogency of such a distinction, and the pressure put on it leads a number of scholars to either reject the reality of mental illness[59] or to reject the hard distinction between the medical and moral. Early Chinese thinkers, who accepted organic views of mind, body, and agency, and who rejected the medical/moral distinction as drawn in contemporary medical science, were particularly well placed to understand the nature of mental illness and its link to community, personhood, and morality. If we consider the basis of the contemporary distinction between medicine and morality, or even between fact and value for that matter, it becomes clearer that the ground we stand on in the contemporary West is far shakier than we believe, and that views like those of early Chinese thinkers make much better sense of key features of human experience. Part of the issue is likely the professionalization and specialization of modern forms of scholarship and knowledge, including medicine. There is increasing awareness of the insufficiency of much of modern medicine in this area. Psychiatry and psychology are the front lines in this regard, as it is most clearly with the notion of mental order, disorder, health, and illness that the medical/moral distinction faces its greatest pressure. Much of the growth today of movements like mindfulness, cognitive-behavioral therapy, and other roughly "moral" approaches to mental health is due to the increasing recognition of the ultimate inadequacy of the hard medical/moral distinction, and the integration of methods and approaches often drawn from cultural contexts in which there was/is greater recognition of the interpenetration of these two categories. Currently, Buddhist methods seem to have the most influence in the West,[60] but perhaps early Chinese methods will also come to enjoy wider adoption in Western medicine.[61]

[59] Szasz 1973; Wakefield 1992.

[60] See Sauer et al. 2011, 1.

[61] Not all early Chinese approaches are equally helpful. We have to keep in mind the diversity of thought in early China (as anywhere and anytime else), but I stick closest to the views I find the most interesting and useful.

Kuang seems to be used in at least two senses in early texts—to refer to excitement or enthusiasm in general, as well as *kuang* as illness. These uses are not completely distinct, however, and there seems some ambiguity as to when one shades into the other. Even the uses of *kuang* as something like "excitement" contains a suggestion of something not quite right or slightly unbalanced about the *kuang* individual. There are uses in the philosophical texts that clearly refer to *kuang* as mental illness or the mentally ill person, however. The most famous of these uses is application of the term to the "Madman of Chu" (楚狂), who shows up in a number of texts, including the *Analects*, *Zhuangzi*, *Hanshi Wai Zhuan*, *Lie Xuan Zhuan*, and *Fayan* (among others),[62] and is a major subject of discussion in Chapter 4. This character is the basis for a major disagreement on madness between Confucians and Zhuangist—one that plays out through at least three texts.

Kuang becomes a major theme in early texts, representing the unformed, malformed, and helpless (among other images). In the *Diankuangbing* ("The Illnesses of Depression and Madness") chapter of the *Huangdi Neijing*, *kuang* appears in this chapter as the quintessential illness of *agency*. One acts in particular transgressive ways that flout ritual and proper action in a visible and communally accessible way. With *dian*, however, while it still involves action, it is an understated and absent action, something that does not present itself as a challenge or alternative to ritual and civilization. As I argue later (in Chapter 3), states such as *kuang* and *kuang* characters were associated by many early Chinese thinkers (and throughout Chinese history) with the wilds, with untamed humanity, nonhuman animals, the overgrown forest, the various barbarians, and activity unshaped by the tools of civilization such as ritual. As we will see, the question of the status of the *kuang* or otherwise mentally ill intersects with that of the status of the barbarian or those who have rejected civilization, such as the "primitivist" Zhuangists and the Proto-Daoist Yangists of *Analects* 18.

Kuang is also sometimes used in the sense of "excited" or "over-eager" in early texts. *Analects* 5.22 and 8.16, for example, speak of people being *kuang* in the sense of eager or energetic (certainly not "mad"). This sense of *kuang* as excited or eager also suggests a kind of ritual infraction. One's attitudes, emotions, and motivations must also be structured by ritual, not only one's visible behaviors. This is the basis of Confucius's claim in *Analects* 2.7 that

[62] There are repetitions of the story of the *Analects* in *Shiji* 47.51, and other stories of the Madman of Chu in *Hanshi Wai Zhuan* 2.21 and *Lienu Zhuan* 2.5. Though the story of the *Zhuangzi* clearly riffs on that of the *Analects*, the *Zhuangzi* version makes a quite different point.

simply taking care of one's parents when they get old is not identifiable with filiality. It is this behavior plus the kinds of motivational and emotional states proper to it that constitutes filiality. Here, we see that a distinction is made between visible behaviors, such as providing clothing, food, and shelter, and publicly inaccessible mental states, such as care, love, or motivation. If the *Analects* presents us with a psycho-physical conception of the self such that motivational states are publicly accessible on the basis of care being defined as behavioral (the idea that certain patterns of action constitute care), then such distinctions are empty. The care/concern Confucius is talking about here must thus be something that cannot be manifest in publicly accessible behavior alone. There is an implicit appeal to the private, mental aspect of the self.

Mental illness is wielded by both Confucians and Zhuangists as either illustration for or against the social conception of personhood. Early Confucians deny the reality of mental illness by either intimating or outright claiming that it is feigned or otherwise under the control of the individual person. Zhuangists, however, deny the reality of mental illness by "normalizing" the mentally ill person. The Zhuangist position is that the mad person is only mad because their characteristic ways of being are outside of the accepted social norms, and that such a person is seen as ill by society simply because of society's inability to think outside of its own strictures. The "mad" person operates free of these strictures and, as such, has access to a deeper understanding of reality. Thus such a person is not ill at all—rather, it is only those stuck in the narrow confines of the socially acceptable who (wrongly) perceive the "madman" as mad.

Both the conceptions of the Confucian and the Zhuangist reduce mental illness to either the result of a character trait or an undeserved slight. How each school views mental illness is instructive for their positions on personhood. This also raises interesting questions concerning why they seem to have seen madness in a different way than the society around them—in different ways, early Chinese texts stressed the moral or the medical aspects of mental illness, without ultimately making a cleft between them.

The mad and rejected are not accorded the seriousness or the consideration of the well-integrated, those persons central to the function of the system of social norms, and who have become part of this very fabric itself. This is perhaps just how we should see the sages. In their mastery of ritual, their action becomes enmeshed with that ritual, such that in successive generations, the actions of these sages are associated with and becomes inseparable from ritual. The patterns of their actions themselves become normative and guiding—such that in following the ritually proper way of the Zhou, one is following the way of Yao and Shun, the way of the Former Kings. Exemplary performers of an art define the parameters of action within it. The mentally ill, mad persons, and other social rejects are not only invisible in such a ritual system, they are unintelligible to it. They are unlike the person who follows the rituals poorly or often fails for whatever reason, the *xiao ren* (petty person) the early Confucians speak of. Unlike the bad piano player who cannot play the standards with the skill and flair of the virtuoso, the *kuang* person is like one who bangs on the keys in a completely haphazard manner, or mashes on the keys with their foot, acting in a way completely unintelligible even as music to the person following the normal standards. There may be a pattern and reason to what seems like the haphazard acts of the *kuang* person, but it is not something the person acting within the conventional standards can make sense of. It presents itself thus as madness, as nonsense.

What defines the mad person as mad is their divergence, rather than the particularities of the divergent pattern they follow. If there is a single way to function properly, following ritual, then there is a multitude of ways to diverge, as any other action is a divergence. But something is wrong here. Not just any divergence from the normal, ritually specified modes of action counts as madness. It is a particular kind of divergence that is perhaps unaware of the norms, or wholly unresponsive to the norms. One who violates ritual standards in the understanding that they are the standards, ought to have some hold on him, and for which he has constructed a story to justify breaking with ritual—this person is not mad. The mad person is one who responds to altogether different standards, unformulated in the ritual tradition. The actions and standards of the barbarians, then, or other "unformed" persons can appear as (and be categorized as) mad.

In contrast to both the Confucian and Zhuangist views of madness (about which we will see much more in Chapters 3 and 4), one strain of thought in early China seems to have seen madness as legitimate mental illness, neither completely determined by social conventions, nor cultivated or feigned on the basis of morally responsible social reasons. In the syncretistic position developed in the Han text *Huainanzi*, as well as in the earliest extant Chinese medical text, *Huangdi Neijing*, dating to roughly the same period, mental disorders such as *kuang* (madness) and *dian* (depression) are clearly understood as illnesses (*bing*). We will look more closely at this shift in thinking about madness in Chapter 5.

Normativity and the Patterns of Nature in Mental Illness

Already, we can see that there is an ineliminable normative element in the concepts of disorder and illness. We cannot construct a useful concept of disease from simply the descriptive facts about what is normal or most likely in the function of human bodies, for example. George Graham uses the example of morning sickness from pregnancy to make the point.[63] Perhaps we should take this as an important and necessary part of the functioning of a human body, but we treat the illness caused in terms of physical discomfort and unwelcome pain. If we could not eliminate this sickness without ending pregnancy altogether, then we might determine that it is a state overall for the good and something that ought to be suffered through.[64] We might imagine different cases as well, in which certain kinds of physical pain or change are viewed as positive based on their effects or overall role in our value structures. Enduring pain was seen as spiritually necessary or even edifying at earlier times in American culture.[65] Variable cultural attitudes toward particular kinds of pain can be seen to have a differential effect on the way those pains are viewed, expressed, and treated (or not) in different cultures.[66] Much the same can be said about our ideas of what is or is not a physical disorder or disease. Perhaps there is no Chinese malaria, Western malaria, or African malaria, but there is divergence in how the symptoms of this virus manifest themselves in different places, and which aspects of those myriad symptoms are relevant in consideration of treatment. In the case of malaria, we can say that there is a virus responsible for the illness, but we do not (and should not) equate virus and illnesses, as there are plenty of illnesses that are not viruses (cancer, heart disease, anemia), and plenty of viruses that are not illnesses (cowpox, endogenous retroviruses).

In order to distinguish the category of *illness* from any of the others we might associate with it, virus, pain, disorder, and so on, we must import

[63] Graham 2013, 99–100.

[64] Graham 2013, 100.

[65] Rey 1998, 53–57. This is particularly relevant today insofar as newer attitudes toward pain and its elimination or reduction have led to the proliferation of prescription pain medication, which has played a role in the opioid addiction crisis in numerous parts of the United States.

[66] Kenneth Sakauye discusses some of these issues in Sakauye 2005.

evaluative concepts. As Graham says, "the notions of bodily health and physical well-being are evaluative or normative through and through."[67] Given this, why would scholars like Szasz or Foucault make the mistake of associating mental illness uniquely with value and normativity? Part of the reason, I think, is that the normative elements of illness are much more prominent in the case of mental illnesses, because the nature of most normative concepts is that they involve evaluation by thinking agents. And agency, by the nature of mental illness, plays a much more important role in mental illness than in nonmental illness. Whether a particular reaction, thought, or behavior is constitutive of mental illness is going to have much to do with the appraised value of those states. States that ancient Maya or other shamanistic cultures would have understood as valuable will be called mentally ill in modern Western culture, because there is no similar social context for these states to be effective—or rather, there *is*, but that context is a medical one. Hospitals and pharmaceutical companies and the field of psychiatry could not exist without mentally ill people, and the thoughts and behaviors of the shaman today would serve the purposes of the medical complex today. Shamanistic goals have been put aside; medical ones have been taken up. Similar points have been made concerning mind-altering drugs. In certain religions (historical and modern), such drugs are used as part of a spiritual exploration, prayer, shamanistic communication, or other religious purposes. In modern Western cultures, for the most part, such drugs are understood primarily in terms of recreation, which creates a different social attitude toward them, and different norms concerning their use (and abuse, and indeed what abuse even *consists* of).

Thus, it is easier to see the normative role in mental illness. This is especially so as cultural constructs are closely tied to our conceptions of agency and behavior, and there may be a larger and more variable set of options concerning acceptable or unacceptable mental states than there are concerning physical states. We can see just this when we find unified accounts of things like malaria in places this virus was a problem, or certain types of cancer. It is much more problematic when we look for symptomatic mental illnesses that are familiar to us in other historical and cultural contexts.

The idea of normativity as part of illness leads most Western thinkers to look to conventional norms, cultural constructs, and other human-dependent constructions in order to make sense of this normativity. The

[67] Graham 2013, 99.

reason for this is the dominance of the fact/value distinction in Western thought at least since the early modern period. We find this implicit in much of modern scientific and philosophical thought. The idea is that the mind-independent world contains no normativity inherent in it, and that value is not properly understood as in the world mind-independently. Value only enters into the picture with human decisions, constructions, emotions—that is, it is a construct of the *mind*. We begin to see why the very idea of mental illness may strike one as problematic when it is determined that value is an ineliminable part of the construction of illness. If value is mind-dependent, and value is a necessary part of constructing illness, then illness is mind-dependent. And *mental* illness is doubly difficult to make sense of on this picture, as the mind-dependency of illness points toward the very thing the illness purports to be of, namely the mind.

The *Huangdi Neijing* texts give us a standard for determining disorder or illness that lies in the effect of particular states on *qi* or *yin* and *yang*. As we see in *Suwen*, chapter 5, mental states such as anger and joy harm the *yin*, *yang*, and *qi*. But what does it mean for these things to be harmed? The *Huangdi Neijing* texts seem to have in mind the idea that there are certain regular patterns of transformation of *qi* through *yin* and *yang*, and that this order represents a *normative* order. It is a pattern that can be found active throughout the world. This is part of what is behind the development of correlative cosmology in the Han. There are certain patterns inherent in the world that we can recognize in the heavens and the "natural world," and these patterns are the source of value. Thus, divergence from these patters signals disorder, a fall from the proper natural order, and this will issue in the accrual of disvalue—whether in pain, suffering, or other negative states. One of the key differences between much of the early Chinese tradition and contemporary philosophy, beginning perhaps from early modern Europe, is the idea that value is built into the natural patterns of the world—it is a descriptive fact about such patterns that they are valuable. Value is not something humans add to the world, but something we discover about the world.

The idea of the *qi* or *yin* and *yang* being harmed, then, that we see in the *Huangdi Neijing* texts, serves as a standard for determining disorder and illness. But these go beyond merely a medical context. The natural patterns can be violated for any of a host of reasons, and there are a number of ways to reestablish these natural patterns. The origins of the philosophical project in early Confucianism and Mohism can be seen as representing one attempt at reestablishing natural patterns. According to the Confucians, the social harmony facilitated through the cultural norms established by the sages (the ritual of the Zhou in this case) represents the proper pattern for human society,[68] and the way to return to this social harmony is the construction of virtue and adherence to ritual.

The idea that the patterns of nature (to which humans are also subject) encode normative value in addition to descriptive content is shared by Daoists and Zhuangists, despite their many divergences from the Confucians and Mohists. The core of the difference between them is their different conceptions of what these fundamental patterns are, not the fact that there are indeed fundamental patterns. While the Confucians and Mohists insist that these patterns include human value and design, the texts of the *Zhuangzi* argues that the normative patterns of nature are broader than what human constructions such as ritual would allow for, and that adhering to these patterns is a matter of understanding *transformation* of things (*wanwu zhi hua* 萬物之化), and the ways in which ritual and all human source of value is contingent on more basic patterns of value rooted in *dao*, which is itself the source of constant change.[69] The Zhuangists are not arguing against the normativity of the patterns of nature, rather they are arguing against opponents that those patterns of nature ever offer one rigid and unchanging structure. Instead, there is an innumerable number of possible patterns that have their basis in an exemplary pattern of the *dao* itself, which cannot be captured directly.

Though this argument is only implicit in the *Zhuangzi*, in the *Huainanzi*, it is brought to the surface. I have argued in other work that the *Huainanzi* is a necessary tool in understanding the texts of the Zhuangzi. A number of scholars have argued, including Harold Roth, that the *Zhuangzi* itself should be seen as a *Huainanist* text, compiled by the authors of the *Huainanzi* in the mid-second century BCE.[70] The various chapters of the *Zhuangzi* almost certainly predate the *Huainanzi*, but their selection and collection into the text as we have it is likely a result of Huainanist concerns. This, of course, problematizes our reading of the *Zhuangzi* as a single text with unified concerns. Even the "inner chapters" story that has been continually told is fraught with difficulty.[71]

[68] For example, *Analects* 3.14.
[69] *Zhuangzi* 4.2; 6.2.
[70] Roth 1991. Esther Klein challenges these views in Klein 2011, 355–360.
[71] Liu 1994; Klein 2011; Roth 1991, 360–361.

Given this, looking to the *Huainanzi* to understand themes of the *Zhuangzi* can be a useful method. Of course, there are numerous places in the chapters of the *Huainanzi* where *Zhuangzi* material is used for purposes clearly at odds with those of the authors of the *Zhuangzi* chapters, such as the material from *Huainanzi*, chapter 2, which is used to offer a cosmogony in the *Huainanzi*, while it is used to undermine claims to our ability to construct truths using language in the *Zhuangzi* (ch. 2).[72] Certain overarching themes of the *Huainanzi*, however, such as its attempt to understand the connection between the overarching (and ultimately ineffable) patterns of the *dao* and the particular patterns of human life, activities, and concerns, are consistent with those of numerous chapters of the *Zhuangzi*, and the *Huainanzi* develops in a more detailed and consistent way what is only hinted at in the chapters of the *Zhuangzi*. It could be that part of the reason the *Zhuangzi* chapters are merely suggestive on this point is that Zhuangist authors thought that no more than this was possible concerning the origination of patterns in the *dao*. This would certainly be consistent with a broader Daoist view (found in *Daodejing* 1 among other places) that *dao* itself is ultimately ineffable, as well as the claims of *Zhuangzi* 2 that any attempt to capture truths about the *dao* using language will ultimately misfire due to the contingent reliance of language on certain transformable patterns not themselves identifiable with the fundamental pattern(s) of *dao*. *Huainanzi* offers us a way of making sense of the pattern of *dao* from which all contingent and changing patterns emerge.

In the *Zhuangzi*, the authors make appeal to the "natural propensities" (*tian li* 天理), arguing in numerous chapters that following these natural patterns is key to success or attainment of value (as discussed in Chapter 1). While this seems to conflict with the radical relativism of the text in general, this can be understood as consistent when we take the natural patterns to represent something ultimately inexpressible and that is the source of the myriad norms and patterns of action individuals follow, which are all in themselves only contingent.

The patterns of nature, in terms of *tian li*, are understood in the *Huainanzi* as the "root" (*ben* 本), associated with *dao*, which cannot be expressed through language, and can be understood but can only be followed through some particular kind of non-*dao* activity. This activity that is linked to and

[72] Even if one disputes my reading of the *Zhuangzi*, ch. 2 material (which is notoriously difficult to interpret), what everyone will agree on is that there it is used for a deconstructive purpose, employed against opponents like the Confucians and Mohists, while in *Huainanzi*, ch. 2, it is used in a constructive purpose in building an account of the origins of the cosmos.

perhaps expresses the *tian li* is referred to as *mo* 末 (branches), and associated with the vastly different contingent and changing human activities, perspectives, and concepts that the *Zhuangzi* argues are limited.[73] While this structure helps to make sense of the *tian li* and how the numerous contingent perspectives can be understood as grounded in *dao*, the question for the *Huainanzi* becomes whether we should understand the norms that ground concepts like harm (violation of the norms) in terms of these *root* patterns or the branch patterns. If it is the root pattern that is fundamental in making this determination, it gives us a universal standard for things like harm, disorder, and thus also illness. However, the *Huainanzi*, like the Zhuangist texts, holds that the root (or *dao*) cannot be directly appealed to in grounding universal norms. At points, the *Zhuangzi* seems to suggest that there can be no such ground. The *Huainanzi* suggests, however, that the root or *dao* that grounds all contingent perspectives, even though it cannot be directly appealed to, can be accessed through these perspectives. Thus, the norms we use to determine things such as pain and disorder are to be found within the individual perspectives (*mo*), but in such a way as to understand them as emerging from the universal patterns of *dao*.

One unique problem that arises from much of the early Chinese tradition connected to the issue of the underlying patterns of nature is that of the possibility of divergence from those patterns. It is, in some sense, a kind of inverse free will problem. Given that there are patterns of nature and that myriad things follow these patterns, how do things or people ever fail to follow these patterns, without the intervention of something that is not pattern structured? Most studies of the issue of freedom or free will in early Chinese texts have tended to begin with the assumption that freedom or autonomy is a good, and then reading the texts as endorsing some conception of freedom.[74] Looking to an instructive section of the *Huainanzi*, however, we can see that this approach is problematic. Freedom or autonomy in the sense prized by early modern European philosophers presents itself not as a clear good in early Chinese thought, but as a *problem* to be solved. The solution to this problem, however, is not simply obedience to superiors or unchallenging conformity to the status quo (if things were only that easy!), because what most early Chinese texts argue that we should conform *to* is not a certain social structure or desire of a ruler, but rather the patterns of nature. And given

[73] *Huainanzi* 20, 27–29. Also see Major et al. 2010, 14.

[74] Chenyang Li (2014a) advances a conception of freedom as "choosing the good."

our ability to stray from these patterns of nature, recognizing and following them will necessarily take work—more than simply "following the leader" or doing what society dictates. The leader and the society themselves have this potential for divergence, and thus they themselves can only be useful guides at best, in cases where they themselves follow the natural patterns. *Huainanzi* 1 offers insight into this:

> 天下之事，不可為也，因其自然而推之；萬物之變，不可究也，秉其要歸之趣。夫鏡水之與形接也，不設智故，而方圓曲直弗能逃也。是故響不肆應，而景不一設，叫呼仿佛，默然自得。人生而靜，天之性也；感而後動，性之害也；物至而神應，知之動也；知與物接，而好憎生焉。好憎成形，而知誘於外，不能反己，而天理滅矣。故達於道者，不以人易天，外與物化，而內不失其情
>
> the affairs of the world cannot be deliberately controlled. You must draw them out by following their natural direction. The alterations of the myriad things cannot be fathomed. You must grasp their essential tendencies and guide them to their homes. When a water mirror comes in contact with shapes, it is not because of wisdom and precedent that it is able to flawlessly reflect the square, round, crooked, and straight. Therefore, the echo does not respond at random, and the shadow does not independently arise. They mimic sounds and forms and tacitly grasp them. That which is tranquil from our birth is our heavenly nature. Stirring only after being stimulated, our nature is harmed. When things arise and the spirit responds, this is the activity of perception. When perception comes into contact with things, preferences arise. When preferences take shape and perception is enticed by external things, our nature cannot return to the self, and the heavenly patterns are destroyed. Thus those who break through to the Way do not use the human to change the heavenly. Externally they transform together with things, but internally they do not lose their genuine responses.[75]

Part of the reason there is divergence from the natural patterns, according to this, is the intervention of the mind in its attempt to "deliberately control" the course of events. This represents a kind of freedom of will, but as we see here (and in the *Zhuangzi*), this free will presents itself as a problem. Free will represents a degradation of an initial state of harmony with natural patterns,

[75] *Huainanzi* 1.5 (Major et al. 2010, 53).

rather than a central and exemplary feature of human nature. In the cosmogony offered in *Huainanzi* 2.1, the authors give an explanation of how this degradation took place—of how we are able to veer from the natural patterns at all.

It is not only in the Daoist/Zhuangist influenced texts that we find such views. The natural patterns emerge in the guise of *ritual* in the Confucian texts and *standard/law* in Legalist texts. Conforming to ritual, for the Confucian, takes us away from the forked path possible with reliance on one's own will. It undermines the deliberate control of the mind. There is only one possible way that a ritually correct action can be in a given situation, and thus adhering to this is to follow a set and natural pattern, rather than one's whims, choices, or will. This is why *Analects* 12.1 insists that "overcoming the self and returning to ritual" (*ke ji fu li* 克己復禮) constitutes humanity (*ren* 仁). The problem of free will in early Chinese texts in general seems to be that we *have* free will, and thus have the ability to act inconsistently with the natural patterns. This is why the variety of responses to the problem do not take autonomy and choice as key components of morality, as we see in Western thinkers such as Kant. The key to following the natural patterns is not simply undermining of our will through conformity to a standard, because there are many possible standards and we may conform with the wrong one (indeed, this seems to be Xunzi's worry about customs in *Xunzi* 19). Rather, we need a way to determine and follow the *natural* patterns—as the patterns of nature themselves, those privileged by nature, are also the right patterns. Their normativity is included.

The *Neiye* chapter of *Guanzi* includes a discussion of the natural state of the mind in conformity with the natural patterns:

> 凡心之刑，自充自盈，自生自成；其所以失之，必以憂樂喜怒欲利。能去憂樂喜怒欲利，心乃反濟。彼心之情，利安以寧，勿煩勿亂，和乃自成。
>
> The form of the mind is spontaneously full and replete, spontaneously born and complete. It loses this form through care and joy, pleasure and anger, desire and profit-seeking. If able to rid itself of care and joy, pleasure and anger, desire and profit-seeking, the mind returns to a good state. The natural feelings of the heart cleave to rest and calm; don't trouble them, don't derange them, and harmony will spontaneously be completed.[76]

[76] *Guanzi* 49.1, Eno trans., modified.

The claim here is that the natural patterns are inherent within the mind as much as anything else, and it is particular emotions or mental states based in desire and will that thwart these patterns. Free will, the problematic concept, is based not primarily in choice, but in emotion. And as we see in *Huangdi Neijing*, *Huainanzi*, and other texts, emotion is a matter of disordered *qi*. The divergence from the natural patterns that comes about on the basis of the (natural?) decline from the initial "grand purity" creates the possibility of willful divergence from the natural patterns, as the transformations in *qi* create the possibility of the arising of certain emotions, desire, and will in the human mind. One of the interesting points here is that these states are not, for the *Neiye* as for other texts, natural states of mind. The states of mind that are natural, according to the text, are just those that result in tranquility (*ning* 寧).

Of course, all of this raises the question of where these other patterns come from and what they are, if they are not natural patterns. How can a nonnatural pattern emerge in the natural world? This is just the problem of free will. How, in a deterministic cosmos in which all things follow patterns, can we ever have divergences from those patterns? How can we explain how alternatives emerge? Whence arises the ghost in the system that can derail the natural patterns? And why are not these very disruptions themselves natural, such that we can say that part of the natural patterns themselves is this tendency to be disrupted, in the creation of multiple possibilities?

While the early texts do not sufficiently answer the earlier questions (and how could they?), there is good textual reason to think that early Chinese thinkers did not, for the most part, see the disruptions of the natural patterns and the emergence of human will and choice as themselves part of the natural patterns. This can be demonstrated in part by the fact that early texts seem to agree that there can be divergence from the natural (and thus also correct) patterns. Given that the naturalness of the pattern also fixes its propriety, as value and fact are merged in this conception of the natural, the fact that there are improper actions, and that these natural patterns can be undermined, shows that the divergence cannot itself be taken as part of the natural patterns.

What makes a pattern part of the natural patterns in this sense is its status as the pattern things would follow without the disruption of elements of human will, such as desire, choice, and so on. This is a very different reading of the earlier tradition than we find in other scholarship, and it is controversial enough that it requires a defense. In essence, I claim here that a prominent early Chinese conception of the person was as transcendent and autonomous entity not (necessarily) subject to the deterministic natural patterns, and thus to this extent "standing outside" of nature. This may seem hard to square with the clearly naturalistic leanings of the early texts, which culminate in later slogans such as "heaven and humanity form one unity" (*tianren heyi* 天人合一). Purely naturalistic readings of personhood in early Chinese texts have missed some important points, however. Of greatest importance is the fact that claims like "heaven and humanity form one unity," as well as the correlative cosmology with human body and action as elements and other naturalistic aspects of early Chinese thought, are primarily *aspirational*, rather than descriptive of how human beings actually are.

This should not be completely surprising to us. As far back as the earliest Chinese philosophical texts, the aim of authors was rarely descriptive or explanatory, but rather was primarily *prescriptive*. Texts from the *Analects* and *Zhuangzi* to the *Chunqiu Fanlu*, *Huainanzi*, and *Huangdi Neijing* had as their primary aim instruction in the best way or ways to attain certain goals. The goals differed by text—the Confucians were concerned mainly with development of virtue and social harmony, the Zhuangists with individual thriving (perhaps), the Huainanists with social cohesion and the concerns of empire. *Huainanzi*, chapter 2, explains that the ideal person will be one who achieves conformity with the natural patterns:

> 得一之道，連千枝萬葉。
>
> They obtain unity of the *dao* and join with its thousand branches and ten thousand leaves.[77]

To fail to follow the natural patterns is to be lost, and to be mad (*kuang*) is to be not only lost, but completely unconstrained. The mad person in early Chinese texts, in terms of *kuang*, is described as being unconstrained by both the normal patterns of action represented in society and the characteristic emotional responses of the normal person. Madness presents itself as an antagonistic mirror, through which the inversion of the norms and patterns of the ordered society present themselves. The madman is thus in some ways the consummate *anti-person*, which on the Confucian view makes him or her a threat—even the most dangerous threat, as it threatens to undermine the Confucian social project itself. Yet we don't see the Confucian terror of madness that we see of sexuality in medieval Christian contexts, which

[77] *Huainanzi* 2.4; Major et al. 2010, modified.

threatened to take one's eye off of the Kingdom of God through the dreaded sin of concupiscence (a concern that did not exist in early China). If madness undermines the very core of the Confucian project, why don't we see an even more forceful response against it? Instead, what we find is a suspicion of the mad person, a dismissal, almost diminutive in its lack of concern. While the mad person must certainly be a threat, they are a threat which seems mitigated by its naming. To be a mad person is a state to which no one would aspire—there is nothing tempting about the state in itself.

There *is*, however, something potentially attractive about the state of the mad person, and in which the mad person can follow the natural patterns, as a result of being unmoved by the usual mental states that become obstacles to following the natural patterns. A passage from *Huainanzi* 21 explains:

> 今夫狂者無憂，聖人亦無憂。聖人無憂，和以德也；狂者無憂，不知禍福也。故通而無為也，與塞而無為也同
>
> Now, mad persons are without grief, and sages too are without grief. Sages are without grief because they harmonize by means of potency, whereas mad persons are without grief because they do not know [the difference between] bad and good fortune. Thus, the non-action (*wu wei*) of those who fully comprehend [the *dao*] and the non-action of those who are obstructed from [the *dao*] are alike with regard to their non-action but differ with regard to the means by which they are non-active.[78]

There is some overlap between features of the madman and features of the perfected person, at least at the level of externally visible behavior. This partly explains the romanticization of the madman that we see in Zhuangist texts, as I discuss in Chapter 4. The following passage from *Zhuangzi* 2 shows the parallels to the earlier passage from *Huainanzi*:

> 至人神矣：大澤焚而不能熱，河、漢沍而不能寒，疾雷破山、風振海而不能驚。若然者，乘雲氣，騎日月，而遊乎四海之外。死生无變於己，而況利害之端乎！
>
> Perfected persons are spiritlike. Lakes can burst into flames and they will not feel hot. The He and Han rivers can freeze over and they will not feel

[78] *Huainanzi* 21.19; Major et al. 2010, modified.

> cold. Furious thunder can shatter mountains while the wind jostles the sea, and they will not feel alarmed. Those who are like this ride the clouds and the air as a chariot, ride the sun and the moon as a horse, and wander beyond the four seas. Even life and death cause no changes in them—how much less then will consideration of benefit or harm?[79]

The perfected person, that is, is akin to the madman in that such a person will not be affected by the usual concerns of the "sane" person. And how the divergence of the madman's actions from the social norms is explained will make a crucial difference in the implications of madness (and mental illness in general) for personhood and agency. There is a sometimes very thin boundary between madness and normality, between conformity to the social norms and their violation. In our daily lives we often fail to notice how closely what we barricade away is to what we do in the open. One can walk two steps in my local coffee shop and close a thin door, and then be completely comfortable using the bathroom. One has not closed oneself away—or barely, at least. One can still hear the voices of the customers and baristas only a few feet away. Yet if one stood just half a foot away used the bathroom there (on the other side of the door), it would be so embarrassing and devastating as to cause physical pain. Just a looking away, a thin veneer is all one needs, to make acceptable something that would be the actions of a madman in even a slightly different context. The lightness and seeming arbitrariness of such norms is often driven home when we see different norms, in different cultural contexts. In some countries, one will see people relieving themselves on the side of the road in full view of passersby. No one is bothered by this, while in the social context of my own home in the US East Coast, such an act would be seen as bizarre at best, and perhaps (depending on the contexts) even a sign of mental illness. The internalized norms and the ignoring of those norms must be seen as part of what is relevant in consideration of mental disorder and illness. Our capacities to operate consistently with norms may be compromised, rather than our action inconsistent with them being the result of a reasoned choice to flout norms, as is sometimes the case.

As we will see in the following chapters, social norms, commitment to them, and the roles of these norms in theories of personhood are key to understanding the variety of views concerning madness and mental illness in general we see in early Chinese texts.

[79] *Zhuangzi* 2.11.

3
Feigned Madness, Ambivalence, and Doubt in Early Confucianism

The Question of "Feigned Madness"

The final chapter of the *Xunzi* ends with a strange story, concerning the final years of Master Xun. Within this short and enigmatic passage, we can find packed much of the Confucian attitude toward madness and other forms of mental illness.

> 為說者曰：「孫卿不及孔子。」是不然。孫卿迫於亂世，遒於嚴刑，上無賢主，下遇暴秦，禮義不行，教化不成，仁者絀約，天下冥冥，行全刺之，諸侯大傾。當是時也，知者不得慮，能者不得治，賢者不得使。故君上蔽而無睹，賢人距而不受。然則孫卿懷將聖之心，蒙佯狂之色，視天下以愚。

> The purveyors of doctrines say: "Xunzi was not as good as Confucius." This is not so. Xunzi was coerced by a chaotic age and threatened with severe punishment. Above, there were no worthy rulers. Below, he encountered the violence of Qin. Ritual and righteousness were not being practiced. Teaching and transformation were not being accomplished. People of humanity were held back and constrained. The whole world was living in darkness. Those with perfect conduct were attacked. The feudal lords were all highly deviant. At that time, the wise did not get to deliberate, and the capable did not get to govern. The worthy did not get to be employed. Thus, lords and superiors were fixated and had no clear vision. Worthy people were rejected and not accepted. However, Xunzi maintained the mind of a sage, but feigned the appearance of madness in order to present the world with a façade of stupidity.[1]

[1] *Xunzi* 32.7, Hutton trans., modified.

The Dao of Madness. Alexus McLeod, Oxford University Press. © Oxford University Press 2021.
DOI: 10.1093/oso/9780197505915.003.0004

This is the only reference in early Chinese literature we find to Xunzi's supposed feigned madness in the later years of his life. And it comes, curiously, after an imagined challenge to the authority of Xunzi's teachings (represented by the text itself), on the basis of his not being as good as Confucius. It's unclear why the author thought that he had to defend Xunzi in this way. Absent some accessible tradition or story that Xunzi indeed went mad (or feigned madness) in his later years, why offer *this* explanation for Xunzi's retreat from society in old age?

There was, we know, a comparable tradition surrounding the greatest of Confucian sages. According to the *Shiji*, toward the end of his life, Kongzi returned to his native town in Lu, frustrated with the failure of rulers and people in power to take up his programs of reform.[2] He spent the final years of his life in literary seclusion, according to the tradition, working on editions of Zhou texts such as the *Chunqiu*. This is also the source of a related tradition that was taken very seriously through much of Chinese history that Kongzi himself wrote the *Chunqiu* and a host of other texts during this part of his life.[3]

There are a couple of possible explanations for the odd story ending the *Xunzi*. First—perhaps Xunzi actually *did* go mad (or at least *appeared* to go mad) toward the end of his life, and this later addition to the text is an attempt to explain this seeming madness away, to make it consistent with Xunzi's sagehood. This is a possibility I consider in the next section. We see in numerous Confucian texts, as I describe later, the view that madness is in some sense (ranging from partial to full responsibility, depending on the text) the fault of the person who becomes mad.

The explanation of feigned madness offered by the author of the *Xunzi* passage earlier offers a key distinction between what Xunzi holds in his *xin* 心(heart-mind) and what he displays in his *se* 色 (visage, face). While he retained the mind of a sage, he *feigned madness* (*yangkuang* 佯狂) in his visage or outward behavior. The author is careful to say here that the madness manifest in Xunzi's outward behavior is not a genuine madness—that is, not a madness that originates in the lack of control of a disordered mind, but a madness in *se* 色 only, controlled and intentionally performed so as to deceive the world into thinking that Xunzi was "stupid" (*yu* 愚). While we might wonder whether feigning madness to

[2] *Shiji* 47.
[3] This is not seen by scholars today as a realistic possibility.

avoid responsibility is the kind of thing we should expect from a sage, the author suggests that it was Xunzi's only alternative. Confucian texts are remarkably consistent on this. At some level of degradation, a society is beyond rectification, and the only option for the sage is to retreat so as not to sully himself.[4] In this passage from the *Xunzi*, the author explains that society in the Warring States was so disordered (*luan* 亂) that knowledge and order had become impossible, and a sage could neither be properly employed nor protected.

Confucian texts tend to be less than clear about the standards (or rather lack of standards) that must be present in a society for retreat to be a viable or necessary option for the sage or learned person. It is unclear whether this signals disagreement within the tradition on this question, or whether there are simply vague standards, dependent on the situation. Loubna El Amine discusses what she sees as a general and ineliminable obligation to serve in government in Confucian texts.[5] Passages criticizing Bi Gan's determination to serve (leading to his gruesome execution) and praising Jizi's decision to feign madness can be found in many Confucian texts, however, including the *Liji*, *Hanshi waizhuan*, and *Xin shu*.[6] This suggests greater flexibility on the matter.

This is, however, the kind of question to which we would expect the Confucian to have a clear answer. We do see a concern with such cases and lengthy discussion of them throughout the early Confucian texts, along with consideration of the *techniques* for escaping society, of which feigning madness is one. The question naturally arises: is escape of society through feigning madness doing different work than other ways of escaping society, such as retreating to one's home to edit texts (as Confucius in the *Shiji* account) or going to the hills to live an agrarian hermit life (as the "Proto-Daoist" characters of *Analects* 18)? For our purposes, this helps us answer the question for the *Xunzi*: why madness? If later followers were constructing a story for Xunzi to explain his lack of influence in political culture, why did they feel the need to make Xunzi's story one of *yangkuang* 佯狂, rather than giving him a "saner" end?

[4] The possibility of such withdrawal is considered in the *Analects* itself, as Confucius considers Weizi, who "abandoned the court" one of the three humane (*ren* 仁) persons, along with Jizi and Bi Gan, discussed later. By the Eastern Han, the theme of the good Confucian who abandons society because it is beyond repair is well established, represented in texts such as Wang Fu's (82–167 CE) *Qianfulun* 潛夫論 (Discourses of a Recluse).

[5] El Amine 2016, 151.

[6] *Liji* 19.44.

Avoiding the Bad Ruler

Kuang 狂 certainly would have given one the kind of freedom attached to being shunned by society. In this way, being viewed as *kuang* would have immediately freed Xunzi of all of his social responsibilities and attachments, at the cost of becoming a social outcast. There are a number of *yangkuang* stories in early Chinese literature, generally having to do with a scholar or minister feigning madness to escape a bad ruler, knowing that they are unable to rectify the ruler. Later thinkers evaluate these cases very differently, showing us the wide range of views within the larger Confucian tradition. In perhaps the most famous example of principled *yangkuang*, we find a contrast between two methods of resisting the bad ruler. The contrasting stories of Jizi and Bi Gan discussed in a number of texts show us evaluations of two possible responses to disorder.

Analects 18.1 mentions Jizi and Bi Gan, along with a third figure, Weizi, praising them all as men of humanity (*ren* 仁). The story we see in a number of texts, including the *Tian wen* 天問 of the *Chuci* 楚辭 and the *Shuo yuan* 說苑, among others, is that Jizi and Bi Gan have two different responses to the viciousness of King Zhou, the final king of the ancient Shang Dynasty. The Shang period was surrounded in myth even during the time of the Warring States and early Han when many of these texts were constructed. We find contrasting stories surrounding these figures, and it is impossible to know the historicity of any of them. The most interesting version we find for our purposes here, however, has to do with the differential responses of Jizi and Bi Gan to the king, and the different outcomes of these responses.

The account of Sima Qian in *Shiji* gives us the basic structure of the story.[7] King Zhou grew increasingly indulgent and neglectful of the conduct of the state, perpetuating vicious actions. This would ultimately lead to the downfall of the Shang. King Zhou's worthy ministers, however, knowing that the king's actions would lead to disaster, remonstrated with him. Weizi, the king's stepbrother, was the first to confront the king, but the king failed to listen and Weizi was forced to flee the state (recall the *Analects* passage discussed earlier). Bi Gan, another of the king's ministers, came to remonstrate with the king next, objecting to Weizi's approach and insisting that it was the duty of a servant to argue even to the death (為人臣者，不得不以死爭), and thus persisting in his remonstration. The king's reaction to Bi Gan further

[7] *Shiji* 3.33.

demonstrates his viciousness. According to Sima Qian, knowing of the Bi Gan's reputation as a sage:

> 紂怒曰：「吾聞聖人心有七竅。」剖比干，觀其心。
>
> King Zhou became angry and said, "I have heard the heart of a sage has seven chambers." He then cut open Bi Gan to observe his heart.[8]

In contrast to Bi Gan, Jizi's response is fearful, and he feigns madness, becoming a slave and finally ending up imprisoned by King Zhou. Jizi's is a curious case, and we don't see much about it in the *Shiji*, or any explanation whatsoever of why King Zhou imprisoned Jizi, how his feigned madness played any role in this, or even why we should think that Jizi's madness truly was feigned. As the *Huangdi Neijing Suwen*, which would have been known at the time of Sima Qian's work, claims, madness results primarily from *emotional* imbalance, with fear and anxiety being the main culprits.[9] Sima Qian points out that the brutal and gruesome execution of Bi Gan caused fear (*ju* 懼) in Jizi—this kind of fear certainly seems sufficient to precipitate madness.

The Warring States and Han texts include numerous discussions of the cases of Bi Gan and Jizi, and comment on these cases became a way of situating one's views concerning responses to danger in the state, madness, and responsibility. The story of the three worthies of Shang (Weizi, Jizi, and Bi Gan) had become a well-known symbol of three differing responses to poor rulership even in Confucius's day. Weizi here represents flight, while Jizi is enslaved (as a result of his feigned insanity), and Bi Gan is executed. Though their responses to disorder were different, all of these men stood on principles and refused to be complicit with the cruel and unvirtuous rulership of King Zhou. Mengzi also suggests that the three were equally virtuous in their responses.[10] This then suggests that Jizi's feigning of madness was an equally legitimate response to the misrule of Zhou as the other responses. So what is the difference?

Edward Slingerland suggests, concerning the *Analects* evaluation, that situational differences between the three accounted for their actions and the propriety of their actions. The reason Jizi did not stand his ground to be executed by the king (and that he was right in this) was that he thought it was

[8] *Shiji* 3.33.

[9] *Huangdi Neijing Suwen* 55.9.

[10] *Mengzi* 2A1. Though Mengzi's evaluation of the three seems to have to do with their abilities *prior* to their break with King Zhou.

possible to be later employed again in the king's service, given that he was his eldest uncle. Family obligations played a role in his choice, which were absent in the case of Bi Gan, who was a younger uncle of the king's.[11] Loubna El Amine builds on this, arguing that the Confucian duty of remonstration in the face of bad rulership depended on one's particular relationships, and that it was not a broad injunction.[12]

If this is right, then it seems the Confucians advocate something like the *yangkuang* response in cases in which salvaging oneself is of utmost importance, where one faces a dangerous situation that will otherwise not allow one to salvage one's own life. Interestingly, much of the discussion of madness and other problematic mental states in early Chinese literature surrounds the analysis of actions in insoluble dilemmas, such as that of Jizi and Bi Gan.

In the *Hanshi Waizhuan*, Jizi is praised as one of true understanding and humanity (*ren*), in part because he understood that the kind of head-on remonstration Bi Gan engaged in would not help to reform the ruler and would only lead to fewer opportunities to work toward virtuous rule (how can one help persuade a ruler when one is dead?). A passage discussing this reads:

> 比干諫而死。箕子曰：「知不用而言，愚也，殺身以彰君之惡，不忠也。二者不可，然且為之，不祥莫大焉。」遂解髮佯狂而去。君子聞之，曰：「勞矣！箕子！盡其精神，竭其忠愛，見比干之事，免其身，仁知之至。」
>
> Bi Gan remonstrated and was killed. Jizi said: "To know that it is of no use and yet still speak is stupid. To be killed would clearly be a disloyal act of enmity to my ruler. These things I cannot do—there is nothing good in that." Thus, he let down his hair, feigned madness, and fled. The ruler heard about this, and said: "Jizi! His spirit is exhaustive, and his loyalty and concern are supreme! Seeing the fate of Bi Gan, he escaped intact. This is the summation of humanity and knowledge."[13]

While we might find the ruler's reaction to Jizi in *Hanshi Waizhuan* puzzling and hardly believable (especially given what he'd just done to Bi Gan), one thing all of the texts seem to agree on is that Jizi *feigned* madness rather

[11] Slingerland 2003, 213.
[12] El Amine 2016, 130.
[13] *Hanshi Waizhuan* 6.1.

than actually being driven mad by the horrific circumstances of the time and his situation. Part of what is behind this seems to be understanding Jizi's actions as intentional—his stupidity (*yu* 愚) and disordered conduct (such as letting down his hair like a barbarian) designed to create the impression of mental disorder or illness. While such madness would have likely saved Jizi from the fate of Bi Gan, it did not stop him from being jailed and turned into a "slave." Presumably King Zhou had his doubts concerning the madness of Jizi; nonetheless, he felt compelled to avoid executing Jizi as he had done with Bi Gan. The texts that discuss the incident imply that it was something about Jizi's choice that saved his life—that this feigned madness played the key role. But it is just as likely, if not more so, that Jizi's relationship saved him—that King Zhou did not execute Jizi because Jizi was his senior uncle. Making this claim, however, would seem to attribute some level of conscientiousness or ritual/filial respect to King Zhou, however, which would seem inconsistent with the texts' painting of him as a completely depraved and selfish individual. Of course, it is possible to make sense of King Zhou's clemency in Jizi's case as a selfish act. Given Jizi's status as Zhou's senior uncle, killing him would have been a clear violation of ritual likely to have deep social repercussions and thus damaging the foundation of Zhou's rule. Thus, refraining from killing Jizi could simply have been a shrewd or necessary political decision. This, too, of course, would conflict with the picture of King Zhou the early texts want us to have—not only was he immoral, but he was a bad ruler. The moral and political are fused in early Chinese texts—the immoral ruler is also thus one who does not properly understand the role of government and is unable to sufficiently order the state.

Jizi's feigning of madness here, clearly, is a relevant feature in understanding the outcome of the situation. And the feigning of madness is an important theme in Confucian evaluations of madness in general. The texts seem to take it for granted that Jizi did not actually go mad and that his madness is an act—a practice they claimed other figures engaged in as well. Nonetheless, madness (or perceived madness) seems to provide the person with an exemption from responsibility. The culpability of madness we find in Confucian texts (discussed later) likely in part arises from this. Given the acceptance of *yangkuang* 佯狂 as a potentially legitimate response to misrule and danger, one often has reason to doubt the authenticity of any given case of *kuang* 狂. And there is the related question of just when *yangkuang* itself is justified, rather than alternative responses such as those of Weizi or even Bi Gan.

There is a discussion of the differences between Bi Gan and Jizi in chapter 11 of the *Huainanzi*, following the general strategy of the text of unification of differing actions and viewpoints. A key passage of the chapter reads:

> 王子比干，非不知箕子被發佯狂以免其身也，然而樂直行盡忠以死節，故不為也。...今從箕子視比干，則愚矣；從比干視箕子，則卑矣
>
> Prince Bi Gan was not unaware of the strategy of disheveling his hair and feigning madness to avoid injury to his person. However, he took joy in maintaining upright conduct and utmost loyalty in dying for his duty; thus he would not do it. [. . .]
>
> Now, if we follow Jizi in viewing Bi Gan, he was foolish.[14] If we follow Bi Gan in viewing Jizi, he was base.[15]

The fact that these situations are evaluated similarly for Confucians is problematized in the *Huainanzi*, which considers perspectival differences between Bi Gan and Jizi. The situational difference is not taken into consideration here, but rather the idea that from within one perspective and given the goals of an individual, the other perspective will appear faulty. Yet the *Huainanzi* makes the general point (and in this case as well) that neither of the perspectives is faulty relative to its aim. Whether feigning madness is the right answer in such a situation is a matter of understanding the proper goals and following with the most effective. *Huainanzi* 11 goes on to explain the purpose of this comparison (and others):

> 譬猶冰炭鉤繩也。何時而合！若以聖人為之中，則兼覆而並之，未有可是非者也。
>
> These standards set against one another are like ice and charcoal, angle rule and marking cord; when will they ever accord? If you take the sage as standard, then he comprehensively covers and completely contains them, so there never can be a "right" and a "wrong."[16]

It is difficult to see what this means for the evaluation of Bi Gan and Jizi earlier in the chapter. Clearly, the sage is able to see *either* of these responses

[14] Or "stupid," following my earlier translation.
[15] *Huainanzi* 11.18; Major et al. 2010, 424.
[16] *Huainanzi* 11.18; Major et al. 2010, 425.

to Zhou's misrule as acceptable given a particular end. But how is one to determine the right end? If there is no right and wrong in terms of ends, then any end is as good (or bad) as any other, and there is simply no way to evaluate ends. The sage then understands the resonance between things such that the sage knows if and how Jizi's actions will lead to the saving of his life and gain of new opportunities for remonstration (for example), but can say nothing about whether that end is preferable to that of Bi Gan. In this way, the *Huainanzi* runs into a similar difficulty as the *Zhuangzi*. If we do away with right and wrong altogether, then the only way to evaluate actions is with respect to some inevaluable goal or end, and if ends cannot be evaluated, we are not particularly better off than we are with no moral theory whatsoever.

There are multiple levels of the basic ethical questions—we might ask "what is the best way to achieve *x*?" which the *Huainanzi* and *Zhuangzi* could answer, but a deeper question "why should I care about/do *x*, rather than *y* or *z*?" cannot be answered. And this latter question seems the more fundamental ethical question. *Zhuangzi* (and in certain parts, the *Huainanzi*) attempts to do an end-run around this question by deferring to the notion of *ziran* 自然 (spontaneity) and the responses of one's nature, but this seems to run into a problem related to that raised in passages like that of the "happy fish" in chapter 17. Given that our indecisiveness, discrimination between alternative choices, and need for guidance is itself natural and can be seen as spontaneous (we don't *train* ourselves to act like this nor does it come from anywhere else), how do we possibly avoid this by cultivating a *ziran* approach? Zhuangzi's only answer to this is to insist that it is possible for humans to be without what essentially makes us human, which is *shi-fei* discrimination.[17] This seems connected to the discussion in chapter 4 about ridding oneself of a sense of self (and the concepts of *xin zhai* 心齋, *zuo wang* 坐忘), but it is unclear how such undermining of identity will solve the problem of competing desires or "forks-in-the-road" in which one can only pursue a limited number of many possible actions. *Something* needs to guide those choices, and unless the elimination of the sense of self the *Zhuangzi* advocates leaves one a complete automaton (and how could it?), the problem will still arise.

This view that feigning madness was a legitimate response and possible choice when presented with a difficult or seemingly impossible situation seems to have played a role in the Confucian suspicion of *kuang* as a general state. We find in many Confucian or Confucian-inspired texts views of *kuang*

[17] *Zhuangzi* 5.6.

as manufactured. But if it was possible to feign *kuang*, then there must have been a genuine *kuang* to be feigned. What of cases such as this? From what we find in early texts, one strain of thought (common in Confucianism) seems to be that where there was actual *kuang*, it was at least in part the result of flaws in the self-cultivation of the individual. Given the dominance of the Confucian conception of personhood as outlined in Chapter 1, it becomes easier to see why this would naturally have been the case.

Madness as a Result of Character Flaw

The Western Han text *Fayan* of Yang Xiong mentions Jieyu, the so-called Madman of Chu, in the context of madness in general and the perceived reasons for it. Following earlier Confucian views, Yang Xiong suggests that madness, in the cases of Jizi and Jieyu, is merely an act, put on in order to escape harm. *Fayan*, chapter 11, reads:

> 聖言聖行，不逢其時，聖人隱也。賢言賢行，不逢其時，賢者隱也。談言談行，而不逢其時，談者隱也。昔者箕子之漆其身也，狂接輿之被其發也，欲去而恐罹害者也。箕子之《洪範》，接輿之歌鳳也哉！

> If the words and actions of the sage do not meet with their proper time, then the sage becomes a hermit. If the words and actions of the worthy do not meet with their proper time, then the worthy become hermits. If the words and actions of the jester do not meet with his times, then the jester becomes a hermit. In the ancient past, Ji Zi covered himself in lacquer and Jie Yu unbound his hair and feigned madness. Both feared meeting with harm and desired to flee. Ji Zi wrote the Hongfan (The Great Plan), and Jie Yu sang "Phoenix!" to Confucius.[18]

The suggestion here is that when the times are not advantageous, this changes the outcomes of certain lives. This view becomes widely held in the Han period. When the sage or worthy person meets with the wrong times, he or she becomes a recluse (like Wang Fu), while if the uncultivated person meets with the wrong times, he or she can become like the *kuang* person. Yang Xiong seems to understand *kuang* as a result of failure in moral development,

[18] Bullock trans.

combined with difficulty of times. There is some uncontrollable element to madness (insofar as there is an uncontrollable element to *every* life), but primarily it can be seen as a character flaw.

Chunqiu Fanlu also characterizes *kuang* as a kind of character flaw. In a passage describing the original nature of the people (*min* 民), the text argues that people are originally flawed or uncultivated, and that reformation is necessary to make them good.[19]

> 弗扶將，則顛陷猖狂
>
> If one does not support it, then one will fall into terrible madness.

Jia Yi's *Xinshu* describes *kuang* as involving moral failure—associating it directly with an intentional failure to do good. Jia Yi's formulation is most forceful, offering a definition of *kuang* as moral failure. The *Dazheng shang* chapter reads:

> 知善而弗行謂之狂，知惡而不改謂之惑，故夫狂與惑者，聖王之戒也，而君子之愧也。
>
> To know the good and fail to do it is called *kuang*. To know the evil and fail to change oneself is called bewilderment/confusion (*huo*).[20] Therefore those who are *kuang* and confused are admonished by the sage, and shamed by the morally exemplary.[21]

This is linked to an early use of *kuang* as seen in texts such as the *Analects* and *Mengzi*, sometimes translated into English as "ardent." Mengzi explains *kuang* as the lack of fit between a person's words and their actions. The words of these people are lofty, suggesting that they know what is right, but their actions do not live up to their claims.[22] This is seemingly a low threshold for madness in the more severe sense considered elsewhere, closer to our "madness." But this use of *kuang* reveals an important feature of the concept operative in all of its cases—*kuang* is a particular disorder that involves the

[19] A view shared with, and probably influenced by, the *Xunzi*, which was the most important Confucian text during the period *Chunqiu Fanlu* was written.

[20] *Kuang* and *huo* are sometimes placed together as part of a single *bing* (illness). The *Xunzi* in particular mentions the two together often in the formulation *kuang huo ji bing* 狂惑疾病.

[21] *Xinshu* 51.2.

[22] *Mengzi* 7B37.

misalignment of one's mental states and behaviors from the proper patterns, where those are sometimes conventionally accepted.

But what then distinguishes *kuang* from simply divergence from natural pattern, or improper action in general? Surely not just *anything* that fails to conform to the proper patterns is an instance of *kuang*.

Kuang, according to Confucian texts, seems to be linked to failure to cultivate oneself attributable to the individual and/or his or her community, or to the failure of the ruler to create the kind of atmosphere (and thus *times* [*shi* 時]) the people need to cultivate themselves. Either way, we can hold some party at fault for the genuine possession of *kuang* by some individual person, although the Confucian is always suspicious that there is ever genuine possession of it. We see Confucian views ranging from the relatively benign, blaming the world or the ruler for the *kuang* state of the individual, to the vehemently moralist, putting full responsibility for *kuang* on the shoulders of the *kuang* individual for failure to cultivate oneself. Either way, *kuang* is a result of specifically moral failure. We see nothing here suggesting illness or nature.[23]

Lest we write this off as simply a feature of a dominant view of mental illness in early China, we can find other sources that treat *kuang* and mental illness in general very differently. While the *Zhuangzi* and related texts celebrate *kuang* as an inversion of standard values, early Chinese medical texts understand *kuang* as a *bing* (illness) in the same vein as physical illnesses such as fever. So we can see that the Confucian view of *kuang* as resulting from moral failure is not representative of all early Chinese views on the subject. The Confucians are taking features of persons such as *kuang* and transforming them into cultivable aspects of character, thus moralizing them. As discussed in Chapter 2, the moral and the medical were in general not separated in early Chinese thought, but there were certainly particular emphases in different literatures. Thus, we find the moral centered in Confucian texts with little discussion of the medical. This would have been a radical turn from earlier (and contemporary) ways of thinking about the person, and it is just this

[23] One might object here that Jia Yi's quote is not offering a *definition* of *kuang* or *huo*, but rather a claim that to fail to do the good even when one knows it is a kind of *kuang* act. If this is the case, however, the second part of the passage is hard to make sense of. The *kuang* and the *huo* person is admonished by the sage—surely this is meant to take into account *kuang* and *huo* people in general, and not just this specific kind of *kuang* and *huo* act? And even if we read the passage as nondefinitional, the knowledge-action disconnect is taken to be *indicative* of *kuang*, such that properly ordering it will resolve or eliminate this madness. Thus, the failure to do so is a failure of cultivation in the individual, for which the individual can be responsible. (I am indebted to personal communication with Andrew Meyer on this point.)

(among other things) that the Yangist and the Zhuangist attempt to resist, in essence offering a "re-centering" of the view of the person away from the (too) strictly moral.

Much of the negative or ambivalent view of the Confucians toward madness likely also has to do with its association with the wilds, with precivilized and "primitive" nature, and thus also with the non-Chinese "barbarians."[24] We find madness associated in a number of texts with acting like the barbarian tribes—the *Shiji*, for example, describes people who leave their hair untied (like the southern barbarians) in order to appear mad (the suggestion that this is only an act).[25] The idea of feigning madness recurs in a number of texts, including Yang Xiong's *Fayan*, *Hanshi Wai Zhuan*, which recounts in a number of places the story of Jizi unbinding his hair and feigning *kuang*.[26] The image of the wilds is a major aspect of the implicit madness theme of the story of Qu Yuan in the *Chuci* as well. Given that the authors or others could not be said to know whether a person had gone mad or not, the idea seems to be that madness is often an act, and when there are independent reasons that would make it advantageous or otherwise compelling to be deemed mad, that apparent madness is indeed feigned. This kind of view on part of the Confucian authors neglects some important facts. First, while certain features of the results of one's actions may be advantageous (being forgiven a wrong, escaping embarrassment, etc.), there would also accrue to a person an enormous amount of social demerit and ostracization. We see from characters in Confucian and Zhuangist texts alike who are taken as genuinely mad, like the famous "Madman of Chu" (*Chu kuang ren* 楚狂人), represented as definitively outside of society.[27] Given this, we might think it plausible that the negatives of being perceived as mad, especially for a Confucian or one with an important position in society, would far outweigh any benefits. Second, the authors do not consider the possibility that these previously normal people were *driven* mad by their difficult circumstances. They seem to have held a view in which people who temporarily lost control of their senses or their behavior were faking madness. Perhaps these people experienced what we today understand as situational mental illnesses, such

[24] "Barbarians" being a roughly equivalent Greek-derived term for the early Chinese use of *yi* and *di*, groups outside of the perceived Chinese world associated with backwardness, nature, and the untamed wilds.

[25] *Shiji* 38; Lewis 2006, 71.

[26] As do other texts, such as *Da Dai Liji*.

[27] Although *Hanshi Wai Zhuan* casts doubt on the legitimacy of the Madman of Chu's madness as well, suggesting it was feigned.

as adjustment disorder, anxiety, acute stress disorder, or posttraumatic stress disorder.

Laurence Schneider discusses the connection of madness to the uncultivated wilds, in connection with the story of the Warring States minister Qu Yuan of the southern state of Chu 楚 (coincidentally the same origin as Jieyu), found originally in the collection *Chuci* (Songs of Chu).[28] In early Chinese imagery, the state of Chu is itself linked to the semicivilized outskirts of society, nearly a barbarian territory itself according to northerners who thought of themselves as the center of civilization.[29] The exotic, untamed, and wild is associated with the south, with shamanism and magic, and the mad. Madness in this sense is linked with the seemingly unrestrained and unritualized (and thus also unpredictable) action of individuals.[30]

This unrestrained "barbarian" activity was for the Confucians the essence of the unritualized and uncivilized. Given that their project centered on the restraint and shaping of human action through ritual in socialization and society-making, the uncivilized was the polar opposite of the Confucian ideal. The Zhuangists and Daoists recognized this, and actively upended this ideal in the *Daodejing* and the "primitivist" chapters of the *Zhuangzi*. This is likely also the reason we see an embrace of such rejected characters as the madman and other social outcasts in Zhuangist texts. The madman (as described in the following chapter) is the quintessentially *useless* person. The Zhuangist appeal to and use of madness can only be effective in light of the robust ritualization and civilization approach to self-cultivation that we find in early Confucianism.

The seeming unwillingness to treat *kuang* as a *bing* 病 (illness) unconnected to cultivational aspects by Confucian authors is consistent with their overall view on character and the cultivability of character, as well as with the implicit connection between medicine and morality. As much as features like honesty, filiality, and humanity, features such as *kuang* involve both behavioral and (seemingly) motivational aspects. As such, the Confucian view of

[28] Schneider 1980, 208. "Madness has been the most dramatic metaphor for self and individuality throughout the Qu Yuan lore. In addition to linkages with the South and southern individuality, in retrospect we can add a final link here with the notion of the barbarian. . . . The idea of madness which developed in the lore is evocative of wildness, eccentricity, and nonconformity. Its opposites are cultivation, civilization, and conformity."

[29] See David Pankenier's discussion of the Chu/Jin war in the mid-seventh century BCE, in Pankenier 2015, 261–263.

[30] Discussing the construction of the *Chuci* in the Han, Cook and Major write: "Han period writers were encouraged to preserve the images and songs of what they remembered as Chu, an exotic shamanistic culture of southern and southeastern barbarians." Cook and Major 2004, vii.

moral development expressed in numerous passages in early Confucian texts would seem to require that *kuang* must also be subject to cultivation, just as virtues and vices.

The Confucian view of the relationship between the individual and society also likely plays a role here. The Confucian suspicion of madness and Confucian claims of inauthenticity or moral failure on the part of the seemingly mad follow the general Confucian worldview that makes the individual, in concert with his or her community, morally responsible for the features of an individual's character. One can be held morally blameworthy for failing to cultivate certain virtues such as *xiao* 孝 (filiality) or eliminate vices such as greed and selfishness. The key to such moral cultivation is provided in *Analects* 12.1: *ke ji fu li wei ren ye* 克己復禮為仁也 ("overcoming the self and returning to ritual is humaneness"). Through integrating our activity and motivations with the specified norms dictated by ritual (whether these are understood in a conventionalist or realist way), we generate the features of character indicative of the morally exemplary person (*junzi* 君子).

The explanation of Xunzi's end in the final chapter of the *Xunzi* thus likely had a number of purposes. First, as mentioned earlier, it explained Xunzi's inability to successfully institute his reforms for the state, giving him a "way out." Second, it allowed for the explanation of seemingly mad activity as a cultivated choice, stressing the valuable aspects of *yangkuang*. Third, it covered for any potential charge of lack of cultivation Xunzi may have attracted for exhibiting the symptoms of madness in his later years. One thing we ought to consider here is that madness (in the catch-all sense of generalized mental disorder/illness) was relatively prevalent in early China (we certainly hear much about it in the texts), perhaps as a result of the numerous traumatic events of the Warring States period. The view on moral self-cultivation of the Confucians entailed that while one could not control external situations due to the times or to *tian*, one could control one's own character and responses to situations. Thus, the cultivated person would respond to chaos with composure, to trauma with compassion and renewed moral vigor.

So why didn't other texts comment on this madness of Xunzi? There may have been many reasons for this. If the final chapter of Xunzi represents an after-the-fact justification for Xunzi's ineffectiveness, surely there would have been far better ways to do this than appealing to *yangkuang*. In the case of Confucius himself, the times (*shi* 時) are blamed, and it's unclear why this couldn't have been imported to Xunzi's case as well, especially given Xunzi's many claims to the importance of the times in determining success.

Madness and Moral Cultivation

More importantly, why might the genuinely mentally ill person present a difficulty for the Confucian picture of moral cultivation? *Mengzi* 2A6 might reveal at least part of what is going on. Mengzi says there that every human being has the heart of compassion such that they would feel a shock and alarm at seeing a child fall into a well. Mengzi here is committed to the idea that there are certain basic mental states that are essential to being human. Certain mentally ill persons, however, can seemingly fail to have these responses. Someone who is a sociopath, for example, might be expected to have no such response at all. It is unclear, of course, that this will constitute much of a problem for Mengzi's position—his position boils down to a claim about what is *natural* for humans insofar as they are human, not one about what every single human being has. One may make a claim that "everyone has two hands and two feet" as a way of expressing that it is part of the nature of humans to have two hands and two feet, without being committed to the extreme view that there is no human without two hands and two feet. Such humans exist, but they diverge from the norms specified in human nature, for a variety of possible reasons (accidents, diseases, etc.).

This is especially the case if we begin with a view of mental disorders such as *kuang* or sociopathy as mental illnesses. Presumably the existence of illness due to natural causes that undermines the existence of what Mengzi thinks of as the sprouts (*duan* 端) of virtue in our nature problematizes Mengzi's view about it as basic. There is an important disanalogy between the "child in a well" case and that of missing hands or feet. Having hands or feet, while it might be part of what constitutes humans, is not a *necessary* feature of humans—that is, there can exist humans without hands or feet. Mengzi's definition of nature (*xing* 性) in his discussion with Gaozi suggests that it is only those necessary features of the human that qualify as being part of our nature—those things without which one is not human. The discussion of the nature of water in 6A2 reinforces this. In addition to requiring necessary features, Mengzi also seems to require that the features are unshared between humans and other things. Breathing, for example, would not count—although no human that lives fails to breathe, there are other animals that also breathe. The "sprout" of compassion represented by the feeling of shock upon the child falling into the well is thus problematized by the failure of certain people to have it, such as the sociopath or other mentally ill persons. Seemingly the only way around this is to show that such people *do* have the sprouts of compassion, but that negative cultivation or other external factors interfered such that their nature has become completely muddied. This response requires that the mentally ill individual has some control over their state. Even if madness is not feigned outright, one is morally responsible for becoming mad, rather than cultivating the sprouts of virtue properly.

We see in the Confucian case a suspicion about the reality of mental illness as such, not for the reasons given in modern works like that of Thomas Szasz, which relies on the difficulties inherent in understanding illness across a purported mind–body/brain divide (as well as on the sociality of mental illness, which the Zhuangist *does* rely on). Rather, the Confucian rejection of mental illness is based on Confucian conceptions of self-cultivation and personhood, which provide little or no room for the possibility of mental illness.

This may be the reason that the idea of "feigned madness" (*yangkuang*) is prominent in Confucian literature, in uses of *kuang* that suggest madness (in distinction from *kuang* as "excited" or "ardent"). As we see in the stories of Jizi and Bi Gan, it is an assumed part of the story that the madness is feigned, in order to achieve some gain that would otherwise be impossible. The *Gaoshi Zhuan* even claims that the famous "Madman of Chu" himself was feigning madness in order to escape his responsibilities.[31] Investigation of the Confucian stories shows that there is something far more consistent with modern views of mental illness in the Confucian understanding than what we find in Western sources all the way until the nineteenth century.

The legal "insanity defense" first developed in France in the 1820s, with Étienne-Jean Georget's suggestion of various mental illnesses as constituting grounds for the decision of *non compos mentis* ("not of sound mind").[32] The idea that madness absolved one of *moral* responsibility for one's actions is of course older than this in the Western tradition, whether madness was understood as possession by spirits (a view common to a number of religious traditions[33]) or as the loss of one's self. In the Chinese tradition as well, as we have seen through consideration of the *Huangdi Neijing* passages, the cosmological/metaphysical explanations given lend themselves to understanding madness as a purely naturally determined phenomenon. Movements of *yin* and *yang* and the effect on *qi* happens independently of self-cultivation or actions of an agent. The feigning of madness would have been attractive,

[31] 見楚政無常，乃佯狂不仕，故世人謂之楚狂。
[32] Pietikainen 2015, 112.
[33] Mark, 2003, 257; Collins 2014.

according to the Confucians, to those seeking to escape moral and social responsibility for their actions. Thus, Confucian thinkers in general seem suspicious of *any* claim to compulsion or lack of agency.

This seems to suggest a general Confucian view accepting both (1) the universal cultivability of traits of behavior or character and (2) the obtaining of moral responsibility even in the absence of full agency. I have argued elsewhere for something approaching (2) for the Confucians, through a consideration of their position on *ren* (humanity) and *li* (ritual).[34] With the Confucian attitude toward madness, we also see evidence for (1).

Culpable Madness

One possibility in explaining the final passage of the *Xunzi* is that Xun Qing actually *had* become mad during the last years of his life, and the passage represents an attempt by Xunzi's later followers to explain away this problematic fact. Why would this *require* such explanation? The clearest explanation is that madness was seen as inconsistent with sagehood. For one such as Xunzi purported to be a sage to become mad in his older age would have been conclusive evidence against claims of others to his sagehood. Thus, the charge this passage begins with, that Xunzi was not as good as Confucius, would have been warranted.

Xunzi would have had reason to *feign* madness, as demonstrated earlier. But given that this strategy of retreating from the world would have been so much more risky than others that would have worked equally as well, the story does have the ring of after-the-fact explanation to it. This passage is the only place in the received early Chinese literature that Xunzi's purported madness is mentioned.[35] Does this in itself show that the madness (or feigned madness) is a wholesale invention of later Xunzian thinkers?

To uncover more of the reasons behind the Confucian ambivalence concerning madness, we have to return to the issue of what madness (and mental disorder in general) is. When we talk about specifically mental illness, we point to certain behavioral disorders rooted in the ways the mind (rather than the brain or the entire organism) works.[36] These behavioral disorders

[34] McLeod 2012.

[35] Hutton 2016, 342n10.

[36] Martha Li Chiu points out the importance of behavioral (or what she calls mental) symptoms in accessing illness (Chiu 1986, 271, 302). Fabien Simonis disputes this, charging her with "reproducing

will necessarily be understood in terms of the proper behavioral norms of a community, and the inability to properly integrate or play a role in a given community on account of the mental features of the ill or disordered person.[37]

Does it make a difference whether we think of *kuang* as a "behavioral" rather than a "mental" disorder? I think it does, as mental disorder suggests an internal ability to recognize and follow patterns that itself may be a behavior (if we are behavioral reductionists), but which early Chinese texts would not have seen this way. The main reason contemporary mental health is sometimes called "behavioral health" (though this is decreasing) is the influence of twentieth-century behaviorists and physical reductionists. Insofar as there is (we now recognize) a great deal of intellectual territory between Cartesian dualism and eliminativist behaviorism, rejection of the former (which most do) certainly does not commit us to acceptance of the latter (which increasingly few do).

If this is right, then *kuang* is mainly defined by the particular violation of norms associated with social disorder. As I showed in Chapter 1, the Confucian position links the person with the community and communal features—thus, this communal disorder associated with the violation of norms is a disorder in individual activity connected to the mind and behavior, understood as *kuang*. And for this reason madness is not only the responsibility of the individual, but that of the society and ruler as well. In a properly ruled and well-ordered society, individuals will not be driven to madness. Just this is suggested by a passage in the *Chunqiu Fanlu* mentioned earlier.

This suggests that the ruler, who has a clear role in ensuring order in society (though not the only one), bears some responsibility for madness in individuals. As we have seen in Chapter 2, however, on a Confucian view of persons, there is no clear-cut way to make a cleft between the responsibility of an individual and that of the community. All of us are comprised of elements of our communities, our personhood determined by roles and relationships. The fact that states like madness may be caused in large part by features of society, then, does not free the individual from culpability for this madness. Indeed, according to some Confucian texts, the possibility of alternative responses to the disordered society further sets the responsibility for the obtaining of madness squarely on the shoulders of the mad individual.

a problematic dichotomy at a lower level" in making such a mental/physical difference (Simonis 2010, 33). I demonstrated in Chapter 1 why this dichotomy is not problematic, despite the lack of complete severing of mind and body in early Chinese texts.

[37] Simonis's account (Simonis 2010, 34) offers a problematic Cartesian dualist view of the mind.

Madness and Grieving

One way we can understand madness is as the constant series of outbursts and infractions of ritual behavior, caused by disorder or illness of one's mind. We can see in a number of texts that the grounds for responsibility is often taken to be the manifestation of behavior, regardless of whether the cause is more or less attributable to the individual (as there is always a confluence of social and individual cause at work). In a number of Confucian texts, we see blame of individuals for outbursts that flout ritual, even where these outbursts are uncharacteristic and would not be attributed (by Confucians or anyone else) to cultivated aspects of one's character. Such outbursts we might see as due to briefly traumatic situations or unusual circumstances that elicit uncharacteristic responses from the individual.

A common theme for such outbursts in Confucian literature is the expression of grief or despair on the death of a parent or other loved one. We see a variety of responses to different forms of ritual infraction on the basis of such grief, some of which are deemed acceptable and some of which are not. One example of unacceptable expression is discussed in the *Kongzi Jiayu* and the *Liji*, in which Confucius's son Boyu has an outburst of wailing after the death of his mother. In both versions of the story, Confucius chides his son for this ritual infraction. One should express grief on the death of a mother, but not the kind of overemotive grief that Boyu expresses. The expectation is that this grief must be properly channeled through the means of ritual, and that Boyu's failure to do so thus demonstrates a key failure to cultivate himself in the right way using these rituals. The suggestion is that had Boyu concentrated on developing himself in the ways Confucius instructed, he would never have come to this point of being unable to properly ritually express his emotions and grief.

> 伯魚之喪母也，期而猶哭。夫子聞之，曰：「誰也？」門人曰：「鯉也。」孔子曰：「嘻！其甚也，非禮也！」伯魚聞之，遂除之。
>
> Boyu was performing mourning rites for his mother, and after the specified time continued to weep. Confucius asked: "Who is that weeping?" His followers said: "it is Boyu." Confucius said: "Agh! This oversteps the boundaries! This is not ritually proper." Boyu, hearing this, stopped weeping.[38]

[38] *Kongzi Jiayu* 42.29.

Of course, there is a relevant backstory here. Boyu, according to what we learn of him in the *Analects*, *Liji*, and *Kongzi Jiayu*, was less than a stellar student, did not put his efforts into self-cultivation, and appears to have been largely a disappointment to his father for these reasons.[39] His ritually improper outburst on the death of his mother then might be seen in terms of an inability to conform to ritual in difficult moments that is ultimately due to Boyu's various failures to apply himself in the cultivation of ritual ability. Though Boyu may very well have no ability to change his actions in the moment, and his spontaneous outburst can be understood in this sense as not directly attributable to his choice, Boyu presumably *is* responsible for the poor choices and insufficient effort that led him to be such that the death of his mother could spontaneously cause such improper outburst. Had Boyu developed himself as his father constantly encouraged him to, the shock and grief of his mother's death would not have led to this infraction of ritual, as Boyu would have cultivated the ability to internalize and properly express such grief.

We can see this kind of response at work in Confucian discussions of madness in general. The culpability of madness comes not from features of the immediate circumstances causing madness, but the cultivation (or lack of cultivation) of character throughout the time leading up to this critical moment. While we see in the *Huangdi Neijing* and other texts the common view that particular situations and emotions lead to madness,[40] the general Confucian view is that self-cultivation involving constraining oneself through ritual enables one to resist these impulses or channel them into more proper behaviors.

The view of culpable madness seems necessary once we take into account features of the Confucian view of self-cultivation via ritual. Ritual operates in part on our dispositions—transforming our behavior through its civilizing effects. Certain emotions, mental states, and character traits without the direction of ritual become vices or disorderly states such as madness. The *Zhongni Yanju* chapter of *Liji* explains:

敬而不中禮，謂之野；恭而不中禮，謂之給；勇而不中禮，謂之逆。

[39] *Analects* 16.13, 17.10.

[40] *Huangdi Neijing Suwen* 46.6; *Huangdi Neijing Lingshujing* 22.

> Being reverent, but not in accordance with ritual, this is called being wild. Being respectful, but not in accordance with ritual, this is called being presumptuous. Being brave, but not in accordance with ritual, this is called being unruly.[41]

In *Analects* 6.3, Confucius praises the (by then late) Yan Hui, saying that he loved learning and that he did not "shift his anger" (*bu qian nu* 不遷怒), suggesting that his ability to control and properly direct his emotions, even in cases when they were aroused, was mainly due to his learning. This learning served then in part as a barrier *not* between madness-inducing situations and the emotions that directly lead to madness, but rather between those emotions and the mental and behavioral symptoms of madness. The cultivated person will still become angry in anger-inducing circumstances, but they will not become *kuang* when anger arises in them. That is, what the Confucians suggest is that the cultivated person will feel the same emotions as everyone else for the most part. The Confucian sage is unlike the Buddhist sage who cultivates equanimity in a broad variety of situations. Part of the reason for this is the *practical* focus of much of early Chinese thought. Confucians were interested primarily in the manifestation of *behavior*. Mental state has a role to play in this, certainly, but many passages show us that the Confucians did not hold that certain mental states had necessary behavioral correspondents. A passage from the *Liyun* chapter of *Liji* further illustrates this:

> 何謂人情？喜怒哀懼愛惡欲七者，弗學而能。

> What are called the human emotions? Joy, anger, grief, fear, love, hate, and desire—these are the seven emotions. One does not learn them yet is able to experience them.[42]

From this, we see that the seven emotions are not themselves cultivated—but this does not yet tell us that they are prone to arise without the direction or assent of our will. It only tells us that we have the ability (*neng* 能) to experience these emotions without learning them. A passage from the *Zhongyong* is complementary here, adding to the picture.

[41] *Liji* 29.1; Ing 2012, 30.
[42] *Liji* 9.18.

喜怒哀樂之未發，謂之中；發而皆中節，謂之和

When joy, anger, grief, and happiness have not yet arisen, this is called centrality (*zhong*). When they have arisen but they are all restrained in the proper way, this is called harmony (*he*).[43]

This follows a general view in early Chinese thought that the emotions are not manifestly negative, even though they can have pernicious effects if not properly integrated and expressed.[44] Doing such is a large part of the role of ritual. As I discuss further in Chapter 4, this is not unique to the Confucians—many other early Chinese thinkers, including Zhuangists, held such a view. While there are certainly major differences between thinkers concerning when particular emotions arise and which behaviors are proper, most early Chinese thinkers would agree that the range of human emotional responses is in general a good or at least neutral thing. Unlike a number of Indian and Western schools and thinkers, early Chinese thinkers resist the view that there are certain mental states that are problematic in themselves in that they directly lead to disorder or suffering.[45]

Outbursts of grief like those of Boyu on the death of his mother are problematic to Confucians not simply because they are infractions of ritual, but because they evince a lack of learning and moral development, of taking the time and effort to internalize the kinds of ritual responses which would cause grief to be manifest in different and more socially acceptable ways. Boyu's failure is not one of weakness or immediate impropriety; rather, it is a lifelong failure of learning and internalization of ritual. The outburst from grief at his mother's death that Confucius laments is merely a symptom of this telling lack.

The outburst based on lack of cultivation for the Confucians is not necessarily indicative of the *xiao ren* 小人 (petty person), though it does suggest a critical failure. The person who becomes *kuang* or engages in other outbursts on the basis of failure of self-cultivation is necessarily different than the

[43] *Liji, Zhongyong* 31.1.

[44] As discussed in Chapter 5, some texts, such as *Xing Zi Ming Chu*, take an even more positive view of emotions and argue that they should *not* be restrained.

[45] Indeed, the problem of suffering as such, connected to mental ease and welfare, is something we do not see much of in early Chinese thought, even while it is at the center of much of Indian thought, including Buddhism. This made for difficulties in the Buddhist "translation" to China in the late Han. The Daoist-Buddhist synthesis that arose in later years has led to numerous scholars reading texts such as the Zhuangzi with Buddhist-like assumptions absent from the thought of Zhuangists. I discuss some of these issues in Chapter 4 of this book and in McLeod 2019.

xiao ren Confucians often refer to. The reason for this is that the *xiao ren* is presented in early Confucian texts as reliably vicious, seemingly possessive of a vicious character, such that their failures are not simply circumstantial, but more clearly global.[46] We find other examples of such outbursts caused not by the possession of a reliably vicious character, but by absences of cultivation that allow circumstances to cause improper behavior.[47]

The kinds of absence of cultivation brought about by failure to adhere to ritual can lead to both vice in general and states such as *kuang*. This makes it somewhat difficult to distinguish between the two categories. Is *kuang* a form of vice akin to other negative character traits of the *xiao ren*, such as selfishness or dishonesty?[48] And how do we distinguish *kuang* from those other states in kind? In some sense, we can indeed say that *kuang* is simply a more extreme form of vice, constructed in the same way and understood the same in kind as other vices. The main evidence for this comes from the various passages about *kuang* in Confucian texts attributing its cause to overabundant emotion, which is connected to failure of ritual cultivation. There are many general statements of the role of ritual in harmonizing emotion, balancing elements of behavior, and other positive benefits. A passage concerning this from the *Zhongni Yanju* chapter of *Liji* reads:

> 子貢越席而對曰：「敢問將何以為此中者也？」子曰：「禮乎禮！夫禮所以制中也。」
>
> Zigong shuffled on his mat and replied, "dare I ask how one comes to find balance (*zhong*)?" Confucius responded, "it is ritual! Ritual! Ritual is the means by which one creates a sense of balance."[49]

Violation of ritual, the passage implies, leads to imbalance, and this imbalance (depending on other crucial traits of the individual) can lead to vice or can lead to madness.

Part of the Confucian suspicion of madness and focus on feigned madness (*yangkuang*), of course, may be due to potential implications of madness for the Confucian view of personhood. If legitimate madness is a personal

46 Amy Olberding discusses this feature of the *xiao ren* in the *Analects* and the difficulty of making sense of moral failure in noncultivated cases in Olberding 2014.

47 This is certainly relevant for the issue of psychological situationism, which has been discussed in connection with early Confucianism by a number of scholars.

48 I am indebted to Heather Battaly for bringing up this point in a discussion of the topic.

49 *Liji* 28.1, Ing trans., in Ing 2012, 31.

failing, such that moral responsibility for it must at least partly fall on the individual who is mad, then the individual's community also bears some level of moral responsibility for the individual's madness—an implication I consider further in Chapter 4, and that forms part of the basis of the Zhuangist challenge to the Confucian views of personhood and madness.

4

The Wilds, Untamed, and Spontaneity

Zhuangist Views of Madness

Inversion of Value and Elimination of Conflicts in the *Zhuangzi*

In this chapter, I consider a very different view of *kuang* and related states, rendering these states not as *illness*, but instead as wellness. In texts such as *Zhuangzi*, there is a focus on the incompleteness and stultification of the value/valueless distinction, in which some nonvalue state is deemed useless or to be rejected. We find argument throughout the *Zhuangzi* that the acts, traits, and states that are valued by most people (such as the Confucians and Mohists) require a devaluation of their perceived opposites. This devaluation renders large parts of the world useless, harmful, or otherwise undesirable, and this leads to inevitable failure of the individual and/or of society to thrive. The way to avoid this harm through devaluation, according to Zhuangists, is to avoid valuation. The process of *shi-fei* discrimination inevitably establishes something as rejected, useless, and negative. Any valuation can only take place along the background of relative devaluation of the noncentered thing. Just as there cannot be a mountain without a valley (to use an image from *Daodejing*), there cannot be value without disvalue.

The *Zhuangzi* presents a number of arguments to show that things conventionally deemed disvaluable, things commonly placed on the *fei* side of the *shi-fei* divide, can have enormous value and be used to facilitate thriving, if only we allow our perspectives to accept these things as valuable, rather than relegating them to the dustbin of the "useless" due to our inability to break out of a particular way of distinguishing between the valuable and disvaluable, our inability to shift perspectives. While it seems in some places that the *Zhuangzi* argues that we should never engage in *shi-fei* valuation and conceptualization,[1] this message is inconsistent with the Zhuangist elevation

[1] *Zhuangzi* 2.4–5, 2.7.

The Dao of Madness. Alexus McLeod, Oxford University Press. © Oxford University Press 2021.
DOI: 10.1093/oso/9780197505915.003.0005

of the disvalued and seemingly "useless" throughout the text. Rather, what seems to be going on is an argument to show that any given valuation or conceptualization of the world is conventional and contingent on perspective, and there is no given perspective that should be constantly or single-mindedly held. Those things deemed "useless" from one perspective are useful from another, and thus the way to maximize the value of our experience is to gain the ability to shift perspectives—to escape being caught within a single narrow perspective that makes it impossible for us to value much of (if not most of) what we encounter in the world, and our ways of being. We find a variety of passages discussing the benefits of the inversion of values through shifting one's perspective. Numerous "useless tree" stories mark sections of the text—the theme being that the tree with wood that cannot be used for the usual purposes (building houses, boats, etc.) has value that can only be recognized when we rethink the value of a tree (as providing shade, etc.).[2] A passage in chapter 1 finds Zhuangzi chiding his friend Hui Shi for his failure to recognize that gourds do not have to be used as bowls, and deeming seeds that grow enormous gourds as useless. Zhuangzi says:

> 今子有五石之瓠，何不慮以為大樽而浮乎江湖，而憂其瓠落無所容？則夫子猶有蓬之心也夫
>
> Now, you have these gigantic gourds—why not consider turning them into large tubs and using them to float down rivers and lakes? Instead you're upset that your gourds diverge from the usual kind? Your mind is full of tangled brush![3]

Following this general view of revaluation and shift of perspective, in the *Zhuangzi* and related texts we find an inversion of Confucian and other "traditional" views of madness, in which the mad person is not presented as flawed or deficient, but rather as superior in understanding to average, non-*kuang* people. This inversion concerning madness takes place in the context of a larger Zhuangist rejection of the notion of the *shi-fei* discriminations of value/nonvalue, right/wrong, and other such dichotomies. When we fail to move between perspectives and evaluate things in alternative ways, not only do we fail to see the possible value of objects such as "useless" trees and enormous

[2] Ex. *Zhuangzi* 1.7, 4.5–6, and the numerous "useless tree" stories of *Zhuangzi* 20.

[3] *Zhuangzi* 1.6.

gourds, we also fail to see the potential value of conventionally undesirable mental states, character traits, and ways of being in the world. This is at the root of the Zhuangist celebration of the *kuang* person and other such conventionally rejected and undesirable characters throughout the *Zhuangzi*.

This Zhuangist reevaluation of the madman both draws on elements of a common image in early Chinese texts and creates a trope that comes to be standard in the later tradition. The wise hermit, madman, or "uncivilized" outsider becomes a common image in Chinese intellectual culture. This is an image with roots in the Daoist and Zhuangist literature of the Warring States period—one that is later bolstered by later Daoist-influenced movements, including Xuanxue (Neo-Daoism), and schools of Buddhism such as Chan. The authors of the *Zhuangzi* in particular played the central role in the development of a romanticized view of madness. As I show in this chapter, there are numerous reasons for the Zhuangist celebration of madness. Put most simply, the focus of the Zhuangists on a particular view of the "natural" as uncultivated, nonagentive, and spontaneous (*ziran* 自然) contributed to their focus on the mad person as ideal, representative of the activity of the natural, or true person—the *zhen ren* 真人. As part of the Zhuangist criticism and subversion of conceptions of developed personhood like that of the Confucians, they elevated figures such as mad, ill, disabled, and socially ostracized people. They developed a conception of the natural and spontaneous exemplified by such figures. Later, I begin with a discussion of the ideas of nature, the wild, and uncultivated, showing how these tie to overarching Zhuangist concerns. I then consider the Zhuangist views of madness and mental illness through investigation of the many appearances of mad characters and reflections on madness throughout the text. I then consider the Zhuangist approach to mental states deemed negative through a consideration of the issue of anxiety in the *Zhuangzi*, arguing that this approach informs the Zhuangist view on mental illness more generally. Finally, I discuss the Zhuangist rejection of the problematic nature of madness in light of Zhuangist views on agency and personhood.

The Wilds, Barbarians, and Unrestrained Behavior—Expressing Our "Nature"

Sarah Allan claims that we do not find a nature-culture distinction in early Chinese texts,[4] and that instead what we find is a distinction drawn between

[4] Allan 2017, 4.

what is so of itself (*ziran*) and what requires human construction (*wei* or *zuo*).[5] She writes:

> There is little evidence that categories denoting "nature" and "culture" (or "wild" and "domesticated") were ever a defining dualism in early Chinese thought.[6]

Part of the way this proceeds, however, is through term matching. Allan claims that there is no single term in Classical Chinese that matches "nature." This is perhaps true, though it alone is not enough to show that there is no concept of nature in early Chinese texts.[7] Part of what I show in this section is that madness is associated with the wild, untamed, and uncivilized in early Chinese texts—both where madness is shunned as well as where it is praised. We see some texts subvert this through a reevaluation of the natural, but the generally accepted position seems to be association of madness with the unhewn, the wilds outside of the reach of culture.

Particular associations, such as with southern states like Chu 楚 of the Warring States period, play a role in conceptions of madness in early texts. It is not a coincidence that the famous "Madman of Chu" is a denizen of the state of Chu, rather than a more central and "civilized" state such as Confucius's native Lu, or even the warlike western state of Qin. Chu becomes associated with the periphery, the wilds, and barbarism in early texts. Chu is an uncultivated beyond to which exiles from civilization are sent, and which thus has particular meaning in terms of the "wilding" of previously civilized people, unlike the also barbarous north. As Laurence Schneider writes:

> the South comes to be associated with deviance and dissent, with eccentricity and defection. The [Qu Yuan] lore begins by showing that the South is a place to which deviants and dissenters are transported. Eventually, it says that the South is the place from which they come. The [Yangzi] River becomes a mythological frontier of experience as well as a geographical frontier.[8]

5 She also argues against understanding *zuo* as "creation" in Michael Puett's sense. Allan 2017, 3.
6 Allan 2017, 4.
7 See Van Norden on the "lexical fallacy" (Van Norden 2007, 22), and McLeod 2015, ch. 1.
8 Schneider 1980, 14.

The association of the wilderness and the madman or the castoff became a major theme of Chinese literature in the Warring States and beyond. Especially prominent in this literature was the theme of the official feigning madness (*yangkuang*) to escape the stultifying or impossible situation of society under an incapable ruler or other corrupted social circumstances. A number of characters in early Chinese literature, whom I discuss later, show us elements of the theme of the connection of madness, wilderness, and the lack of civilization.

The "primitive madman" theme can be seen in stories of scholars coming across strangely wise hermits in the countryside. Such figures are often represented as farmers or fishermen. Fishing motifs figure in a number of texts with hermit characters encountering good officials or Confucians in trouble. We see the example of the fisherman (*yufu* 漁父) in the *Zhuangzi* and *Chuci* chapters of the same title, featuring Confucius and Qu Yuan, respectively. The hermit fisherman character is set against the structures of the world of civilization, government, social norms, and order. The fisherman is not *only* flouting society by being a solitary hermit in the wilderness but also is rejecting the norms of this human society, the kinds of norms dictated by the *li* of the Confucians, for example. This propriety can only happen within community, within the system of roles in a larger social structure. This is just what the fisherman does not have—he is a lone figure sustaining himself on his own, uncontextualized, and thus like the Proto-Daoist hermits of the *Analects*, without full personhood. To learn from the hermit fisherman is to be tempted by madness, by the untamed wilderness. In early texts madness was associated with the rural, the rustic and uncivilized, in opposition to the urban and civilized.[9] Not only does the familiar theme of the hermetic rustic madman follow this, but the association of such madness with the state of Chu 楚, through figures such as the infamous Jieyu, "Madman of Chu," and Qu Yuan, among others. Chu, as numerous authors have commented, was by the Han period seen as the quintessential raw, wild, and semibarbaric countryside.[10]

The shamanistic association with Chu and its perceived falling outside of the ritual and social norms of the "civilized" northern states is also part of the picture here in the association of Chu, wilderness, and madness. Not

[9] Laurence Schneider points this out in Schneider 1980, 13–14.

[10] Schenider 1890, 13. Cook and Major 2004, vii: "Han period writers . . . remembered as Chu, an exotic shamanistic culture of southern and southeastern barbarians."

just *any* wilderness is a mad wilderness. We do not find the same associations with the northern barbarians such as the Xiongnu, for example, despite their seeming strangeness and the wild or unruly acts often attributed to them.[11] One of the differences between the Xiongnu and the state of Chu by the Han Dynasty would have been that Chu was a distant memory of a people definitively associated with the Han, with the empire itself, a kind of semimythical "barbarian within," while the Xiongnu were not only a live problem but also a more clearly distinguishable "other," despite the porous and diffuse nature of Han (or more properly Zhou) civilization and identity.[12]

To be mad in this conventional (Confucian) understanding was to wander outside, to flout the norms of society, whether on purpose or because forced to. Thus we might connect *feigned* madness (*yangkuang*) to a kind of *kuang*. *Yangkuang* for the early Chinese tradition was not *merely* a kind of "malingering."[13] In choosing to leave the binds of society, one also chose to take on the kind of wildness and malformation of the outside, of the barbaric untamed wilds. One did not simply keep one's cultivation and civilization intact and bring it with one into the woods—rather, in an important way one *became* the wilds. If we look back at the Confucian (and roughly conventional) conception of the person discussed in Chapter 1, we can see why an abandonment of civilization for the untamed wilds would require a kind of transformation of the essence of the person. One could not leave society without a critical transformation of oneself, constituted in part by the person's integration into this new, wild, and ultimately *kuang* asocial situation of the forest. This is how we might understand Confucius's horrified injunction in *Analects* 18.6 that "one cannot follow the way of the birds and beasts." Unconventional characters who flout or otherwise fall outside of the conventional bounds of society are found in the wilderness in early Chinese literature. It is hardly ever in the village, in the court, in ordinary society that we find such madmen and hermits. Part of the explanation for this is the *transitory* nature of the madman. While Confucius and his students, *ru* scholars, good ministers, or

[11] Accounts of the Xiongnu are found in the *Shiji*, *Han shu*, and *Houhan shu*. Honeychurch 2015, 223.

[12] Such individuals as Liu Yuan (d. 301 CE), a Xiongnu rebel who fought the Jin and considered himself the king then emperor of a new Han state, represent this ambiguity. Liu had been educated and raised in a Chinese manner. Knechtges and Chang 2010, 544.

[13] Thomas Szasz infamously discusses the distinction between malingering and illness and changing conceptions of this in Szasz 1973, 12–13.

village folk stay in their place, adhering to their roles and performing consistent, if not mechanical rituals, the madman's failure to be contextualized by these roles and rituals renders him unpredictable, wavering, abrupt, and meandering, just like the parts of the world that have been untamed by human touch, working, and integration.

Perhaps this is part of the allure of the image of the fisherman in discussions of the hermits and madness (as discussed further later). Where fish seem to dart from place to place inexplicably, following some invisible logic or pattern indiscernible to the human mind, the madman who inhabits the wilds follows this same unhewn pattern. We see here an echo of the Daoist injunction to follow the patterns of nature, in distinction from following the patterns of the human. Throughout texts such as the *Daodejing* and *Zhuangzi* we find discussions of the insufficiency of the (merely) human way and calls to instead follow the way of the nature. With madness associated with the natural or at least nonhuman way in numerous texts, this already seems to commit the Daoist to a positive or romanticized view of madness.

Confucian texts, however, come down squarely on the side of ordering and human society. Confucius and Zilu in *Analects* 18.5–7 express their shock and disdain at the prospect of leading lives like those of the hermits they encounter, who have, according to Confucius, abandoned the human way and chosen instead to follow the way of the "birds and beasts." Xunzi is even more forceful in his rejection of such a way.[14]

The one possible exception to this for the early Confucians is Mengzi, who presents us with a difficult case. Though he, like the other early Confucians, accepts that a uniquely human-ordered way is the proper way, he understands this way as implicitly included within our inborn characteristics in a way that suggests that given our unstinted growth, we will develop along the lines of the human way. Thus people like the Daoist hermit or the madman develop in the ways they do because of injury to their nature, veering off the path on the basis of some insult to the system. This is important for our purposes because Mengzi's position seems to suggest a kind of *reversal* of the dominant view associating madness with the raw, wild, and untamed. Another possibility, of course, is that what we see in Mengzi shows us that we should be careful connecting the wild and untamed with the *natural*. What we see here offers us an alternative—connection of the natural state with the cultivated

[14] For example, *Xunzi* 21.15: 若夫非分是非，非治曲直，非辨治亂，非治人道，雖能之無益於人

and ordered human state, with the wild and untamed a divergence from this natural state.

After all, there is an inherent instability in any appeal to the "natural" in terms of the way things should or otherwise would be without interference from some (nonnatural?) source. As in the case of appeals to "Natural Law" in Western traditions, any claim that the nature of humans contains certain content is open to the objection that things falling outside of this content are equally, if not more, easy for humans to possess or perform. If what is natural is what is inborn in us in a way that suggests effortless manifestation or possession without cultivation, then it looks like we will have to concede that *everything* we do is natural. If it is a human tendency to fall away from the Confucian path, for example, for whatever reason, then in what sense can we call all of those things that cause this fall "unnatural"? One way we might go about this, as the Confucians do, is to make the claim that the function of one specific kind of thing, such as the human, is understood in a certain way, and the reason such a thing may fail to function in the natural ways is due to the influence of other things on that thing. Of course, this move requires also accepting the position that part of the nature of the thing in question is its ability to be so influenced by outside objects and events. In which case, we are back to the original problem that any feature possessed by or action performed by the object in question must be, in some sense, in its nature.

We might see just this difficulty as one of the central insights of the early Daoist tradition, discussed in texts such as the *Daodejing* and *Zhuangzi*, which challenge the concept of the *ren dao* 人道 (human way) as the uniquely privileged or uniquely natural way for humans to follow. The *Zhuangzi* in particular emphasizes the point that the range of possible human actions is far broader than what the "human way" of the Confucian and others allows, and that all of these actions can be seen as consistent with nature, understood in the right way. The *Zhuangzi* and related texts such as *Huainanzi* suggest a radical revision of the concept of nature. We can see similar reasoning behind their reevaluation of states such as madness.

In the numerous madman/hermit stories we find in early literature, we see a close link between madness and the wilderness. This is only subverted with texts such as the *Zhuangzi*, in which both madness and wilderness are praised as among the highest of values, and an ironic reevaluation is made in which social contextualization and the "human way" are seen as truly mistaken, cross-purposive, and thus "mad" in the sense non-Zhuangist thinkers usually conceive of it.

In early China, just as in Western contexts, people associated transgressive activity with barbarism and lack of civilization, which was/is in turn associated with the wilds, with nature, with the untamed. We see this association still today in the West, in the sometimes well-meaning but ill-considered association of Native American groups with "nature"—the idea of the primitive "savage" (even though not many still use those words, the idea endures) as closer to nature or even a part of nature, unlike the "developed" or "civilized" Euro-American. This is part of what leads some to prize Native cultures as a kind of antidote to civilization, a way of undoing or moving away from the problems inherent in civilization, such as alienation, loss of meaning, a sense of isolation from the nonhuman world, and so on. Interestingly, this is very similar to the strain of what is often called "primitivism" in the *Zhuangzi*, in which numerous arguments are made that the project of civilization (and government most of all) injures our nature, and that the only way to thriving is to ultimately reject this project and instead live a life closer to our "nature." There are tricky and thorny questions lurking here that must be worked out, and I attempt to do some of that in this chapter.

First, we must distinguish questions concerning "nature" and human development in the (modern) Western context and that of early China. For all their similarity, there are fundamental differences between these conceptions that will make it the case that any attempt to understand the early Chinese understanding through our Western conception of nature will yield problematic results. And in this case it is particularly crucial that we understand these divergences *because* these conceptions of nature and human development are so similar. They are so close to one another that it becomes easy to see in early China the same issues concerning nature and development that we find in the modern West unless we are cautious. Where early Chinese concepts and views are clearly or radically different from our own, we are less apt to make the mistake of simply attributing familiar Western views to early Chinese thinkers.

In the Western tradition, the concept of nature that developed early in the period at the beginnings of modern Western science in the seventeenth century is one commonly used today, which creates a dichotomy between nature and technology or nature and humanity (and human artifice).[15] Interestingly, it is this conception of nature that is closer to the Zhuangist

[15] See Brown and McLeod 2020, ch. 1.

understanding than a conception of nature with greater antiquity in the West, that found in ancient Greece, through the medieval period in Europe and the Islamic world—the conception of nature and the natural as the essential and proper features of a thing. We find such a conception developed in the work of Aristotle, who holds that nature is an internal principle of rest and change,[16] within a particular thing. This sense of nature is still understood in the English term, when we say things like "it is the nature of a bird to fly," and this sense of nature is echoed in some ways in the early Chinese conceptions of *zhi* 質 and *xing* 性.

The concept of nature of the early modern West, which we generally use to translate the cluster of concepts associated with this idea in early China, was seen as oppositional to the conception of human artifice and creation. Thus, human technology or society and its norms serve as a counterpoint to "nature." It is this we see in the discussion of the "state of nature" in philosophers such as Hobbes and Rousseau. Though they have different conceptions of the content of this state of nature, they agree that it is a state completely devoid of the artifice of human society, which is needed in order to rectify certain developments either within the state of nature or based on moving away from this state of nature.

Michael Puett has discussed a similar conception of the development of ritual (*li*) in early Chinese thought, with *li* understood as human artifice (constructed by the sages) necessary to rectify negative patterns that arose in humanity as a result of straying from the most natural state (this being closer to Rousseau's picture of nature than that of Hobbes).[17] He captures the ambivalence concerning human culture in this understanding of ritual, arguing that though ritual was seen as necessary, it also caused its own problems in human life in part as a result of this artifice, which then required the construction of new rituals to rectify it. We see such an understanding of ritual in a number of places in early Chinese literature, perhaps nowhere more prominently than in the *Huainanzi*. Part of the reason for the prominence of this point in the *Huainanzi* is the syncretic nature of the text. Providing arguments for the necessity of Confucian ritual, it also looked to defend Daoist and Zhuangist views of the insufficiency and corrupting nature of ritual. Thus, though the text argues that ritual and the other artifices

[16] *Physics* 1.2.
[17] Puett 2015.

of culture only exist because of decline from the original state of "grand unity" (*tai yi* 太一), ritual is still necessary to soften this decline, to bring humanity back toward this state as much as is still possible.[18] In this way, there is resonance between the *Huainanzi*'s story (and other early Chinese accounts) and Abrahamic accounts of the fall of humanity from an original state of perfection and the subsequent necessity of laws (although in the Abrahamic religions these laws are said to be of divine rather than human creation).

There are difficulties inherent in the Confucian concept of ritual when it is associated with inborn human characteristics. The early Confucians attempted to build ritual into human inborn characteristics (*xing*) or nature more broadly understood, in part as a response to Yangist and Daoist (and later, Zhuangist) criticisms of ritual as artificial and thus injurious to the human. A view like this is even suggested in the *Mengzi*, in Mengzi's discussion with Gaozi in *Mengzi* 6A1. This may be the reason that ritual has far less emphasis in the *Mengzi* than it does in texts like the *Xunzi*, in which a much less rosy view of human inborn characteristics grounds the view that ritual (even if conventional) is a necessary corrective. According to Xunzi, ritual constrains and shapes human desire and behavior, with the idea that given our "natural" inclinations, in the absence of such constraint, our desires will grow unwieldy and inevitably lead to the construction of vicious character.[19] This echoes a number of claims of the *Analects*, in which Confucius and his students claim that ritual is necessary in the formation of character.[20] In the *Analects*, it is much less clear than it is in the *Xunzi* that ritual constitutes a largely human technology, something seen as opposed to "nature" in roughly the dichotomy drawn by early modern European philosophers.

Ritual is associated by all of the early Confucian philosophers with civilization (*wen*), community, and government. And it is this entire complex of concepts that Yangists, Daoists, and especially Zhuangists see as problematic, in part because they are seen as violating or cutting against natural human responses, and thus disordering patterns of action that can be found in "nature," whether understood in terms of *xing* (one's own inborn characteristics) or *tian* (the natural characteristics of the rest of the world). The early Daoists

[18] See *Huainanzi* ch. 11, *Qisu*, and the introduction to ch. 11 in Major et al. 2010.
[19] *Xunzi* 19.1–2.
[20] *Analects* 1.12, 2.3, 12.1.

and Zhuangists use the concept of *li* 理 (pattern, propensity) to capture this idea. Proper action, natural action, follows from observing and going along with natural patterns (*tian li*), rather than following the dictates of artificial and nonnatural rituals.[21]

The early Daoist concept of *ziran* (self-so, spontaneity) is connected to this idea of the proper human activity as the unregimented, uncultivated, and unforced—the *natural*. In Han texts and into Neo-Daoism in the Wei-Jin period, this concept of *ziran* is combined with that of inborn characteristics (*xing*) to express the idea of the natural behavior of a thing, in terms of its development absent the constraints of things like ritual. In the late Han, Wang Chong develops a view of *ziran* as the principle of development of things—in his case, in order to avoid the view of purposive and guided development of elements of the nonhuman world and even human fate or allotment.[22]

The early Daoist and Zhuangist view of *ziran* comes closest to the expression of the natural, unforced, and uncultivated action that cuts against the kind of purposive shaping of Confucian ritual and other guided forms of self-cultivation. "Natural" responses are ones that occur of themselves and without training. Indeed, the fact that certain behaviors and responses require training shows in itself that these are not natural human responses. We might think, given this, that the Daoists cannot make sense of the fact that humans learn behavior and language, but there is a way around this. Certain patterns of learning and adoption of behavior are not strictly purposive, but humans simply find themselves in situations such that they spontaneously and without intention adopt particular mental states.

This Yangist/Daoist/Zhuangist conception of natural human responses is not completely alien to other early Chinese traditions. The *Mengzi*, perhaps influenced by Yangist and Daoist views, held a very similar view, but made it consistent with Confucian ethical positions by building the kinds of basic behaviors and attitudes ritual activity expresses as part of the inborn characteristics (*xing*) of human beings, and thus attempting to undercut the Daoist

[21] *Li* is a difficult concept in early Chinese thought, and it is more familiar in its Neo-Confucian context. While early conceptions of *li* played a role in the development of Neo-Confucian conceptions (along with Buddhism), the idea of *li* as patterns of nature opposed to manufactured patterns of human artifice (such as ritual, according to Daoists) is more prominent in early texts. Brook Ziporyn discusses the development of this concept in the first volume of his two-volume study of *li* (Ziporyn 2013). Ultimately I think his interpretation fits certain Neo-Confucians better than it does the early texts, in which something like "natural pattern" is at work.

[22] *Lunheng* 54. Also see McLeod 2018a, 216–219.

objection to Confucian self-cultivation that such cultivation violates our nature, making it impossible to spontaneously express our inborn characteristics, and thus impossible to be truly human (a goal the Confucians claim to be centrally concerned with).[23] The Daoist position is certainly blunted by this move of the *Mengzi*, but the position saddles Mengzian Confucians with new difficulties. It is perhaps in part for this reason that the role of ritual is deemphasized in the *Mengzi*, being mentioned along with *yi* in a number of passages, and seemingly disparaged in some places it is mentioned, such as 4A17.[24] In that passage, Mengzi offers an objection to ritual standards that one might expect from a Yangist or Daoist, arguing that the inherent human responses and the emotions that lead to them ultimately ought to be followed, suggesting that these are the surest guide to proper action. If this is so, however, then why is ritual necessary at all? That is, in his focus on *yi* alongside *li* as perhaps the more important concept, Mengzi seems to vitiate ritual and undermine any need we might have for it. The most ritual could be is a kind of ethical shorthand. But if this is what ritual is, then why shouldn't we think that the cultivated person is one who uses ritual as a heuristic early in their development before the generation of ethical expertise, and who discards it as they become more sensitive to *yi*? That is, why would a morally developed person ever have need of ritual?

This is clearly different from what we see in texts like the *Lunyu* and *Xunzi*. There are passages of the *Mengzi* that suggest that this move was at least in part intended to respond to Daoist concerns that may have found purchase in Confucian students.[25] I consider the Mengzian response further later, investigating whether or not it could have provided an adequate response to the Zhuangist challenge on the issue of mental and behavioral divergence, madness, and natural action.

Confucians such as Xunzi, as well as most other early Chinese Confucianism beside the *Mengzi*,[26] took the "natural" responses enjoined

[23] *Analects* 18.5–7.

[24] The famous passage in which Mengzi challenges the ritual against men coming into physical contact with women for its rigidity.

[25] *Mengzi* 7B26 describes the natural progression in movement between the schools, suggesting that people begin with Mohism, and rejecting it move to Yangism, and rejecting it finally move to Confucianism.

[26] The popularity and centrality of the *Mengzi* in the Confucian tradition did not happen until the mid-Tang Dynasty, and with the rise of Neo-Confucianism in the work of thinkers like Zhu Xi. During the Pre-Qin and the Han periods, the *Xunzi* and similar texts held a much more central place in Confucianism—Xunzian Confucianism would have been "orthodox" or mainstream. Watson 2003, 10; Zhao 2015, 182.

by the Zhuangists as in themselves unformed, uncivilized, and transgressive. In texts such as *Liji*, *Hanshi Waizhuan*, *Chuci*, and many others, we find an association made between nature, the natural, the unconstrained, and transgression. Madness plays a key role in this, and the madman character is often associated with the wild, the uncivilized, the rustic, and outside of nature.

A common theme in early Chinese literature is the hermetic escape of the thwarted minister—usually a virtuous figure deemed to have been wronged by a bad ruler. We find such an image in Qu Yuan of the *Chuci*, and by the Eastern Han this image had become such a well-established trope as to be used as a literary theme to clearly express a particular image, in texts such as Wang Fu's *Qianfulun*. By Wang's time, the figure was a well-worn literary type. This figure, though common, presented problems for the early Confucian approach to self-development. Early Confucians in general were committed to the view that self-development could only happen in community, as community and commitment to it formed the basis of human identity.[27]

The connection of the themes of madness, the wilds, and uncultivated human activity in early Chinese texts clearly influenced Zhuangist thinkers, who used the opportunity to invert these themes in their celebration of uncultivated spontaneous action following the "natural patterns" (*tian li* 天理) of human behavior. From the Yangist background, Zhuangist texts playfully and skillfully deploy characters associated with the wild, uncultivated, and mad, raising them as moral exemplars in ways surely intended to be shocking to traditional readers. Throughout the *Zhuangzi*, we find presentation of characters inverting the values of the Confucians, in which Zhuangists praise the efficacy of the behavior and attitudes of these characters. Perhaps the clearest example of this is the character of the "Madman of Chu" (*Chu kuang ren* 楚狂人), who echoes the words of the same character in Book 18 of the *Lunyu*, but offering a Zhuangist position and emerging as the hero rather than the foil. Examining these characters in the *Zhuangzi* can tell us much about the Zhuangist view of the person, and the ways in which they reject the Confucian position. It also helps us understand the kind of "deconstructive" view of *kuang* on offer in the *Zhuangzi*, which later texts attempt to undermine.

[27] *Analects* 18.5–7, 4.1, 4.7. See also McLeod 2012.

Transgressive, Ill, Wild, and Mad Characters in the *Zhuangzi*

The *Zhuangzi* offers up a panoply of characters falling outside of the bounds of proper society, social norms, ritual, and "civilization." These are intentionally transgressive characters, presented by the Zhuangists as a challenge to the rigidity of perspective of Confucians, Mohists, and other positive moralists. It can be useful here, for an understanding of Zhuangist views of (and re-envisioning of) illness and disorder, to look to a number of important examples of such transgressive "ill" characters in the *Zhuangzi*.

Certain passages of the *Zhuangzi* claim the unknown value of states such as *bing* 病 (illness). The ill are deemed conventionally useless, like the useless tree, such that they will not be harmed in the way that conventionally "useful" things will. In chapter 4, we see discussion of the three kinds of thing that are not to be used for sacrifice, according to the traditional view—oxen with white heads, pigs with high noses, and people with the illness of piles. And it is just because they have these seemingly negative features, according to the text, that these things avoid sacrifice and go unharmed. This is what the *shen ren* 神人 (spirit person) understands.

In chapter 6, the character Ziyu becomes ill (*bing*) and explains this to his colleagues as a boon. When asked if his illness bothers him, Ziyu explains that, on the contrary, it can be seen as a good thing. He says, when asked if he dislikes the fact that he is ill:

> 亡，予何惡！浸假而化予之左臂以為雞，予因以求時夜；浸假而化予之右臂以為彈，予因以求鴞炙；浸假而化予之尻以為輪，以神為馬，予因以乘之，豈更駕哉！且夫得者時也，失者順也，安時而處順，哀樂不能入也。此古之所謂縣解也，而不能自解者，物有結之。且夫物不勝天久矣，吾又何惡焉？

> How could I be upset by this? If I were to fall into calamity and take my left arm to be a rooster, I would then use it to mark the time of the night. If I were to fall into calamity and take my right arm to be a crossbow, then I would use it to shoot an owl and have a feast. If I were to fall into calamity and take my butt to be a wheel and my spirit to be a horse, then I would drive them around—how much better could I possibly drive? Just when one obtains it is its season, when one loses it is when it should go. Grief and joy then cannot enter. This is what the ancients called untying the cord. But

> you cannot untie yourself when things keep you bound up. It's long established that things cannot defeat nature (*tian*)—how then could I be upset by this?[28]

Ziyu's rejection of the idea that he is distressed by his illness is based on his acceptance of the transformation of things, as well as his rejection of the idea of the self (*ji* 己)—that is, any particular commitment to the kind of thing he has to be or wants to be, on which his thriving hinges. Whatever transformation Ziyu encounters, whatever situation in which he finds himself, whether it is illness or being a horse or a cart, he can make use of this situation and find value in it. Finally, when death comes, this transformation, too, can be the source of value as long as one is able to accept the myriad transformations.

> 已化而生，又化而死，生物哀之，人類悲之。解其天弢，墮其天袠
>
> Things transform and (a person) is born, they again transform and a person dies. Living things mourn this, and it causes humans grief. But it is just untying the natural bow, the discarding of the natural scabbard.[29]

For purposes of considerations of madness in this chapter, I do not differentiate between chapters of the *Zhuangzi* on the basis of "Inner," "Outer," or "Miscellaneous" groupings (or any other for that matter). I take it as a given that the compilers of the received *Zhuangzi* (whether this was the authors of the *Huainanzi* in Liu An's court or some other group[30]) selected the material for the text on the basis of shared views and a coherent theme, which for the most part we find between the chapters (with some notable exceptions). Certainly on the issue of madness and the value of transgressive states, the various chapters of the *Zhuangzi* offer a consistent view. Thus, I draw in the discussion later from the entire text, to reconstruct a "Zhuangist" view of madness and its role in activity and self-development (of which the Zhuangists have a particular conception, even though they reject Confucian and Mohist self-cultivational approaches).

[28] *Zhuangzi* 6.5.
[29] *Zhuangzi* 22.5. There are a host of other passages in the text making a similar point, including *Zhuangzi* 2.11, 3.5, and 6.1 (as well as throughout chapter 6), among many others.
[30] See Roth 1991; Klein 2011.

Jieyu, the "Madman of Chu"

The most common and clearly "mad" character found in the *Zhuangzi* is the infamous Jieyu, "Madman of Chu," who appears in chapters 1, 4, and 7. Interestingly, he is only discussed in the so-called Inner Chapters, and if we accept the view of Liu Xiaogan, A. C. Graham, and Burton Watson, among others,[31] that the Inner Chapters represent the earliest texts of the *Zhuangzi* collection, then it may be that the figure of Jieyu was the standard representation of the mad and transgressive outsider or hermit for Zhuangists of this early period (or the author of the inner chapters), but that the character's image lost its power for the authors of the Outer and Miscellaneous chapters.[32] We certainly find the Madman of Chu discussed in a wide range of texts across the Warring States and Han—from early Confucian texts such as the *Lunyu* and *Xunzi* to Han Confucian and Daoist texts, and the Han histories. In texts from the Han, however, discussion of Jieyu is usually based on references to earlier texts such as the *Lunyu*, although we do seem to find a "new" Jieyu story in the *Lienu zhuan*. Jieyu's appearance in Book 18 of the *Lunyu* appears to be a foundational reference to which many of the later accounts (including those of the *Zhuangzi*) refer, either directly or indirectly.

This link to the *Lunyu* is also likely part of the explanation for the power of the character as a key transgressive example for the authors of the *Zhuangzi*. Jieyu appears in that text as an antagonist to Confucius, expressing something like the view some refer to as "Proto-Daoist" or Yangist,[33] enjoining Confucius and his students to abandon the project of attempting to morally rectify the world. Such a situation fits Zhuangist uses perfectly, as Confucian methods and conceptions of personhood and sagehood come in for criticism. Jieyu is even given a speech in the *Analects* fairly consistent with the Zhuangist views.[34] The *Zhuangzi*'s adoption of the character then may be an attempt to claim (or reclaim) this very Zhuangist character from the midst of the Confucians. We find that one of the appearances of Jieyu in the *Zhuangzi* plays directly on the Jieyu passage from *Lunyu* 18, expanding his speech about the *feng* bird on his meeting with Confucius.

[31] Graham 2001; Liu 1994; Watson 1968. Also see Ziporyn 2009, ix.

[32] Esther Klein, however, convincingly challenges this "Inner Chapters" story in Klein 2011.

[33] See Hansen 2000, 163, 195.

[34] The view that these "Proto-Daoist" passages are so charitable to the Daoist/Zhuangist view that they may have been later Daoist additions to the text is mocked by Brooks and Brooks 2001, 183.

The passage echoing that of *Analects* 18 comes in chapter 4 (*Renjianshi*), which is itself an extended criticism of Confucian notions of personhood and moral self-cultivation.[35] While the madness of Jieyu, in both the *Analects* and the *Zhuangzi* 4 versions of the story, is muted, the message of his poem is strikingly similar, although extended in the *Zhuangzi* version. Let us look to the both passages:

[*Analects* 18.5]
楚狂接輿歌而過孔子曰：「鳳兮！鳳兮！何德之衰？往者不可諫，來者猶可追。已而，已而！今之從政者殆而！」孔子下，欲與之言。趨而辟之，不得與之言。

Jieyu, the Madman of Chu, passed by Confucius, singing: "Phoenix! How have you lost your virtue? What is gone cannot be reproached, (but) what is to come can still be pursued. Enough! Those who follow after proper governance today are in danger!" Confucius came down (from his horse), desiring to have a word with him. (The Madman of Chu) hurriedly fled the scene, and Confucius was not able to speak to him.

[*Zhuangzi* 4.8–9]
孔子適楚，楚狂接輿遊其門曰：「鳳兮鳳兮，何如德之衰也！來世不可待，往世不可追也。天下有道，聖人成焉；天下無道，聖人生焉。方今之時，僅免刑焉。福輕乎羽，莫之知載；禍重乎地，莫之知避。已乎已乎，臨人以德！殆乎殆乎，畫地而趨！迷陽迷陽，無傷吾行！吾行卻曲，無傷吾足！」

山木自寇也，膏火自煎也。桂可食，故伐之；漆可用，故割之。人皆知有用之用，而莫知無用之用也。

When Confucius went to Chu, Jieyu, the Madman of Chu, was wandering near the entrance (to Confucius's room), and said: "Phoenix! How have you lost your virtue? Ages to come cannot be waited around for, (and) ages gone by cannot be pursued. When the world possesses the way (dao), the sage is completed therein. When the world lacks the way, the sage is born therein. As for today's age, one can only avoid punishment therein. Prosperity is as light as a feather, yet no one knows how to carry it. Enough! Enough of coming close to people through virtue! Danger! In marking the earth then hurrying on! Bewildering the light, yet my travels are unharmed. My travels are backward and meandering, and my feet are unharmed!" A mountain

[35] See McLeod 2011; Chong 2016, 25–27.

> through its trees crowds itself. Grease used in a fire fries itself. The cinnamon tree can be eaten, therefore it is chopped down. The lacquer tree is useful, therefore it is carved up. Everyone knows the use of the useful, but no one knows the use of the useless.

In the *Zhuangzi* 4 version of the Jieyu and Confucius story, there is an inversion of the image of madness. Rather than Jieyu, Confucius is meant to appear to us as the truly "mad" person—engaged in a social struggle he himself knows he cannot win, and committed to his own harm and decline for seemingly no reason other than to demonstrate his moral beauty at the expense of others (as discussed earlier in the chapter in the conversation between Confucius and Yan Hui). While the Confucian version of the meeting in *Lunyu* 18 leaves Jieyu appearing as an example of a duplicitous person who cleverly uses the appearance of madness to shirk their responsibilities, the *Zhuangzi* 4 Jieyu turns the tables, wielding then dogged Confucian commitment against them. While the conventional-minded or the Confucian reads Jieyu as mad, it is the Confucians, chapter 4 suggests, who are truly mad. Just as the overarching theme of the chapter is to invert the Confucian notion of personhood itself (thus the cleverly jabbing title *Renjianshi*—"In the World of Persons"), in the chapter 4 appearance of Jieyu, madness is being inverted. The madman, like the useless tree, is the one who makes his way through the world unharmed, while the Confucian insisting on rectifying the world and generating virtue and social harmony only ends up securing his own demise (as Confucius warns Yan Hui earlier in the chapter).

The appearance of Jieyu in chapter 4 is clearly meant to be a comment on *Lunyu* 18, and the purported "madness" of the character is peripheral to the main point. The selection of this *Lunyu* passage, however, may be in part based on the madness of Jieyu, as we find other passages surrounding the Jieyu passage in *Lunyu* 18 that may have otherwise worked just as well to make the Zhuangist point. Indeed, we find one of these stories turned into an extended reflection in the *Yufu* chapter of the *Zhuangzi*. Chapter authorship questions aside, the inclusion of Jieyu in *Zhuangzi* 4 suggests a specific focus on his "madness" as redemptive and the source of true wisdom—a kind of wisdom that cuts against the fruitlessness and façade that Zhuangists see as inherent in the Confucian project.

A number of features can be associated with Jieyu from his *Zhuangzi* 4 appearance. (1) Jieyu recognizes the transformation of things, as well as the need to move between perspective because of this constant transformation.

His criticism of Confucius early in the passage demonstrates that he thinks Confucius's main problem is that he is unable to recognize the proper time for activity and to allow for differing activity for differing times. (2) Jieyu is able to make his way through the chaotic and changing world without being harmed, primarily due to his lack of desires and concerns. (3) Jieyu recognizes the "use of the useless" discussed toward the end of the passage, having the ability to follow the natural patterns, and to shift perspectives so as to enable valuation of any given thing. (4) Finally, Jieyu himself, as mad person, *represents* the conventionally useless—the individual with no seeming talent or role in society, and whose uselessness goes even beyond not having a context within society, but even representing a *problem* for society. The mad person does not only fail to fit within the conventional norms, but such a person's action presents a challenge to them—not a silent problematic piece, but one that threatens to take others out of their place, who plays an active undermining role.

While this challenge of conventional norms is consistent with much of what is said about the Zhuangist sage elsewhere in the text, the perfected person (as distinct from the mad person) is sometimes characterized as completely silent and withdrawn in a way the mad person is not.

The two other appearances of Jieyu in the *Zhuangzi*, especially that of chapter 1, more clearly reference aspects of his thought and character associated with madness. In chapter 7, Jieyu explains to Jian Wu the fruitlessness and backwardness of the (Confucian) conception of virtue, continuous with Jieyu's response to Confucius in chapter 4. In the chapter 1 passage, we gain a glimpse into Jieyu's own character and actions, in a discussion about him between Jian Wu and Lian Shu. Jian Wu is a character[36] who appears four times in the *Zhuangzi*, and in two of his appearances is linked to Jieyu. In all of his appearances, he is connected to the rejection of Confucian conceptions of rulership found in Jieyu's message.

The discussion of Jieyu in *Zhuangzi* 1 begins with Jian Wu's description of Jieyu's words, and he and Lian Shu go on to discuss their meaning.

> 肩吾問於連叔曰：「吾聞言於接輿，大而無當，往而不反。吾驚怖其言，猶河漢而無極也，大有逕庭，不近人情焉。」連叔曰：「其言謂何哉？」曰：「藐姑射之山，有神人居焉，肌膚若冰雪，淖約若處子，不食五穀，吸風飲露。乘雲氣，御飛龍，而遊乎四海之外。

[36] Jian Wu was understood as a spirit *xian* 仙, one of the immortals.

其神凝，使物不疵癘而年穀熟。吾以是狂而不信也。」連叔曰：「然，瞽者無以與乎文章之觀，聾者無以與乎鍾鼓之聲。豈唯形骸有聾盲哉？夫知亦有之。是其言也，猶時女也。之人也，之德也，將旁礴萬物，以為一世蘄乎亂，孰弊弊焉以天下為事！之人也，物莫之傷，大浸稽天而不溺，大旱、金石流、土山焦而不熱。是其塵垢粃糠，將猶陶鑄堯、舜者也，孰肯以物為事！…

Jian Wu asked a question of Lian Shu: "I heard the words of Jieyu—they were large and failed to hit the mark, and when they were finished he didn't return to them. I was startled and frightened by his words, which were vast like the galactic disk and without limit. They were large and went past understanding, not connecting with the essence of persons." Lian Shu asked: "what is it that he said?" Jian Wu replied: "he said: 'far away on Guye Mountain, there is a spirit person (*shen ren*). His muscle and skin are like ice and snow, gentle and delicate like a virgin. He did not eat the five grains, but instead inhaled wind and drank dew. He rode the clouds, driving a chariot with flying dragons, and wandered beyond the four seas. His spirit was concentrated, causing things to be without decay and each year's grains to be abundant.' I thought his words were mad (*kuang*) and couldn't believe them." Lian Shu responded: "This is so—the blind can't see beautiful figures, and the deaf can't hear bells and drums. How could deafness and blindness be only of the body? Knowledge also has these features. You can tell this from your words. Of that person, and his potency—fills all things, and allows the current day to be disordered. How could be concerned with the affairs of the world? This person—nothing can harm him. In the greatest floods, reaching up to heaven, he would not drown. In the greatest droughts, hot enough to metal and rock and burn the earth, he would not feel hot. From the dust and chaff, he could form a Yao or Shun—why would he bother himself with the affairs of the world?"[37]

In addition to his own words being outside the bounds of the accepted and usual, Jieyu also describes a nameless *shen ren* (spirit person) with similarly transgressive activity that nonetheless has almost supernatural power. Jieyu's *kuang* words are here contrasted with the blindness (*gu*) and deafness (*long*) of the non-*kuang* or conventional person. This feature of Jieyu

[37] *Zhuangzi* 1.5.

thus allows him an ultimately more accurate perception of the world, rather than one channeled through artificial human conventions.[38] There is also the power of Jieyu's understanding of the *shen ren* Jieyu describes to Jian Wu in the latter's recounting. There is a relevant question here of what makes Jieyu a madman, what makes him transgressive. In other literature, Confucian authors make the assumption that Jieyu was not mad at all, but represented a case of *yangkuang*, feigned madness, in which the madman character was affected so as to help Jieyu avoid social responsibilities.

Jieyu's words, Jian Wu notes, are far outside the boundaries of what is normal, as vast as the cosmos itself, likened to the galactic disk lying beyond the planets and stars.[39] It is the madman's transgression, his failure to be captured in the limited perspective or within the limits of acceptable activity, that here represents his ability to move outside of the confines within which those like the Confucians are trapped. Jieyu, like the "spirit person" he discusses, is vast and contains multitudes. His activity thus appears to those stuck within narrow perspectives as nonsensical, useless, or even terrifying. The activity and thought of the "madman," for the Zhuangists (with the scare quotes here suggestive of the way in which they re-envision madness as order rather than disorder) is only made intelligible from outside the boundaries. It is the very transgressiveness of the madman in this case that makes the case for his expansiveness.

But we might challenge the Zhuangist here. Transgression alone, we might think, is insufficient to show that one has a broader understanding of the world that is unconstrained by a particular perspective. The unconstrained Zhuangist sage who can move between perspectives certainly would be a transgressive figure, and may be seen as a madman by those without understanding, but a transgressive figure or a madman is not necessarily a spirit person who can move with ease between perspectives. Thus, is the Zhuangist here guilty of drawing too close a connection between madness, transgression, and the spirit person's ability to move between perspectives? It does appear as if the claim is made not only that the spirit person will *appear* to others as mad, but that the spirit person in some important sense *is* mad. Madness here is in part constitutive of this ability. In explaining Jieyu's words

[38] I am indebted to a reviewer who pointed out this issue concerning defective perception in the *Zhuangzi*.

[39] The path of the plane of the Milky Way across the sky was a common sight for people in the ancient world (unlike many of those alive today, living in heavily light polluted conditions). Its distance as beyond the planets and stars was apparent to the ancients, as the planets moved over top of it, and stars could be seen against it as background. Pankenier 2015, 383–384.

to Lian Shu, Jian Wu says that "they seemed mad and unfixed (*bu xin*)." Lian Shu does not disabuse Jian Wu of this notion; instead, he agrees with this evaluation, responding "it's true! (*ran*)." What is true here is not that these vast words *seem* mad, but are truly sane or wise, but that they *are* mad. This much is consistent with what Zhuangists maintain elsewhere in the text. The mad, ill, and transgressive characters we see throughout (as I discuss further later) are not skilled despite their deviance, but because of it. It is Jieyu's madness (and the spirit person's madness) that allows them to roam outside the boundaries and see the value of acting in ways the nonmad would never consider.

But if this is case, what does this mean for the mentally stable and nonmad readership of the *Zhuangzi*? If madness (or something like it) is required for the perspective and abilities the Zhuangists enjoin us to develop, then most can never hope to achieve it, unless there is some reliable way to make oneself truly mad. Leaving aside for now the *Huangdi Neijing*'s implicit claim that there *are* such ways, namely the possession of excessive emotional disturbance (whether positive or negative), this problematizes the position the Zhuangist is seemingly committed to here.

It may not be the case, however, that *all* of the features associated with madness are associated with the spirit person, the Zhuangist "sage." As the *Huainanzi* later explicitly claims, mad people and sages are alike in some key ways in their behavior and even mental states, with the critical difference being the *reasons* for those behaviors and states.[40] The claim in *Huainanzi* is that for the sage, these behaviors and states result from knowledge, while in the case of the mad person, they do not (along with the suggestion that the mad person has no choice, while the sage does).

Jieyu, and the spirit person he discusses in chapter 1, represents the perspective beyond that of the conventionally bound. Like the blind person unable to see things of value (such as the visually aesthetically pleasing), the cicada and student dove of chapter 1 (who cannot understand the vastness and transformability of the fish/bird Peng), and the scholar who laughs at the *dao*,[41] the conventional-minded person is unable to recognize the expansiveness of the mad person who wanders outside the bounds of the conventional perspective. The *Zhuangzi* does not exclusively use the mad in this connection, of course. The text also discusses other transgressive figures such

[40] *Huainanzi* 21.19.

[41] *Daodejing* 41: 下士聞道，大笑之。"when the worst scholars hear of *dao*, they laugh at it."

as the ill,[42] the mutilated (such as the amputees discussed in chapter 5), the conventionally useless (as in the numerous "useless tree" stories[43]), and the barbarian-like or uncultivated as having this perspectival advantage over those bound in the conventional. It seems to be the transgressiveness of madness in part that makes for its value for the Zhuangists.

Madness, however, has a particular power perhaps not available (or as obvious) to other transgressive cases. The discussion between "Knowledge," "Non-Action," and "Hunched Madness" in *Zhuangzi* 22 gives us some sense of the particular knowledge and ability available to the mad person as a result of or part of their madness itself.

"Hunched Madness" and Knowledge Wandering in the North

The beginning of chapter 22 of the *Zhuangzi* sees the character "Knowledge" wandering in the north, traveling to a number of metaphorical locations to ask questions of metaphorical characters. At the "mysterious waters," Knowledge meets with "Non-Action" (*wu wei*), whom he asks three questions about *dao*, concerning how we gain knowledge of *dao*, how we become at ease in *dao*, and how we follow and obtain *dao*. Non-Action remains completely silent and doesn't answer the questions. Knowledge then moves south, to the "pure waters," and there encounters "Hunched Madness" (*kuang qu*). Knowledge puts to Hunched Madness these same questions about *dao*, who replies:

> 唉！予知之，將語若，中欲言而忘其所欲言。
>
> Ai! I know the answer to these, and I was about to tell you, but just as I wanted to speak, I forgot what it was I wanted to say![44]

Knowledge finally consults Huang Di, who gives him answers to the three questions. Knowing the *dao* comes through nonthought and nonconcern, being at ease in the *dao* comes through nonoccupation and nonservice, and following and obtaining the *dao* comes through nonfollowing and

[42] Such as the wise hunchbacks of *Zhuangzi* 6.5 and 19.3.
[43] *Zhuangzi* 4.5, 20.1.
[44] *Zhuangzi* 22.1.

noncommitment. Further, it turns out that Non-Action and Hunched Madness have a fuller understanding of *dao*, Huang Di says, than either he or Knowledge has, because true understanding of the *dao* is not spoken—"those who know it do not talk about it, and those who talk about it don't know it" (*fu zhi zhe bu yan, yan zhe bu zhi* 夫知者不言，言者不知). Huang Di continues on to give a long diatribe about *dao* (thus demonstrating that he doesn't *fully* know it), in which he offers what seems like an apophatic understanding of *dao*, which lies behind and is not fully capturable through our concepts or intentional activity.[45] Huang Di explains this in terms of human inability to capture the *dao* in terms of concrete conceptualization or being made a particular subject of discussion— "the *dao* cannot be made an object" (*dao bu ke zhi* 道不可致).[46]

Huang Di instructs Knowledge that the sage recognizes that all things should be valued as one—both that conventionally deemed useful or valuable and that conventionally deemed useless or harmful—that one who understands the *dao* will understand this. Non-Action is closest to this understanding, as he did not speak at all, and Hunched Madness is a close second, because even though he prepared to say it, he forgot the words. If we connect this activity with features of madness as a disorder, we find that the view seems to be that the disorder itself, the ways that it disrupts the usual functioning of the human mind, is in such a case an advantage. Humans have some natural predilection for valuing and devaluing, for making *shi-fei* distinctions concerning the world,[47] and madness gets in the way of this, a veritable wrench thrown into the works of human conceptualization. It is key here that Hunched Madness had the desire to explain the *dao* to Knowledge, but was stopped from doing this because he forgot the words. Due to circumstances outside his control, Hunched Madness was unable to perform the act of speaking he otherwise would have happily engaged in. His madness—that which led him to forget—stood between his intention and his action, like a bulwark against the enemy.

This gives us some sense of what the Zhuangist sees as valuable about states like madness. The difference between the mad person and the complete sage, the *zhi ren* or *shen ren*, is that in the latter case, intention and action have been unified. The spirit person, like Non-Action in chapter 22, does not speak because they do not desire to speak—and the suggestion is

[45] Franke 2018. Also Brown and McLeod 2020, chs. 9, 10.
[46] *Zhuangzi* 22.1.
[47] See Zhuangzi and Hui Shi's discussion of the essence (情 *qing*) of humans in *Zhuangzi* 5.6.

that it would not even occur to them to speak. Their following of the *dao* is complete—their recognition of the unity of value of all things leads them to reject the very idea of engaging in *shi-fei* distinction making. In the case of the mad person, it is some disorder that disrupts their usual discriminative ability that puts them in a state somewhat like that of the fully realized and nonactive person, but without a unified intention. The mad person is close to the *dao* because such a person achieves the proper response to the world, but without the proper intention.

This is reminiscent of the passage from the *Huainanzi* (mentioned earlier) discussing the distinction between the sage and the mad person. The sage's fearlessness, according to the passage, is based on an understanding of the world, on recognition of *dao* and a grasp of the reasons for fearlessness. We might call this stance a "rational fearlessness." It is distinct from the fearlessness of the mad person, which is a result of the disorder of certain natural human capacities that generally result in fearfulness when faced with difficult situations. This leaves the mad person in much the same situation as the rationally fearless person—that is, in a state of fearlessness—but the suggestion in *Huainanzi* is that this state is not yet the perfected state, and lacks something crucial. The *Zhuangzi* 22 passage discussed here makes a similar point. While the mad person has an advantage over the nonmad, and it is features of madness itself that make this so, the mad person should not be seen as the Zhuangist ideal. Madness is one way that the *shi-fei* discriminative faculty that often gets in the way of full understanding of *dao* might be broken or undermined, but a more effective way of undermining it is through the rational undermining of our commitment to this faculty.

An important passage in *Zhuangzi* 4 demonstrates the Zhuangist commitment to rational or intentional deconceptualization, connected to the concept of *zhi* (intention, will). Explaining the so-called fasting of the mind to Yan Hui, the Zhuangist parody version of Confucius says:

> 若一志，无聽之以耳而聽之以心，无聽之以心而聽之以氣。聽止於耳，心止於符。氣也者，虛而待物者也。唯道集虛。虛者，心齋也。

> Be as if unified in intention (*zhi*). Don't listen with the ears, but listen with the mind (*xin*). Don't listen with the mind but listen with *qi*. Listening stops with the ears, and the mind stops with signs. As for *qi*, it is empty and waits

for things. Only the *dao* collects in emptiness. This emptiness is the fasting of the mind.[48]

We see here that it is unified intention that Zhuangists recommend as a way of generating the "fasting of the mind" that involves deconceptualization. While madness may cause states that resemble to some extent those of the person who has engaged in such intentional "fasting," madness is not generally recommended as a route for achieving these states. Might this be due to a view (like the one prevalent in our own society) that mental illness is at least in part a matter of intrinsic natural features (such as genetic predisposition, on a contemporary account, or *xing* on an early Chinese account), and so cannot be the kind of thing that a text can encourage or facilitate in readers? This *might* be so, but if Zhuangists in this period accepted anything like the *Huangdi Neijing* view that held extreme emotion and heightened states as the primary causes of madness (which Confucians of this period and earlier seem to have assumed), then this position would not be available. Given that the *Huangdi Neijing* view appears to be consistent with other views of madness and its connection to emotions at the time,[49] and the fact that the *Zhuangzi* nowhere contains an argument against this view or even a claim of disagreement with it, suggests that it was accepted or assumed by the Zhuangists as well. This then suggests that the Zhuangists viewed intentional or rational deconceptualization as superior to deconceptualization via madness, regardless of whether this madness was brought on intentionally or not. Even if madness can bring one somewhat close to understanding the *dao* (if not all the way to it, as claimed in chapter 22), the intentional deconceptualization we attain through processes like "fasting of the mind" are superior, as they bring a more complete understanding of the *dao*.

Such a position explains why we see arguments in the *Zhuangzi* at all, such as the intricate anti-language arguments of chapter 2, rather than simply encouragements to have experiences that bring about extreme emotions and thus lead us to eventual madness (in the causal relationship discussed by *Huangdi Neijing*).[50] But one major question remains: why should we prefer intentional or rational deconceptualization, rational fearlessness, and so on to deconceptualization or fearlessness caused by madness or other

[48] *Zhuangzi* 4.2.

[49] Unschuld 2003, 155. The key development of the *Huangdi Neijing*, as I discuss in Chapter 5, is the use of the concept of *qi* as psychophysical explanation for mental illness (and illness in general).

[50] *Huangdi Neijing* 46.6.

nonrational disorders or incidents not linked to intention (or not linked *in the right way* to intention)?

Chapter 22 suggests an answer to this—namely, that madness is not fully *reliable*. "Hunched Madness" desired to speak about the *dao*, and the suggestion is that he would have, had he not forgotten what he wanted to say. Were he to regain his memory, he would say it. "Non-Action," on the other hand, presumably stayed silent because he understood why it was best to stay silent, and memory or the ability to speak would not change this. Non-Action is responsive to reasons in a way Hunched Madness is not. Recognition and proper reasons are, contrary to some readings of the text,[51] central to the *Zhuangzi*. The mad person then is not *perfect*, does not qualify as the spirit person, the genuine person, or the perfected person (at least on account of their madness), but their madness does give them an advantage in perspective over those stuck in a conventional understanding of the world.

Hong Mang and Yun Jiang in the East

In chapter 11, a story expresses the connection and likeness between the mad person and nature itself, a transforming process not held in check by the boundaries of ritual, intention, or regularities of order. The *Zhuangzi* here contrasts the actions and understanding of the mad person with the ordering (*zhi* 治) desired by those involved in government. The description of Hong Mang at the beginning of the passage presents him as manifesting classic symptoms of *kuang*—wild, unconstrained, and outlandish action, hyperactivity, lack of social sense, and confusion. Indeed, Hong Mang describes himself in the dialogue as *kuang*. It will be helpful here to include the extended passage:

> 雲將東遊，過扶搖之枝，而適遭鴻蒙。鴻蒙方將拊髀雀躍而遊。雲將見之，倘然止，贄然立，曰：「叟何人邪？叟何為此？」鴻蒙拊髀雀躍不輟，對雲將曰：「遊。」雲將曰：「朕願有問也。」鴻蒙仰而視雲將曰：「吁！」雲將曰：「天氣不合，地氣鬱結，六氣不

[51] See Hansen 2014: "Traditional orthodoxy understood Zhuangzi as an anti-rational, credulous follower of a mystical Laozi." Although numerous scholars did hold something like this view, Hansen is mistaken to associate mysticism with "anti-rational" sentiment. Also, "For Zhuangzi, reason proves too crude to capture the variety, nuance, and texture of the world through which we navigate" (Carr and Ivanhoe 2000, 55). This reading may be influenced by the later Zen tradition, which clearly has Daoist/Zhuangist elements, and its "anti-rationalism."

調，四時不節。今我願合六氣之精，以育群生，為之奈何？」鴻蒙拊髀雀躍掉頭曰：「吾弗知，吾弗知。」雲將不得問。又三年，東遊，過有宋之野，而適遭鴻蒙。雲將大喜，行趨而進曰：「天忘朕邪？天忘朕邪？」再拜稽首，願聞於鴻蒙。鴻蒙曰：「浮游不知所求，猖狂不知所往，遊者鞅掌，以觀無妄，朕又何知！」雲將曰：「朕也自以為猖狂，而百姓隨予所往；朕也不得已於民，今則民之放也。願聞一言。」鴻蒙曰：「亂天之經，逆物之情，玄天弗成；解獸之群，而鳥皆夜鳴；災及草木，禍及止蟲。意！治人之過也！」雲將曰：「然則吾奈何？」鴻蒙曰：「意！毒哉！僊僊乎歸矣！」雲將曰：「吾遇天難，願聞一言。」鴻蒙曰：「意！心養。汝徒處無為，而物自化。墮爾形體，吐爾聰明；倫與物忘，大同乎涬溟；解心釋神，莫然無魂。萬物云云，各復其根，各復其根而不知。渾渾沌沌，終身不離；若彼知之，乃是離之。無問其名，無闚其情，物故自生。」雲將曰：「天降朕以德，示朕以默，躬身求之，乃今也得。」再拜稽首，起辭而行。

Yun Jiang was wandering in the east, where he was carried by grasping onto a meandering branch, and he happened upon Hong Mang, who was slapping his butt and skipping around like a sparrow. Yun Jiang stopped to watch, standing reverentially before Hong Mang. He asked: "good elder, who are you, and why are you acting like this?" Hong Mang slapped his butt and skipped around like a sparrow, answering: "I'm wandering!" Yun Jiang said: "I have a question for you." Hong Mang raised his head and looked at Yun Jiang, then said: "Gaaah!" Yun Jiang said: "the *qi* of heaven is not unified, and the *qi* of earth is tied in knots. The six forms of *qi* are not properly in motion, and the four seasons are not regulated. Now I want to unify the essence of the six forms of *qi*, to give life to the multitude—but how can I do this?" Hong Mang slapped his butt and skipped around like a sparrow, and shaking his head, said: "I don't know! I don't know!" Yun Jiang never got an answer to his question. Three years later, when he was wandering in the east, passing through the fields of Song, he again happened upon Hong Mang. He was happy to see him, and quickly approached him, saying: "has heaven forgotten me? Has heaven forgotten me?" He bowed his head, wishing to hear what Hong Mang had to say. Hong Mang said: "I drift and wander, not knowing what I seek, wild and mad, not knowing where I'm going. Wandering with my reins, I see that nothing is wrong in the world—how then should I have knowledge?" Yun Jiang replied: "I am also myself as if wild and mad, yet all the people follow me where I go. Now, as the people do

> with me, I would like to hear from you." Hong Mang said: "Disordering the works of heaven, turning away from the essence of things, the mysteries of heaven failing to be completed—this lets loose of the animals, the birds all chirp at night, is a catastrophe to grass and trees, a calamity to insects. This is the misfortune of bringing people into order." Yun Jiang said: "if this is so, then what can I do?" Hong Mang said: "you will only poison them! Now I have to return to the place of the immortals.: Yun Jiang said: "securing this meeting with heaven has been difficult—I would like to hear one more thing from you." Hong Mang said: "Nourish the mind. If you follow the way of staying in non-action (*wu wei*), then things will transform of themselves. Let go of your concern for the body, get rid of your focus on intelligence, forget about your relationships with things, and be like the vast waters. Let loose your mind and liberate your spirit, not doing, as if without a soul. The myriad things are legion, and each returns to its root. Each returns to its root, but does not know it. Turbid and confused, but in the end never departing, as if they always knew it—just like this they depart. Don't ask its name, don't search for its essence, and things will gain life of themselves." Yun Jiang said: "heaven has given me this reward, and shown me its stillness. I've long been seeking this, and now have finally obtained it." He again bowed his head, then rose and traveled onward.[52]

We see here an endorsement of madness and another claim (aligning with that of chapter 22) of madness as involving forgetfulness, particularly a kind of forgetfulness of expression in language. The mad person does not seem to forget the proper kinds of activity or how to spontaneously follow their nature. What the mad person forgets is how to put the knowledge that they seemingly have into words—how to explain through conceptualization or some other means the knowledge that in some sense they seem to have. And they must have some form of knowledge even in their forgetfulness, as in this passage and others like it, mad persons are praised because of their unique understanding.[53] In this passage, the mad person's understanding is linked to the spontaneous and nonintentionally active (無為 *wu wei*)[54] following of

[52] *Zhuangzi* 1.4.

[53] This may be connected to the "greater knowledge" (*da zhi* 大知) of *Zhuangzi* 1.1, 2.2, and other chapters. See Sturgeon 2015.

[54] *Wei* is negated here as specifically intentional activity, so that *wu wei* refers to a nonintentional action rather than nonaction. The fact that *zi sheng* (self-generation) is discussed only a few lines after this warrants this reading, as such self-generation is often understood as opposed to intentional generation, and an example of *wu wei* activity.

dao in terms of "return to the root" (*fu* [*qi*] *gen* 復其根). Lack of knowledge here is connected with spontaneity and self-generation (*zi sheng* 自生).

Hong Mang, as the mad person, is also associated with nature itself (*tian*), his spontaneous and nonintentional action likened to the activity of *tian*, in which things are self-generated and not intentionally constructed. Unrefined nature, as wild, uncivilized, untamed, has a major role to play in Confucian literature as well as defining what falls outside of the human *dao*. Confucius charges the "Proto-Daoist" hermits in *Lunyu* 18 of being akin to the "birds and beasts,"[55] suggesting that the failure of these hermits to commit to the social project commits them to being wild, outside the human conventional standard, untamed, akin to not only the barbarians but even that which fails to meet the basic requirements of humanity. We might ask the question, however—how are madness and spontaneity or nonintentional action linked? How are madness and uncultivated and unshaped nature linked? The activity of *kuang* persons, while it may be quite transgressive and seemingly automatic, need not be understood as any more spontaneous or natural than nonmad activity. Indeed, our responses to questions and our investigations into nature or virtue often involve a kind of spontaneous ease. And the activities of the mad person also often involve (in fact possibly always or *necessarily* involve) resistance, hesitance, lack of spontaneity, and agency. The Zhuangist seems to make the common mistake here (often found in our own culture) of complete denial of agency to the mentally ill person. Insofar as one acts in particular ways as a result of or relatedly to one's mental illness, this is often seen as mutually exclusive with agentive or intentional activity. One might be inclined to think this because a disordered or dysfunctional rational functioning (or whatever it is the proper functioning of which constitutes sane or healthy mental function) seems to entail that the disorder itself has some causal function—that one is caused to act (and think) as they do on the basis of this disorder. But when we consider what this amounts to, we see that this renders the mad person no more prone to deterministic necessity than the healthy person—in fact, it seems to do the exact opposite! That is, insofar as a human is functioning properly, then they follow a particular pattern of functioning. Anything that diverges from that pattern, then, can be considered disordered, and thus there should be far more possibilities for disorder than there are for order. As the first line of Leo Tolstoy's classic novel *Anna Karenina* put it: "happy families are all alike; every unhappy family is

[55] *Lunyu* 18.6.

unhappy in its own way." Disordered functioning then can be more easily squared with agency (insofar as agency requires ability to choose, something like free will) than can ordered functioning. That is, insofar as one is functioning in the *proper* ways, aren't particular processes determining their activity?

The mad person, in this sense, can be understood as less constrained and more free than the properly functioning person. There is an inherent tension here in the Zhuangist view, as in numerous points in the text, they argue that the person with greatest understanding is one who follows the "natural patterns" (*tian li*),[56] while at other points, as in the discussions of madness, they suggest that the person with greatest understanding and ability is one who is seemingly unconstrained by particular conventions or ways of being, and can "wander free and easy."[57] Perhaps one way of squaring these two positions is to take the determination of activity by the natural patterns as radically different from the determination of activity by human-created social convention or moral norms. The "freedom" then that obtains on following the natural propensities may be that such activity outstrips that of the activity possible by following the narrowly human way. Freedom, that is, may simply be a matter of the range of activities possible given different ways of constraining or determining human activity. Given that our activity must be chained to *something*, determined by *something*, such determination by the natural patterns leads to a more expansive and effective activity that can mirror and move along with the transformation of myriad things than activity determined by particular perspectives, which do not have the same sensitivity to change. True freedom is always a kind of "wandering in the cage." [58] The largest cage, perhaps, is that of *tian* itself.

"They Act Wild and Mad"

In chapter 20, the character Yiliao, a state official, has a discussion with the Marquis of Lu concerning the latter's continual failures to achieve order, and his meeting with "disaster" (*huan* 患). Yiliao explains to the Marquis that it is commitment to the kind of social project he is engaged in that is the root

[56] *Zhuangzi* 3.2, 15.2, 29.2.
[57] The 逍遙遊 of *Zhuangzi* 1.
[58] *Zhuangzi* 4.2.

of disaster. He discusses various people who meet with disaster and explains that it is commitment to the self that is the Marquis's main problem. Ridding himself of desires and a mind clouded by them is the key to avoiding disaster, and Yiliao enjoins the Marquis to "wander in the open country that is without people" (*you yu wu ren zhi ye* 遊於無人之野). He then explains what the people of the best state are like, a state to which he encourages the Marquis to move:

> 南越有邑焉，名為建德之國。其民愚而朴，少私而寡欲；知作而不知藏，與而不求其報；不知義之所適，不知禮之所將；猖狂妄行，乃蹈乎大方；其生可樂，其死可葬。吾願君去國捐俗，與道相輔而行。」
>
> There is a region in the south within the state of Yue called the State of Established Potency. Its people are dull-witted and simple, they have little selfishness and few desires. They know [how to put forth] effort, but do not know [how to] store things up. They give away without seeking anything in return. They do not know what righteousness calls for, and they do not know what the rules of ritual enjoin. They act wild and mad, thus their feet trod the great path. When born there is rejoicing, when they die there is proper burial. I wish you could abandon the common and go to this state, (and protect yourself and act along with the *dao*).[59]

Following the *dao* (here the "great path") is associated with the wild and mad action of the people of the state of Established Potency. There is a causal connection drawn here—it is *because* they act wild and mad that they are able to trod the great path. This madness is connected to their wandering, to their abandonment of self. Being like these people, according to Yiliao, will help one avoid disaster.

The "Perfected Person" (*zhi ren* 至人)

In chapter 19, we see a description of the "perfected person" (*zhi ren* 至人) that may help explain some of this, while opening up new difficulties. The character Zibian Qingzi explains to Sun Xiu the features of the perfected

[59] *Zhuangzi* 20.2.

person, which echo the features of the mad person we see throughout the *Zhuangzi* and considered earlier.

> 子獨不聞夫至人之自行邪？忘其肝膽，遺其耳目，芒然彷徨乎塵垢之外，逍遙乎無事之業，是謂『為而不恃，長而不宰』。

> Have you alone not heard how the perfected person acts? He forgets his liver and gallbladder, abandons his ears and eyes. Muddled as if restless/indecisive beyond the trodden earth. Wandering, he is engaged in the business of no business. Thus it is said "acting yet not depending on it, leading yet not dominating."[60]

We see a number of relevant features of the perfected person here—in particular, three characteristics that the various chapters of *Zhuangzi* also attribute to the mad person: forgetfulness or lack of propositional knowledge, transgressive activity connected with "wandering" outside the bounds of ritual norms, and (less clearly in this passage) determination by the "natural patterns" (*tian li*), rather than intentional goal-directed activity. All of these features the *Zhuangzi* associates with the perfected person are also associated with the mad person, but it is unclear whether the *Zhuangzi* authors thought that mad persons possessed any additional problematic features or other features that distinguish them from the sage. That is, the prescriptive claim of the *Zhuangzi* is clearly for us to become more like the mad person, but whether we should ourselves become mad persons, or merely adopt those features of the mad person that the mad person shares in common with the perfected person, is not as clear (as I discuss later, in connection with the *Huainanzi*). In chapter 20 we even find the explicit connection of the mad person and the perfected person, with the claim of the perfected person that "his actions attain [to the way] but he does not gain renown for it—simple and commonplace, it seems as if he is mad."[61]

The perfected person appears to have similar properties to the mad person in a host of other ways. Such a person is not moved by the calamities that take place in the world, and thus is not harmed by them either. A passage in chapter 2 explains:

> 至人神矣：大澤焚而不能熱，河、漢沍而不能寒，疾雷破山、風振海而不能驚。

[60] *Zhuangzi* 19.14.
[61] *Zhuangzi* 20.4 (得行而不名處；純純常常，乃比於狂).

> The perfected person is spiritlike—the great lakes can be aflame and they will not feel heat, the He and Han rivers can be frozen and they will not feel cold. Massive thunder can shatter the mountains, and vicious winds can shake the seas, and they will not feel alarmed.

The perfected person, we see here, shares features attributed to the mad person both in the *Zhuangzi* itself and the likely related *Huainanzi*. Although the *Huainanzi*, as we will see, distinguishes between the mad person and the perfected person on the basis of the differing *causes* of their lack of bothered response to things in the world, the resulting states of the perfected person and the mad person are in this way the same. The perfected person, like the mad person, does not pursue a reputation or "name," nor does either person hold onto positions of power. Both of these would get in the way of "wandering," which is a key feature (as explained later) of the perfected person and the mad person. Once one has a reputation or power, one becomes forced into a particular identity, a particular perspective, a role from which one must always act. This not only makes freedom impossible, but more importantly makes "going beyond" impossible. One cannot wander, in the sense of wandering as transgressing or swerving outside the boundaries governing roles and other norms, if one is committed to and will be communally held to a particular role or identity by the community and oneself.

Propositional Knowledge

Lack of propositional knowledge, particularly in the form of forgetfulness, is a key feature of the perfected person and the mad person. We saw earlier in the case of "Hunched Madness" that his lack of knowledge was based on his forgetfulness—his wandering and flightiness of mind being similar to that of his behavior in general. The perfected person is described in a number of places in the *Zhuangzi* as lacking a particular kind of knowledge, a "storing up" of facts or descriptions or propositions about the world. A passage from chapter 7 describes this process and the alternative process used by the perfected person:

> 至人之用心若鏡，不將不迎，應而不藏，故能勝物而不傷。

> The perfected person uses the mind like a mirror—it doesn't reach and it doesn't obtain. It spontaneously resonates [with things] and does not store

things up, and thus the perfected person achieves victory over things and remains unharmed.[62]

The knowledge of the perfected person is understood in terms of a following or mirroring of the activity of things or nature itself—which we can link with the process of "following the natural patterns" discussed in a number of *Zhuangzi* chapters.[63] The lack of propositional knowledge in the perfected person is based on a lack of concern with distinction making, tied to the issue of valuation. For the Zhuangists, every act of distinction making (*shi-fei*) comes with a valuation—a *shi* that is valued and a *fei* that is disvalued—and the primary purpose of engaging in *shi-fei* distinction making is to create valuations.[64] A distinctive feature of the perfected person is that such a person refrains from such distinction making in a number of cases because they are unconcerned with the valuations that lie behind such distinction making. The perfected person, as suggested in *Zhuangzi* 2.11, does not "know" the difference between benefit and harm (or value and disvalue), not because the perfected person has no discriminative ability, but because the perfected person is not concerned with obtaining or avoiding. The perfected person does not prefer one option over the other in terms of any possible distinction. As the passage reads:

> 死生无變於己，而況利害之端乎！
>
> [Even] death and life do not change the self [of the perfected person], so how could considerations of benefit or harm begin to do so?[65]

Because such considerations of benefit and harm are of no import to the perfected person, such a person has no underlying reason to engage in the kind of *shi-fei* distinction making intended to distinguish between benefit and harm, right and wrong, "this" and "not-this." Since such value considerations cannot move or change (*bian* 變) the perfected person, such a person does not make the kinds of distinctions on which statements (*yan* 言) rely—this is how we can account for the numerous examples of the silence of the

[62] *Zhuangzi* 7.6.
[63] *Zhuangzi* 3.2, 14.3, 15.2, 29.2. 順天之理 and other formulations.
[64] Fraser 2015.
[65] *Zhuangzi* 2.11.

perfected or fully knowledgeable person (insofar as such a person possesses "greater" rather than "lesser" knowledge).[66]

"Wandering" and Transgressive Activity

Another shared feature of the perfected person (and the sage-like in general in the *Zhuangzi*) and the mad person is that they are understood to "wander" (*you* 遊) beyond the boundaries of normal activity within the narrowly human perspective. The concept of wandering here may at first glance seem to cut against the third key feature I point out of the perfected person and the madman, namely determination by the natural patterns, but given a proper understanding of the use of *you* in the *Zhuangzi*, we can dissolve this difficulty.

While wandering is often associated with a freedom and lack of constraint (which is certainly true in the sense of lack of constraint from perspective-bound determinations), it is also very much consistent with constraint of a different kind—by the natural patterns themselves. Insofar as constraint is contrasted with self-direction in terms of goal-directed activity, then wandering itself can be a kind of constraint. It is not, however, constraint in itself that bothers the Zhuangists—rather, it is constraint by one's desires and goals, by perspectives that don't correspond continually to the natural patterns (because unchanging). Constraint by the natural patterns can also be understood in terms of constraint by our nature (*xing*)—something with which Zhuangists have no problem and that is associated with wandering. David Chai writes, of "wandering":

> To wander is . . . to leave things undetermined such that our conscious will is blocked off, allowing our instinctual dance with Dao to commence. Faced with this situation the outcome of our wandering creates itself while never deviating from being in accordance with our inborn nature; to be otherwise would be unnatural and in conflict with the oneness of all things.[67]

This nature, necessarily connected to the natural patterns as itself a manifestation of the patterns through *tian*, allows us to transform and shift

[66] For an argument that "lesser knowledge" is statement or proposition based, while "greater knowledge" is skill or conduct based, see Connolly 2011.

[67] Chai 2019, 161.

perspectives, to wander.[68] Guo Xiang's prefatory commentary to *Zhuangzi* 1, stresses this component of wandering, in which "each thing acts corresponding to its nature" (*ge ren qi xing* 各任其性).

In chapter 14, the authors discuss the "perfected people of ancient times," writing:

> 假道於仁，託宿於義，以遊逍遙之虛，食於苟簡之田，立於不貸之圃。逍遙，無為也；苟簡，易養也；不貸，無出也。古者謂是采真之遊。
>
> [they] rested in benevolence and made a stayover in righteousness, and they wandered in the emptiness of the beyond (*you xiao yao zhi xu*), ate in the fields of lack of concern, and stood in unloaned gardens. Going beyond is non-action.[69] Lack of concern is easy nourishment. Not lending is to not go outside [the bounds]. The ancients called this the wandering (*you*) that collects truth (*zhen*).[70]

The combination of wandering (遊 *you*) with "going beyond" or "rambling beyond" (*xiaoyao* 逍遙) is common in the *Zhuangzi*.[71] The title of the very first chapter of the text, *Xiaoyao you* (Wandering to the Beyond) sets the tone for the entire volume. The "beyond" of *xiaoyao* is crucial here for establishing my point. This concept is translated differently by a number of other scholars. A. C. Graham translated *xiaoyao* in the title of chapter 1 as "without a destination,"[72] while Burton Watson translated it as "free and easy."[73] Brook Ziporyn comes closest to what I think is the right understanding of it when he translates *xiaoyao* as "far and unfettered."[74] The association of *xiaoyao* (as well as *you*) with going beyond the usual or the boundaries of the narrow perspective is supported by the content of chapter 1, ranging from the enormous fish who transforms into a bird flying vast distances, who is misunderstood by the small cicada and dove stuck in the forest, to the example of Liezi, who according to the text could ride the wind and soar above heaven and earth.

[68] Zhuangists may not in the end be consistent about this view. They ultimately determine that such capacities as *shi-fei* distinction making are part of our nature or essence (*qing*).

[69] Or, more accurately spelled out, "non-intentional action."

[70] *Zhuangzi* 14.5.

[71] Luminita Balan refers to the *Zhuangzi*'s conception of "the kind of wandering that defies temporal and spatial limits." Balan 2001. Guo Xiang's commentary connects *xiaoyao* to action based on nature. *Zhuangzi Jishi*, vol. 1, 1.

[72] Graham 2001, 43.

[73] Watson 1968, 23.

[74] Ziporyn 2009, 3.

A key aspect of "wandering," in its discussion through much of the *Zhuangzi*, is the sense in which it takes one beyond the usual or expected path. Various passages in the text link wandering with going outside or passing boundaries. The text contains numerous instances of the connection between wandering and going outside or beyond (*wai*): "wandering in the unbounded" (*you wu qiong* 遊無窮),[75] "wandering beyond the four seas" (*you hu si hai zhi wai* 遊乎四海之外),[76] and "wandering beyond the dust and dirt" (*you hu chen gou zhi wai* 遊乎塵垢之外).[77] This wandering lacks the kind of goal-oriented determination of activity of cultivated activity. Wandering, in addition to its connection with the beyond or outside, entails independence of goal-based consideration and activity. The wanderer goes where they do not through any intentional design, but through the vagaries of nature. One who wanders allows oneself to be taken along by the myriad things in the world—in this sense, to have their action determined by those natural patterns inherent in the world. A number of characters throughout the text happen upon key insights or knowledge as while wandering in the sense of non-goal-directed activity. These characters don't travel seeking out wisdom, and thus they find it. Yun Jiang was carried into the east where he met Hong Mang by drifting with a branch.[78] Nanbo Ziqi's wandering brought him into contact with the "useless tree," whose wood is so mangled and bent that it could never be used to build anything, but thus unlike other more "useful" trees it lives out its life and achieves an enormous size.[79] Jieyu, the "Madman of Chu," wandered through the countryside leading to his encounter with Confucius. The footless Wang Tai (whose wisdom is connected to his deformity)[80] is followed by a number of "wanderers" attracted to his seeming unconventional sagacity.

Wandering is contrasted with planning (*mou*) in chapter 5. After a discussion of various deformed people who represent potency and ability, we find the following passage:

> 聖人有所遊，而知為孽，約為膠，德為接，工為商。聖人不謀，惡用知？

[75] *Zhuangzi* 1.3.

[76] *Zhuangzi* 1.5, 2.11.

[77] *Zhuangzi* 2.12.

[78] *Zhuangzi* 11.4. Also see earlier.

[79] *Zhuangzi* 3.6.

[80] In addition to madness, a host of other usually alienating features are celebrated by the *Zhuangzi* and associated with wisdom, such as deformity (loss of one's feet was generally due to criminal punishment.), illness, ugliness, and other conventionally "useless" features.

> The sage has that in which he wanders, and sees knowledge as a disaster, agreement as balled up glue, virtue as connectivity, and effort as a business tool. The sage makes no plans—what use could such a person have for knowledge?[81]

The "knowledge" discussed here is likely the "lesser knowledge" (*xiao zhi* 小知) discussed in a variety of places through the text, as "greater knowledge" is not rejected in this way by Zhuangists. The "lesser knowledge" dismissed here is presented as the result of goal-directed activity, the culmination of plans or a path of self-cultivation. Whatever we understand "greater knowledge" to be, it results not from intentional or planned activity, but from wandering. The kind of wandering in which the sage engages does not aim at knowledge or any other end, and the sage sees such knowledge as injurious. The knowledge the sage comes by or happens upon, insofar as it can be called knowledge, is not the knowledge that results from intentional development or goal direction (and this is thus an aspect of "greater knowledge").

In chapter 7, the Confucian concerns of *ren* 仁 (humanity) and *yi* 義 (righteousness) are posed as obstacles to wandering, as rigid norms that chain us to certain ways of acting that disallow a following of the constant transformation of the world fixed in the natural patterns. Xu You, here representative of the Zhuangist sage, explains to Yi Erzi, who has come to him to seek advice, that the exhortation to humanity and righteousness Yi Erzi has received from the "sage king" Yao[82] will hinder Yi Erzi, particularly in his ability to wander "bathing in the beyond" (*yao dang* 遙蕩). Xu You says, of Yao's teaching of humanity and righteousness:

> 汝將何以遊夫遙蕩、恣睢、轉徙之途乎？

> How then will you be able to wander bathing in the beyond? How will you gaze unconstrained, and follow the way of divergent motion?[83]

[81] *Zhuangzi* 5.5.

[82] A figure to whom Confucians often refer, generally as a standard or exemplar. Yao and Shun are often treated as perfect exemplars, sages who achieved perfect expression of the Confucian (and human) way.

[83] *Zhuangzi* 7.8. Brook Ziporyn renders the passage: "How can you ever roam in the far-flung and unconstrained paths of wild, unbounded twirling and tumbling?" Ziporyn 2009, 48.

This lack of constraint and divergence is suggestive of the transgressive nature of the wanderer (both the mad person and the perfected person). The actions of such a person, from within a conventional perspective, can be seen as violating norms, as disordering certain human and humane regularities. The mad person, both in appearances in the *Zhuangzi* and consistent with understandings of madness of contemporaries of the authors, is marked by the transgressive nature of his or her activity. Perhaps mad persons were known for spontaneous outbursts in general, but it is not spontaneous ritualized or prosocial activity that is remarked on in discussions of mad persons, but spontaneous activity that represents radical infraction or even seeming flouting of such activity. Thus, we find Hong Mang slapping his butt and skipping like a sparrow, "Hunched Madness" forgetting how to speak, and other such stories in the *Zhuangzi*. In the *Analects* and *Mengzi*, we find *kuang* associated with overexcitement and frenetic abandon that lead to infraction of ritual (in addition to madness, as in the case of Jieyu).[84] In the *Xunzi*, we see *kuang* associated with loss of one's mental faculties and lack of control.

This violation of norms that the mad person represents is, for the Zhuangists, an opportunity for freedom in terms of transformation and shifting of perspective. To be constrained by a normative system is to be constrained by a perspective, and plagued by *shi-fei*, by the valuable and useless. To get outside of such a system (to *wander* outside) is to escape or otherwise transcend constraint by normative systems—although there are questions here as to whether the Zhuangists think that we can ever achieve a perspectiveless, conceptless, or normless perspective (a perspective of the *dao* itself, if you will), or if instead the perfected person transcends normative systems by being able to move back and forth between different perspectives, each with their own conceptual and normative systems.[85] With this wandering ability, as discussed earlier, comes freedom from determination by intentions and goals, and the abandonment of goal-directed activity in some important sense. But this "freedom" does *not* entail lack of determination. Indeed, one becomes more fully determined, not by one's intentions or by perspectival norms, but instead by the patterns of nature themselves. This is the "following of natural propensities" discussed throughout the *Zhuangzi*—an activity the mad person and the perfected person are able to engage in.

[84] *Analects* 5.22, 8.16, 13.21, 17.8, 18.5. *Mengzi* 7B37.
[85] See Mou 2005; Mou 2017; Ziporyn 2013, 194.

Determination

Chris Fraser argues that the Zhuangist view is that we should restrict the focus of agency to a certain category of things, and that this leads to a kind of "flexible" agency that is able to adapt to circumstances. This is how he reads the Zhuangist notion of following the patterns and "riding along with things" (*cheng wu* 乘物). I think we can show that something more radical than this is going on in the *Zhuangzi*. The Zhuangists do not mean for us to *restrict* or focus the scope of our agency, but to eliminate it altogether. The discussions of the virtues of mad persons and their resemblance to the perfected person (among other parts of the text) show that the Zhuangists hold a view in which the perfected person follows the natural patterns (*xun tian zhi li* 循天之理) because they have undermined agency such that they have no choice; they simply automatically and spontaneously act in ways that mirror the natural patterns. A discussion of *ziran* 自然 (spontaneity, self-so-ness) and its connection to *wu-wei* 無為 (nonintentional action) and *zhi* 志 (intention) is also necessary in this section to make the case.

A number of passages in the *Zhuangzi* recount the Zhuangist sage's ability to use or follow the natural patterns, and the efficacy of doing so for accomplishing any action. In the story of the excellent butcher Cook Ding in chapter 3, Ding explains that rather than seeing an ox, he "relies on the natural patterns" (*yi hu tian li*) when he cuts, allowing the knife to move through the empty spaces. It is not any preconceived notion of what an ox is supposed to look like, or what parts of an ox along which one is supposed to cut, that guide's Ding's hand.[86] He does not rely on such conventional or perspective-dependent norms. His ability to rely on the natural patterns themselves (empty and filled spaces, rather than ox parts) depends on his ability to deconceptualize his experience, to fail to see an ox. Lesser butchers see oxen when they carve and follow norms for carving oxen. Perhaps this has some effectiveness, but such butchers do not reach the height of skill of Cook Ding. What Cook Ding is able to do, however, relies not on his own knowledge or even technique, but rather on his ability to be determined by the natural patterns themselves.

In a discussion of "perfected music" (*zhi yue* 至樂) in chapter 14 (*Tianyun*), Huang Di describes the effectiveness of such music by reference to its following of the natural patterns (*shun zhi yi tian li*), as well as its spontaneity,

[86] *Zhuangzi* 3.2.

resonance (*ying* 應),[87] potency, harmonization, and spontaneity of activity (*ziran*), all features associated with the determined patterns of nature. The perfected person, according to chapter 1, has no self (*ji*),[88] comparing such a person to the spirit person, who has no achievement (*gong* 功), and the sage, who has no renown (*ming* 名). The "self" being denied of the perfected person here is discussed in a number of places throughout the *Zhuangzi* and itself seems to have to do with goal-directed and intentional commitments on the part of the individual. A discussion at the beginning of chapter 2 between Nanbo Ziqi and Yancheng Ziyou suggests the connection of *ji* (self) to agency in terms of self-impetus. The winds of nature are caused to blow of themselves and complete of themselves (*shi qi ziji ye, xian qi zi qu* 使其自己也，咸其自取), suggesting that there is no outside influence or direction, but that the activity is impelled only by what is internal to the thing itself. What the perfected person lacks, then, is not a self in terms of a subject of experience (indeed, how could one lack this?), or even something like "selfish desires" (as Zhu Xi reads *ji* in the *Analects*),[89] but self-directedness in terms of agency or goal-directed activity. The perfected person is able to follow the natural patterns precisely because such a person is not following the *ji*—is not impelled to act on the basis of intentions and goals.

A passage from chapter 11 expresses this well, in discussion of the "great person" (*da ren* 大人), likely an alternative Zhuangist allusion to the perfected person and sage. This passage clearly presents the great person as both determined and without a *ji* (self) and seems to draw a connection between this lack of *ji* and the great person's determination (via lack of agency).

> 大人之教，若形之於影，聲之於響。有問而應之，盡其所懷，為天下配。處乎無響，行乎無方。挈汝適復之撓撓，以遊無端，出入無旁，與日無始，頌論形軀，合乎大同，大同而無己。無己，惡乎得有有！睹有者，昔之君子；睹無者，天地之友。
>
> The teaching of the great person is like the shadow cast by a physical thing, or the sound of a voice. When there is a question, the great person answers it, to the point of exhausting that within his mind. He blends with the world, remaining still and without sound. His actions are without location.

[87] "Resonance" is understood largely in terms of the effect of one thing on another through indirect or harmonious means based on similarity or type. Major 1993, 66.

[88] *Zhuangzi* 1.3.

[89] Gardner 2003, 79–80.

> He assists you in going and returning without disturbing. His wanderings are without a trace, his leaving and entering without similarity, like the motions of the sun, without a beginning. We can praise and discuss his form—he is unified with the great entirety. Being the great entirety, he has no self. Having no self, how could he obtain things?[90]

In lacking a self, the great person (seemingly merged with the myriad things of the world) does not "obtain things"—which seems to suggest also a lack of goal-directed activity, of the aiming at things that the text associated with intentional activity.

Although there are passages in the text that suggest that a single unified intention is behind the activity of the perfected person (such as in the discussion of *xin zhai* 心齋—fasting of the mind—in chapter 4), the activity of the kinds of person the Zhuangist sees as ideal throughout the text (the perfected person, the sage, the spirit person, the mad person) is characteristically non-goal-directed and nonintentional, connected to wandering, absence of self in terms of agentive direction, and lack of even the basis of such direction, which requires the kind of propositional "lesser knowledge" the Zhuangist rejects.

The Image of the Fisherman

We find in a number of early Chinese texts the motif of the wandering fisherman as a mysterious and sagely figure of unconventional wisdom. The fisherman appears not as an expected or a usual exemplar, but rather as an example of the kind of person praised throughout the *Zhuangzi*—the wandering hermit, outside the boundaries of normal society, unconstrained, and wild. It is an important part of the motif that the fisherman appears in the wild, in the unconstructed backways of the land, in forests and along meandering rivers. The fisherman, like the seas and rivers with which they are connected, comes and goes seemingly at random, unimpeded by regularity, without regulations and regularities guiding his action. In this way the fisherman is transgressive, but adheres to the patterns of nature, insofar as they themselves change and move and wander.

As associated with nature, the fisherman also represents the wild, the untamed, and (in an important sense) uncivilized, with which texts like the

[90] *Zhuangzi* 11.5.

Zhuangzi also associate the mad person, who is unconstrained by human norms and determined by the patterns of nature just as is the wild overgrowth that imposes on the human world, but is not bothered or altered by human attempts to regulate it—attempts that are always ultimately thwarted.

Chapter 31 of the *Zhuangzi* is devoted to the character of the fisherman (漁父 *yufu*). Fittingly, this stock character is contrasted with the Confucius, who appears in the chapter as in a number of other places in the *Zhuangzi*, as a counterpoint to and parody of the Confucius of early Confucian texts. At the beginning of the chapter, we find Confucius wandering (*you* 遊) in the forest—already a sign that something unexpected and oppositional is going on here. The Confucian version of Confucius is not one who would be expected to wander—indeed, Confucius represented, for the Confucians, the very opposite of a wanderer: one with strong intentions and a dogged commitment to shape the world in a certain way and get exactly where he intended to go.

The setup of the chapter plays on the events of *Analects* 18, in which we find Confucius and Zilu in the countryside between states on their journey, encountering "proto-Daoist" hermits. Toward the beginning of *Yufu*, Confucius and his followers encounter the fisherman, who stands off in the distance listening to Confucius playing his *qin*. His description in the chapter expresses his wild, uncivilized, wandering, and transgressive nature. The clothing of the fisherman is described as haphazard and unorganized (a stark contrast to the ritually proper attire and organization of the Confucian "exemplary person"). His hair is untied (and uncombed). The fisherman emerges from a boat on the nearby lake in disheveled and soiled state, wild and unrefined as this nature itself from which he comes forth. The fisherman, speaking to Zilu and Confucius's other followers, chides Confucius, as we would expect, for following a way of life divergent from the (true) *dao*.

Where the unexpected turn in the chapter comes is after Confucius's students approach him to tell him what the fisherman in the distance told them. On hearing this, Confucius declares that the fisherman is a sage and goes off to find him. Once he catches up with the elusive fisherman, Confucius entreats the fisherman to instruct him. The fisherman instructs Confucius about a number of topics, including *zhen* 真 (truth, genuineness). He explains to Confucius that the aim to bring about righteousness, commitment to ritual, and social harmony is misguided, and that it represents a desire to step into a position that is not Confucius's own.

While the specific content of the fisherman's teaching in this chapter is of relatively little import for my purposes here, it interestingly diverges somewhat from what we find in earlier chapters of the *Zhuangzi*. We here find a criticism of the Confucian way not on the grounds of their commitment to a particular perspective and neglect of the potential of different perspectives grounded in transformation and revaluation, but instead on more conventional grounds. There are certainly differences between what we see here and in the Inner Chapters and related chapters. One feature the *Yufu* chapter shares with the chapters considered so far, however, is the image of the wild, uncivilized, and transgressive outsider as representative of a wisdom surpassing that of Confucius and those "in the world." The transgressive outsider here is connected to the image of the mad person, the character of the wandering and unrooted fisherman as advisor. The story of *Yufu* is reminiscent of the mad characters of Hong Mang and "Hunched Madness" in previous chapters. While madness itself is not the dominant motif here, the fisherman is, like the madman, a symbol of the wilds, the uncultivated and wandering. In this, the fisherman shares many of the same features that make the madman worthy of praise for the Zhuangist.

The image of the wandering fisherman in the countryside connected with Zhuangist-like ideals, like that of the madman, recurs in a number of late texts throughout the Chinese tradition, including perhaps the most famous appearance such a character in early Chinese literature, in the Han Dynasty text *Chuci*, in which a wandering fisherman laughs at Qu Yuan for fleeing society in anguish because of his insistence on virtue and remaining without moral blemish in a corrupted world.[91]

Problematic Emotions in the *Zhuangzi*

As explained in *Huangdi Neijing* and assumed elsewhere, madness can result from excess of emotion, precipitated by situation. One area of agreement between the Zhuangists and Confucians is on the possibility of disastrous emotional responses that lead to ineffective or catastrophic behaviors. The main difference between the Confucian and Daoist/Zhuangist reading of these situations is that for the Confucians, it is understood as a matter of ritual transgression and of moral failure, and for the Daoists and Zhuangists it is a matter of

[91] *Chuci, Yufu*: 漁父莞爾而笑，鼓枻而去.

effectiveness of behavior at securing particular goals and thriving in general, independently of a fixed moral standard or values. Like the Confucians, the Zhuangists do not advocate eliminating or otherwise undermining human emotions and other mental states that can be problematic.[92] Rather, the Zhuangists argue that *any* emotion and/or mental state considered in its proper contexts can be understood as possessing (relative) value. This is the case even for states that generate madness, or madness itself. A large part of the Zhuangist problem with Confucian morality is that it is based in *shi-fei* (this/not-this) discrimination, a major component of which is valuation and devaluation.

Particular emotions connected with the generation of *kuang*, such as fear and terror,[93] are not, like other states, rejected by the Zhuangists. The *Huangdi Neijing*, in its *qi*-based explanation of mental and physical states, associates states like fear (that precipitates *kuang*) with a certain quality of *qi* collected in particular parts of the body. *Qi*, according to the text, is of *yin* and *yang* quality, depending on the region of the body the *qi* inhabits. In the medical texts, *yin* and *yang* have their more familiar general meanings, associated with qualities of the low, dark, yielding (*yin*) and the high, bright, powerful (*yang*). Here, they are connected with particular parts of the body, and the *qi* that collects in these parts will determine behavior and physical and mental states of the individual. Chapter 62 of the *Huangdi Neijing Suwen* associates the collection of *qi* in the *yang* parts of the body with fear and *kuang*.[94] Wang Bing comments on this idea, quoting *Suwen*, chapter 30:

> When the *yang* is replete in the four limbs, one turns mad. *Suwen* 30 states: "The four limbs are the origins of all *yang*. When the *yang* is abundant then the four limbs are replete. If they are replete then one can climb on summits and sing. The *yang* abundance causes heat abundance in the body. Hence one throws off one's clothes and wishes to run." All this happens because the *yin* cannot overcome the *yang*.[95]

The Zhuangists are in a somewhat difficult position concerning states like *kuang*, and their connections to problematic emotions. They clearly want to accept that there are certain problematic emotions and states—or rather,

[92] A very different approach to problematic emotions than we find in much of ancient Indian and Hellenistic philosophy.
[93] *Huainanzi* 1.14.
[94] *Huangdi Neijing Suwen* 62.7; Unschuld and Tessenow 2011, 74.
[95] Wang Bing, Unschuld and Tessenow 2011, 74.

contexts in which these states are problematic.[96] The discussion of *xin zhai* 心齋 (fasting of the mind) in chapter 4 seems to have something to do with undermining certain kinds of situationally problematic emotions that arise from the commitment to a self as defined by roles and position. The issue they have seems to be with devaluing these states as a whole, universally and across perspective. Confucius's description of *xin zhai* to Yan Hui in chapter 4 can be understood as advocating the control and even elimination of certain mental states (indeed, it is unclear how else this could be read):

> 若一志，无聽之以耳而聽之以心，无聽之以心而聽之以氣。聽止於耳，心止於符。氣也者，虛而待物者也。唯道集虛。虛者，心齋也。
>
> As if with a unified intention, do not listen with the ears but listen with the mind. Do not listen with the mind but listen with *qi*. Listening stops at the ears, while the mind stops at signs. As for *qi*, it remains empty and waits on things. Only when *dao* is collected is there emptiness. This emptiness is the fasting of the mind.[97]

Part of what we are told to empty ourselves of in this process is the focus on *xin* (mind). The mind is both the instrument that engages in *shi-fei* conceptualization[98] and the source and regulator of emotions. In chapter 5, the concept of *qing* 情 is discussed in a way translatable as both "essence" and "emotions"—two senses the term generally has. *Qing* is contrasted with *xing* 形 (form), referring to the contents of mind in general, or those aspects of the person not associated with the physical form, *including* the emotions. A number of translators and commentators discussed this issue, and we see contrasting positions. A number of the traditional commentaries take *qing* in the sense of "emotion,"[99] and many English translations translate the term as such (or a closely related term/terms).[100] A. C. Graham argues that this is an incorrect reading, and that "essence" is a better translation of the term in

[96] For example, *Zhuangzi* 15.2.

[97] *Zhuangzi* 4.2.

[98] *Zhuangzi* 2.4. This *shi-fei* is also the "essence" of persons.

[99] Brian Bruya argues that this use, though found in pre-*Mencius* texts, comes to the fore with the *Mencius*. Bruya 2003, 151–154.

[100] Victor Mair as "emotions," Burton Watson as "feelings," Feng Youlan as "affections," and Brook Ziporyn as "the characteristic human inclinations." Wang Bo understands it as 情感 (emotion). See Bruya 2003 for a historical overview of the concept.

chapter 5 of *Zhuangzi*.[101] Kim-chong Chong argues that we should understand *qing* in the *Zhuangzi* as "facts," with the ambiguity of the term such that it can refer to facts about the emotions or/and other human characteristics, depending on the context.[102]

While I think Chong is right that there are numerous senses of the term in play, I think it is misguided to look for a single unifying sense of *qing* as offered in the *Zhuangzi*.[103] If we read *qing* in chapter 5 as including *all* of the possible senses of the term at the same time, we can make best sense of the passages. This interpretation is also consistent with the wordplay we find throughout the *Zhuangzi*. Chong argues convincingly that the number of senses of the term in the text and other texts of the period, including identification with *xing* 性 (inborn characteristics or human nature) show that it is unlikely that emotion is the *only* sense of the term in chapter 5. But Chong argues that we should not read *qing* as "emotions" in the *Zhuangzi*, because he holds that it is a central theme in the text that grief and mourning are unnatural.[104] This would be inconsistent with injunctions against "violating one's *qing*" (*bei qing* 倍情) in the text. However, I think it is incorrect to understand the *Zhuangzi* as rejecting grief and mourning as unnatural and to be avoided. This would conflict with another clearly major theme of the *Zhuangzi*, which could arguably be said to occupy the main position of many of the chapters (if not all of them)—the avoidance of valuation through *shi* and *fei*, and the rejection of valuation and the inevitable devaluation that comes with it. In many of the chapters, Zhuangists are eager to push back on the notion that there are universal values and disvalues, including things that we must always reject. Rather, these judgments can be made only from a perspective, and perspectives, just as the myriad things, ought to continually change (a theme of the first three of the inner chapters). This seems to be just what is suggested by the statement *shun tian* 順天 (following nature),[105] likely not coincidentally constructed similarly to *dun tian*.

[101] Graham 1967, 33. A number of scholars reject this view, including Kwong Loi Shun (Shun 1997, 7). I side with Graham on this issue.

[102] Chong 2010, 23–24.

[103] Chad Hansen also argues for a single sense of *qing* more broadly accepted throughout early Chinese culture (Hansen 1995). My own view is closer to that of Michael Puett, who disputes this, arguing that "*qing* has a broad semantic range, including such meanings as basic tendencies, inclinations, dispositions (including emotional dispositions), and fundamental qualities, and that this breadth of semantic range is precisely why the term came to be so important in early Chinese thought." Puett 2004, 42.

[104] Chong 2010, 29. Chong reads the statement that certain kinds of mourning are examples of *dun tian bei qing* 遁天倍情 demonstrates that the authors hold that "grief and mourning are inappropriate and unnatural reactions toward death."

[105] Sometimes in the construction *shun tian zhi dao* (順天之道), "following the way of nature."

In following nature, one does not rid oneself of emotion, but rather feels emotions without forcing them, without directing the mind in a certain way to experience certain emotions. One is able to have the emotion proper to a circumstance and within the right perspective, but is not *caught* in this perspective, akin to the cicada and student dove of chapter 1,[106] or the "wandering within a cage" of chapter 4.[107]

If we should thus read *qing* in the *Zhuangzi* then as emotion and essence both—the two being intertwined—then how do we square the earlier interpretation with the conversation between Zhuangzi and Hui Shi concerning ridding oneself of *qing* in chapter 5? There is a quite plausible way to make sense of these passages in ways that do not take them to be enjoining us to rid ourselves of emotional responses. Indeed, as I argue further later, I think that this reading of the *Zhuangzi* is mainly due to the influence of Buddhism and Indian thought on Chinese philosophy, and that the text gives us most reason to accept a different view of the Zhuangist claims.

The first mention of *qing* in chapter 5 comes during a consideration of some physically deformed characters who nonetheless enjoy massive influence and reverence from important historical dukes of the Spring and Autumn Period.[108] This leads to a discussion of the sage-like person (*sheng ren*),[109] including that such a person is without *qing*. The key part of the passage reads:

> 有人之形，無人之情。有人之形，故群於人；無人之情，故是非不得於身。
>
> [The sage] has human form, but lacks the human *qing*. Having the human form, he can be classed among humans. Lacking the human *qing*, *shi-fei* can obtain no place in his person.[110]

[106] *Zhuangzi* 1.1.
[107] *Zhuangzi* 4.1.
[108] The text mentions Duke Ling of Wei and Duke Huan of Qi. The choice of these two may have been intended to further emphasize the point—Duke Ling was famously homosexual, with the suggestion that he would have had a particular appreciation for male beauty, yet still looked on this deformed man as one of normal form. Duke Huan of Qi (reigned 685–643 BCE) was the first of the *ba* 霸 (hegemons) of the Spring and Autumn Period, and one of the famous *wu ba* 五霸 (Five Hegemons). There was inconsistency in the use of this term, with texts such as *Mengzi* claiming five Spring and Autumn figures, with Duke Huan as the first, as the Five Hegemons. Later figures, such as Du Yu (222–285 CE), commentator on the *Zuozhuan*, claimed a different five, beginning with a figure from the distant (and semimythical) Xia Dynasty (~1700 BCE). On either reading, Duke Huan was the first *ba* of the Spring and Autumn.
[109] Using a term common to the Confucians.
[110] *Zhuangzi* 5.5.

Zhuangzi further explains that *qing* here should be understood as *shi-fei*, the distinction making and conceptualization that leads to the artificial construction of "things" (物 *wu*), which make it impossible to follow the natural propensities (*tian li*).[111] Here, while we can understand *qing* as including both emotion and essence—indeed, the human essence in terms of *zhi* 質 will necessarily include emotion and other affective states—it cannot be seen as merely emotion, for even if we are able to rid ourselves of all emotion, thus being without human *qing*, we will still have the ability and inclination to engage in *shi-fei* conceptualization.

For certain, there are certain emotional states that the Zhuangists find problematic. But the problematic nature of these emotions is not something to be found in the nature of the emotions—rather, it is that they are deployed in the wrong places, at the wrong times. Here, we can see a connection between the *Huangdi Neijing* and other medical literature and the *Zhuangzi* (as well as Confucian texts). Emotions such as fear, anger, joy, or grief are not in themselves problematic. The various emotions, according to the text, have no significance in themselves, and are likened in chapter 2 to music-less instruments:

> 喜怒哀樂，慮嘆變慹，姚佚啟態；樂出虛，蒸成菌。日夜相代乎前，而莫知其所萌。
>
> Joy, anger, grief, and happiness—hesitation, admiration, mutability, and fixedness—repose, indulgence, volition, and restraint—are like music issuing from empty pipes, mushrooms created from water vapor. Day and night they come forward to replace one another, yet we don't know from what source they spring.[112]

The problem becomes when we improperly direct these emotions, when they arise on the basis of ignorance or our action contrary to the natural patterns. The famous story of the monkey keeper in chapter 2 illustrates the problem with such generation and direction of emotion—the monkeys given three nuts in the morning and four at night are angry, while an arrangement giving them four in the morning and three at night makes them happy. Zhuangzi explains:

[111] Two distinct phrases used to capture this idea in the *Zhuangzi* are *shun tian zhi li* 順天之理 and *xun tian li* 循天理.
[112] *Zhuangzi* 2.2.

名實未虧，而喜怒為用，亦因是也。

The name and actuality were no different (between the two offers), but the they elicited different reactions of happiness and anger. This is just what is meant.[113]

While the author here is certainly being reticent, as Zhuangists are wont to do, *part* of what the author means is that these emotional responses were improper, in that they did not track any differences either in actuality (*shi* 實) or name (*ming* 名). This shows that at least one of the emotional responses of the monkeys was inappropriate, or that perhaps there was no proper link between the events and emotions at all. Even if the latter is the case, however, it cannot be that the Zhuangists are calling for the elimination of emotion. We see numerous passages in the Zhuangzi in which particular emotional states are seen as good and even necessary things. One famous example is the scene in chapter 18 in which Zhuangzi is found by Hui Shi after Zhuangzi's wife's death, singing and banging on his drum. When Hui Shi upbraids his friend for expressing joy after the death of his wife, Zhuangzi explains:

是其始死也，我獨何能無概然！察其始而本無生，非徒無生也，而本無形，非徒無形也，而本無氣。雜乎芒芴之間，變而有氣，氣變而有形，形變而有生，今又變而之死，是相與為春秋冬夏四時行也。人且偃然寢於巨室，而我噭噭然隨而哭之，自以為不通乎命，故止也。

When she first died, could I alone not respond [in grief] as is usual? But then I investigated her beginning, and the origin of her birth. Without following, she had no birth, and in the origin had no body. Without following, she had no body, and in the origin had no *qi*. In the blending of things, there was a change and there became *qi*, then this *qi* changed and there was form. This form changed and there was birth, and now there is another change and there is death. It is just like the movement between the four seasons, spring, autumn, winter, and summer. Humans lie down to sleep in the great chamber [of earth]. To shout and cry about it would be to fail to understand our natural allotment—thus I refrained.[114]

113 *Zhuangzi* 2.6.
114 *Zhuangzi* 18.2.

This shows that while *grief* may be the inappropriate (or at least less ideal) emotion to feel in this situation, it is understandable, and it is also much more valuable to feel the kind of joy that comes from delight in the transformation of the myriad things. That is, it is not emotion that is the problem here—in fact, Zhuangzi endorses certain emotional responses. When we think of this in terms of ridding oneself of *qing*, then, we should take *qing* to be both "essence" of *shi-fei* conceptualization, and the improper or less-than-ideal emotions that arise on the basis of these problematic *shi-fei*. In the earlier passage, Zhuangzi's sadness was due to his improper understanding of life and death. It was not that his grief and crying were negative things in themselves; rather, it was that they resulted from improper or incomplete understanding of the *dao* and its operation. When he came to properly understand it, his emotional responses changed as well.

Of course, this shift in one's emotional responses on proper understanding of the *dao* and natural propensities will not always be toward what we deem valuable or "positive" emotions. Sometimes the proper response from understanding natural propensities will be a state like fear, anxiety, or hate. It is keeping with the *Zhuangzi*'s general position that we should give up *shi-fei*, including valuation and devaluation, that we refuse to devalue states such as fear or anxiety as wholly negative or useless. It turns out that the various "disordered" persons in society are also understood as having an unrecognized and unique value.

The "Problem" of Anxiety in the *Zhuangzi*

Reduction of psychic distress, the elimination of affective states seen as problematic, such as anxiety, restlessness, and other states that "disturb" the mind are often taken by scholars to be features of the *Zhuangzi*. There have been numerous interpretations of the *Zhuangzi* that argue that one of the main purposes of the Zhuangist program is to eliminate "negative" mental states like anxiety. This can be seen in even recent work on the *Zhuangzi*. Steve Coutinho writes:

> Like the [Pyrrhonian] Skeptics, Zhuangzi also seems to aim for emotional tranquility. He is concerned with how to cultivate an emotional state that

enables us to deal with life's difficulties, no matter how dire, without emotional turmoil.[115]

William Theodore de Bary offers a very similar view, writing: "Zhuangzi seeks to free us from the life-depleting anxiety wrought by an overwrought insistence upon *you-wei* action."[116]

Even scholars who reject such a view, such as Paul Kjellberg, generally reject it on the grounds that it is false because attaining peace of mind is "not all he [Zhuangzi] is after,"[117] not on the grounds that Zhuangzi is not concerned with peace of mind at all.

It turns out that there *is* a problem concerning anxiety in the *Zhuangzi*, and because the views most familiar to us when considering the problem of anxiety, such as the views of the Stoics or the Buddhists advocating elimination of "problematic" mental states, we overlook the different problem of anxiety in the *Zhuangzi*. In addition, because of the influence of Buddhism in China and the use of Daoist and Zhuangist ideas to express Buddhism in an East Asian context, even Chinese thinkers became prone to understanding the problem of anxiety in the *Zhuangzi* as one of problematic emotions. Here is a place where comparative work leads us astray. But it is also through careful comparison that we can unravel the bind that has kept us from sufficiently appreciating this important aspect of the *Zhuangzi*. We should not, the Zhuangist enjoins, spend our time and energy attempting to get rid of mental states like anxiety, fear, and dread. Rather, in understanding *dao*, in grasping the patterns manifest in the world, we can come to gain an understanding of when anxiety is called for and when it is not. And we can then learn to employ it where it is effective, and let it go where it is not. If there is a major goal for the Zhuangist, it is *efficacy* and its role in thriving, rather than the elimination of certain mental states.

Justin Tiwald writes, in a recent article on well-being in Daoism:

> Zhuangzi thinks . . . that our thoughts, feelings and behaviors are moderated by the heavenly point of view even as we appreciate human obligations,

[115] Coutinho 2014, 180.

[116] De Bary 2011, 82.

[117] Kjellberg 1996, 10. Justin Tiwald adds, concerning Kjellberg's claims: "As Paul Kjellberg has pointed out, of the many uses of skepticism depicted in the *Zhuangzi*, anxiety and emotional disturbance are sometimes the least of the author's concerns, and peace of mind is frequently a means to other ends" (Tiwald 2015, 63).

> purposes, and concerns well enough to pursue them. Zhuangzi illustrates this combination in several different stories, often featuring people who outwardly conform to inherited social customs but inwardly maintain a cool, dispassionate attitude toward them—the sorts of people who participate in mourning rituals but don't have feelings recognizable as grief or sorrow, or who strive to master some profession but do not truly care whether they succeed or fail.[118]

Tiwald references a number of stories in the *Zhuangzi* to support this position.[119] I think there are better ways to understand what is going on in these passages, which have nothing (or little) to do with ridding the mind of disturbances and unease, and more to do with effective action, spontaneity (*ziran* 自然), and the "genuine" (*zhen* 真). The reading of these and other stories in the *Zhuangzi* presenting them as offering a picture of how we eliminate or dampen problematic affective states and attain a dispassionate attitude is in essence a Buddhist reading of *Zhuangzi*. While such a reading has a deep history in Chinese scholarship, dominant since the rise of Buddhism and the adoption of Daoist concepts to understand Buddhist doctrine (a process that continued long after the explicit use of terminology called *geyi* in early Chinese Buddhism),[120] this reads Buddhist concerns into Zhuangism where they do not exist. The Zhuangists were not, I contend, concerned with reducing unpleasant or disturbing affective states as themselves problematic. Indeed, Zhuangists seemed to have readily admitted that states such as madness, which they praise throughout the *Zhuangzi*, can sometimes (or perhaps even often) be unpleasant.[121] Rather, they were concerned with effective and genuine action, mirroring the *dao*. Sometimes, according to Zhuangists, such action requires elimination or dampening of obstructing affective states. But sometimes it requires *creation* of such states. In those passages

[118] Tiwald 2015, 62.

[119] Ch. 3: 52–53; ch. 6: 88–89; ch. 19: 205–206.

[120] Victor Mair challenged the idea that *geyi* was ever a major organized attempt outside of a few individuals (Mair 2012), but the influence of Daoism in Chinese Buddhist thought cannot be reduced to direct translation of Sanskrit Buddhist terms in Daoist terms. Conceptual similarities between Chinese Buddhism and Daoism are abundant and clear, and Daoist *ideas* pop up with great regularity in Buddhism in its Chinese context, especially the Chan tradition. Indeed, Buddhism and Daoism are linked as similar in spirit and message as early as the Han Dynasty, in what is one of the first mentions of Buddhism in Chinese literature, Xiang Kai's memorial at the court of Emperor Huan, in which the teachings of "Futu" (Buddha) and those of "Laozi" are mentioned as having the same ends.

[121] Think of the example of "Hunched Madness," discussed earlier, who *wants* to speak, but whose madness will not allow him to.

of the *Zhuangzi* where there is endorsement of elimination or dampening of states like fear, anxiety, and dread, it is never because there is something problematic about these mental states in themselves. Rather, the problem is that for one who has failed to understand and mirror the *dao*, such affective states can arise *where they don't belong* and serve as obstacles to the kind of genuine, spontaneous, and ultimately effective action exemplified by that of the sage. While we can find in the *Zhuangzi* passages in which states such as anxiety are rejected, the Buddhist reading of *Zhuangzi* is too quick to determine this as due to a view on which a Zhuangist goal is the reduction of mental disturbance.

This view is problematized by passages in the *Zhuangzi* in which we find *endorsement* of states we might find problematic, such as fear, anxiety, and even madness, or sometimes *neutral* positions on these states. Such passages tend to be neglected in interpretations of *Zhuangzi*, in part because they do not fit with the Buddhist interpretation. If the *Zhuangzi* enjoins us to attain equanimity or peace of mind, then how can we make sense of apparent claims that the genuine person or Daoist sage sometimes feels anxiety or unease as part of their effective and genuine action?

Readings of the *Zhuangzi* as similar on this issue to Indian and Hellenistic views are not completely unmotivated or unjustified, as there are many striking similarities between these traditions and the Zhuangists in related areas, including their view of the best kind of life. According to Diogenes Laertius, the Stoics aimed to "live consistently with nature" and held that such a life would issue in "a smooth flow of life, whenever all things are done according to the harmony of the *daimon* in each of us with the will of the administrator of the universe."[122] This echoes the position on action consistent with *dao* that we find in the *Zhuangzi*. While there is no appeal to a divine agent anywhere in Daoist literature, *dao* does play a similar role to the "administrator of the universe" in Stoicism. And it is certainly action in accord with nature, including human nature, that the Zhuangist argues will lead to thriving. *Dao* is associated with nature in a number of passages in the *Zhuangzi*, including one I look at more closely later, 5.22–24, in which Zhuangzi tells Hui Shi: "*Dao* gives him this appearance, *tian* gives him this physical form."[123] It is also the case that we should follow or attempt to live in some way in adherence to this *dao* associated with nature. Zhuangzi in 6:10

[122] In Inwood and Gerson 1998, 191–192.
[123] 5.23 (Ziporyn trans.).

claims that the *zhen ren* 真人(Genuine Person) does not use the mind to resist or move away from *dao*.

These parallels are largely shared between Zhuangism and Buddhism as well, and I think this is a large part of the reason that the *Zhuangzi* is read as also sharing a position concerning anxiety and equanimity with Buddhism. I have argued in other works for the wider adoption of what I call an "analogical method" of comparative philosophy to clarify difficult points in historical texts,[124] but I think we must also be careful in drawing analogies between traditions where there is evidence of divergence. We also have to be aware of where traditions or texts that parallel each other in some ways diverge, and why.

In the *Zhuangzi*, where we see most concentration on anxiety is not in consideration of mortality, but in considerations of seemingly unavoidable dilemmas, in which there will be a bad result no matter which path one takes. This should right away tip us off to the fact that the interest with such mental states in the *Zhuangzi* has less to do with their role in mental disturbance or peace of mind than with their role in effective and genuine *action*. While the *Zhuangzi* is certainly a unique text and there is much disagreement between Zhuangists and other early Chinese schools and thinkers, one point on which the Zhuangists agree with the Confucians and Mohists is that thriving is not a matter of having or lacking certain affective mental states, but of both reliably producing effective action and having proper motivations and attitudes. The questions of pleasure versus pain or disturbance versus ease receive relatively little attention from early Chinese thinkers, in comparison to those of Indian and Hellenistic traditions. This is one of the main stumbling blocks for Westerners approaching these texts. We tend (perhaps because of our own influence by soteriological systems) to understand texts enjoining self-cultivation as having to do with creation or maximization of pleasant mental states and elimination of unpleasant ones. In the *Zhuangzi*, however, as in other early Chinese texts, consideration of anxiety based on seemingly impossible decisions is taken as difficult and problematic not because of its contribution to mental disturbance, but because it makes a precarious situation in which the greatest care and concentration are required even harder to navigate successfully.

The seemingly impossible decision is discussed at a number of points throughout the *Zhuangzi*, but it comes up most often in chapters 3 and 4. We see particularly problematic anxiety reveal itself throughout the *Renjianshi*

[124] McLeod 2018b; McLeod 2015, xvi.

chapter of *Zhuangzi*. In one of the vignettes of the chapter, Zigao, having been given an official mission by the king, comes to see Confucius (or the Zhuangist version anyway), looking for advice. He says:

> 王使諸梁也甚重，齊之待使者，蓋將甚敬而不急。匹夫猶未可動，而況諸侯乎！吾甚慄之。[. . .] 吾食也，執粗而不臧，爨無欲清之人。今吾朝受命而夕飲冰，我其內熱與！吾未至乎事之情，而既有 陰陽之患矣；事若不成，必有人道之患。是兩也，為人臣者不足以任之，子其有以語我來！

> The king has given me a heavy mission. The people of Qi treat envoys with great respect but are slow to make any concessions. Even the ordinary folk there are unbudgeable—how much more so the feudal lords! I am quite terrified. [. . .] I am a man who has no special dietary needs, and even when drinking a steaming broth I normally have no need for a cooler, but look at me now: I got my orders this morning and already I am sucking on ice chunks this evening, as if my insides were on fire! I have not yet begun the actual task and already my yin and yang are out of whack. And if the mission turns out to be a failure, I'll surely be menaced by the people around me. Given these two problems, it is just not worth it to be employed as someone's underling! Please give me some advice![125]

Here is a particularly debilitating anxiety, occasioned by being given a seemingly impossible task. Throughout the *Zhuangzi*, it is suggested and sometimes explicitly claimed that part of the problem with action in the project of civilization is that society doesn't have the individual's interest at heart, and to be employed in the project of civilization is to be used as fodder, ground up, faced with impossible choices. How do we possibly get free of the kind of inability to act that such anxiety leaves us with?

The response given to Zigao here suggests that anxiety in the face of situations like this is *acceptable* and ought somehow to be used to make one's way more effectively through such difficult situations rather than be reduced or eliminated. In a sense, Zhuangzi is telling Zigao "anxiety isn't your problem—your problem is your inability to *see past* this anxiety, so as to see how to effectively *use* it!" Zigao's inability to see past the anxiety is due to his failure to give up the kind of conceptualization, the process of *shi-fei* 是非

[125] *Zhuangzi* 4.3; Ziporyn 2009, 28.

(this/not-this, right/wrong, etc.) that the Zhuangzi expresses as problematic throughout the various chapters.

What happens, however, when one stops engaging in the process of *shi-fei*, which is continuous with "sitting and forgetting (*wang* 忘) the self" and "fasting of the mind" (*xin zhai* 心齋) discussed in chapters 3 and 4? Zhuangzi's version of Confucius tells Zigao that what he should do is simply concentrate on performing the task, and not on the self, a reward, or a particular conceptualization of the way things *should* be.[126] The idea here seems to be that it is the *inability to act* that is the problem, rather than the anxiety. In certain situations, anxiety may be the *proper* response. The Zhuangist spontaneity (*ziran* 自然) cannot be carelessness. The key is to be able to channel this anxiety into the kind of care that is necessary if one is to hope to navigate these seemingly impossible situations.

The conversation between Yan He and Qu Boyu later in chapter 4, concerning a prince whom Yan He has been employed to instruct, offers a similar lesson. Yan He describes his own impossible situation, similar to that of Zigao, involving the attempt to train his intransigent pupil. He's likely to be crushed whatever he does, because if he allows his student free reign, his vicious character will result in disaster to the state, while if he constrains the student, he puts himself in danger. Here is a critical trade-off—one's life or the welfare of society?[127]

Qu Boyu, interestingly, advises *caution* (*shen* 慎). What Yan He needs to do, he suggests, is to engage in external compromise while maintaining inner harmony. That is, he can most effectively act by following along with the natural propensity (*tian li* 天理) of his student's action, guiding him without confronting him, redirecting him efficiently. This compromise has to remain hidden, according to Qu, or one is in danger. There is a focus here on *care* or *caution*, but notably not on *ease*. The task of navigating through impossible situations is one that can be done, but it takes skill and extreme care. This itself is the kind of thing that could cause anxiety. Qu likens the skill of dealing with rulers to taming tigers—one has to understand and use the natural propensities of the tiger's behavior, avoiding arousing their bloodlust by giving them live animals to eat, for example.

Of course, the application of caution in itself may not entail that we should be expected to have states such as anxiety. According to the Stoics, the state of

[126] *Zhuangzi* 4.3.
[127] *Zhuangzi* 4.4.

fear is an irrational one that becomes caution when rationality is applied and our emotions are controlled. The Stoics certainly thought it was possible to be cautious while without fear or anxiety, whether they were correct or not. But what this passage (as well as the previous one) *does* seem to show is that the emphasis in the *Zhuangzi*, at least here, is squarely on efficacy of action rather than dissolution of unpleasant or otherwise problematic mental states. Zhuangzi's version of Confucius is silent on the fear/terror (*li* 慄) of Zigao, and whether this can or should be undermined.

Elsewhere, however, the *Zhuangzi* seems more clear in expressing the position that even the sage is not completely free of anxiety, and should not be. The clearest example of this is in the famous story of Cook Ding in chapter 3. Even Cook Ding, close to the Zhuangist ideal if anyone is, and one who in his own words has "gone beyond skill" and gained the ability to avoid conceptualization (*shi-fei* 是非), admittedly feels anxiety when he acts. And the suggestion in the passage is that this anxiety is somehow *necessary* to the efficacy of his action.

In his explanation of his amazing ability to carve oxen without ever replacing his knife, Ding first gives his account of how he does not see oxen at all, but rather the natural joints, and allows his knife to take up the empty space such that the meat falls apart as if on its own. This is where most accounts of Cook Ding's skill stop (as my own used to as well!). But Ding's account does not end here. He discusses what happens when he reaches a difficult point in the carving:

雖然, 每至於族, 吾見其難為, 怵然為戒, 視為止, 行為遲.

When I reach a difficult point, and I see it will be difficult, I anxiously (*chu ran*) employ caution (*wei*), my vision comes to a stop, my movement slows.[128]

This shift enables Ding to make his way through the difficult spot with but a subtle motion of the knife, thus maintaining the sharpness of his blade. Part of what seems to be expressed here is the view that anxiety can be *effective* at helping us achieve certain goals. It is part of the explanation of Cook Ding's ability that he *anxiously* employs caution. He does not just employ caution. That is, at least, if the author is being careful here, and *chu ran* isn't simply a

[128] *Zhuangzi* 3.2.

throwaway comment or something meant to serve as emphasis for the seriousness of the situation.

It seems unlikely that this would be an insignificant comment, given that the author could easily have ended the passage where many discussions of it end, at the seemingly natural point after Ding explains how he does not see oxen. But the author continues here to explain what happens in *difficult cases*. Connecting this to the passage earlier concerning Zigao and the recalcitrant prince, it seems that a common theme that emerges in the *Zhuangzi* is the generation of anxiety or dread in cases in which one faces difficult circumstances in the way of completing one's actions, or in which one's actions have a high probability of failure. In the Zigao passage, there is no suggestion as to whether or not the mental state of fear is one we ought to aim to undermine, but in the Cook Ding passage, the suggestion is that the anxiety one feels on beginning a difficult task is part of the explanation of the skill of the sagely person, which Ding certainly is intended to represent.

The suggestion here seems to be that the kind of caution that gets one through the seemingly impossible situation (tutoring the tyrannical prince, cutting through an ox without dulling one's blade where no empty space presents itself) *requires* anxiety. So clearly we are not dealing here with something like the Upanishadic notion that the anxiety attached to the problems it aims to solve will be dissolved with these solutions—a position echoed in the Buddhist tradition that grows out of the intellectual background of the *Upanishads*.

The term translated here as "caution," *jie* 戒, occurs in a number of other passages that can also help to make the case that Zhuangzi sees anxiety as a necessary part of such caution in certain cases. It is linked with adherence to actions based in *ming* 命 (allotment, destiny) and *yi* 義 (righteousness, appropriateness) in the story of Zigao and the recalcitrant prince in chapter 4, which, as we have seen, is connected to anxiety and fear. It is also raised in the conversation between Yan He and Qu Boyu directly.

The term I translate as "anxiety" here, *chu* 怵, occurs only a single time in the *Yangshengzhu* chapter (chapter 3) that contains Ding's story. It only appears one other place in the inner chapters, in *Yingdiwang*, in the context of an imagined conversation between Yang Ziju and Lao Dan (a story copied in the *Tiandi* chapter). There, *chu* is described as something undesirable or negative. The only other use in the *Zhuangzi* as a whole that seems to come anywhere close to that in *Yangshengzhu* is in the *Daozhi* chapter.[129] Thus we

[129] *Chu* is a rare term in the *Zhuangzi* as it is, with only five occurrences in the entire text (counting those of *Yingdiwang* and *Tiandi* as a single occurrence, given that one is a duplication).

can see that *chu* is not in general seen as a desirable or acceptable state (unlike rational states such as caution for the Stoics), and there are indeed passages in which the Zhuangist author(s) enjoin us to get rid of it. The same construction is used in the *Yingdiwang* chapter and the *Tiandi* chapter (from the so-called Outer Chapters): 勞形怵心者也 (one with toiling in body and anxiety of mind). In both cases, such persons are seen as lacking understanding. *Chu*, or anxiety, is not then an unqualifiedly good or useful thing according to the Zhuangists. It is for this reason that we cannot simply liken *chu* to a less unpleasant form of a more acceptable kind of anxiety akin to the pain that the enlightened person still feels, according to the Buddhists, or the "caution" rather than fear that the wise person feels, according to Stoics. But at the same time *chu* should not be rejected as a wholly negative and "useless" state either. The Cook Ding passage suggests this, but further support can be found in a general position that the *Zhuangzi* adopts concerning the "use of the useless."

The *Renjianshi* chapter closes with a general claim concerning those things that are conventionally deemed useless or disvalued:

> 山木自寇也，膏火自煎也。桂可食，故伐之；漆可用，故割之。人皆知有用之用，而莫知無用之用也。
>
> A mountain through its trees crowds itself. Grease used in a fire fries itself. The cinnamon tree can be eaten, therefore it is chopped down. The lacquer tree is useful, therefore it is carved up. Everyone knows the use of the useful, but no one knows the use of the useless.[130]

The Zhuangists here are emphasizing a point they argue for throughout the text of the *Zhuangzi*. When we value things and devalue other things (the two inevitably go together), we render ourselves incapable of seeing the possible value of the disvalued things. Because the world is undergoing constant transformation (*wanwu zhi hua*), standards are constantly changing—what is useful at one time in one place is not useful at a different time and place. Everything, then, has some value, but the only way we become able to see the value of a thing is to be able to shift perspectives. That which we deem "useless" is "useful" from some other perspective (or in some other situation).

[130] *Zhuangzi* 4.9.

The problem, according to Zhuangzi, is not that we have the wrong things or that we strive for the wrong states, but rather that we have the mindset so as to discriminate things into right and wrong, useful and useless, in the first place. The *Zhuangzi* focuses on the way in which rejection of the "useless" leads to our missing the hidden value of things.

This suggests just the kind of position toward states such as anxiety that we see in the Cook Ding passage and others mentioned earlier. To reject anxiety as something to be avoided, to be eliminated completely in exchange for the "peace of mind" at the center of the Indian and Greek schools discussed, would for the Zhuangist be a kind of *shi-fei*, and rejection of the state as wholly useless. This would, of course, be to miss the ways in which these states themselves can be useful (*yong* 用). One of the key features of the Zhuangist program is that things (*wu* 物) can only be deemed useful or useless from within some perspective, and there is nothing that is useful or useless from every perspective. There is no universally valuable or valueless thing or state, including anxiety. To hold that there is would fundamentally undermine the Zhuangist message that dogged commitment to certain things and values and wholesale rejection of others (a mistake made by Confucians, Mohists, and others) inevitably undermines one's own projects and makes true thriving impossible.

The stories concerning things that are "useless" comprise the second half of the *Xiaoyaoyou* chapter (chapter 1), concerning Jieyu, the "Madman of Chu," Hui Shi's enormous gourd, and the so-called useless tree, Zhuangzi takes pains to point out that the reason certain things are deemed useless and rejected as having value is the valuation of things we insist on making, and our inability to get outside of the perspectives created by those valuations. Hui Shi sees no use for the enormous gourd because he's stuck in the perspective that takes gourds as only useful to drink from or hold liquid. Likewise the tree is deemed useless when one is stuck in the perspective of seeing trees as useful only for timber. We can generalize this to other areas, including mental states such as anxiety. To see anxiety, even neurotic anxiety, as something we need to get rid of is to devalue it absolutely, engaging in the kind of *shi-fei* that takes anxiety as valueless and the lack of anxiety, or ease, as valuable, always and forever. But it is just this kind of thinking, according to Zhuangzi, that blinds us to the *tian li* (natural propensities), gets in the way of efficient action, and leads to "impossible situations" like those of Zigao, Yan Hui, and Yan He in chapter 4.

Rejection of the Problematic Nature of Madness in the *Zhuangzi*

This rejection of the idea that there are universally problematic emotions informs a broader Zhuangist notion of the rejection of the view that states such as madness are problematic in any universal or perspective-independent way. The positive characterization of such people as the madmen and transgressive characters discussed in this chapter demonstrate not only an unwillingness to reject *kuang* as a disorder or illness, but a willingness to point out the *benefits* of states like *kuang*, understanding that it can only be determined valuable or disvaluable from within some perspective and never perspective-independently. If the *Zhuangzi* more often points out the virtues and efficacy of the *kuang* person and other "rejects" like them, it is not because Zhuangists find these people more valuable than others or uniquely effective, but because, as we find in chapter 4, "everyone knows the use of the useful, but no one knows the use of the useless."[131]

Madness as such is not then a problematic state according to Zhuangists. Indeed, the mad person sees the world from a perspective that nonmad people are often unable to see it. The text focuses on such "useless" or rejected characters as a way of demonstrating the value of the conventionally useless. But what, we might ask, do Zhuangists see as potentially valuable about madness? And the additional question—if such states of mind as *kuang* can be (within certain perspectives) valuable, does this show that *kuang* is not a disorder or illness at all? The evidence from the text suggests just this, as this reduction is also made in the case of physical disorders, in particular "deformity." In the Zhuangists' desire to undermine *shi-fei* distinction making, they often collapse the distinctions between illness and health, ugliness and beauty, villain and sage, value and disvalue. The inversion of any kind of valuation one might make through *shi-fei*, whether positive or negative, is always possible.

The Zhuangist view concerning *kuang* then seems to reject the reality of mental illness (as with physical illness). The Zhuangists reconceptualize illness, through shifting of perspective akin to what they recommend for the reader. From the right perspective, what is conventionally useless, including "negative" mental states such as anxiety or "illnesses" such as madness, can be understood as possessing value. Thus we find in the *Zhuangzi* a stress

[131] *Zhuangzi* 4.9.

on an alternative kind of self-cultivation, standing in contrast to other familiar methods. Being in a state like that of the mad person is an aim of the *Zhuangzi*, at least in terms of the properties of the mad person discussed earlier. While we find in the *Zhuangzi* rejection of the kind of self-cultivation enjoined by Confucians and Mohists, the text is not without a conception of self-cultivation. Indeed, the process of undermining the "self," transcending knowledge (at least in terms of "lesser knowledge"), and ability to shift between perspectives is itself a skill developed through a process of development involving techniques such as "fasting of the mind" (*xin zhai* 心齋) or "sitting and forgetting" (*zuo wang* 坐忘). While the Zhuangists do not systematize this method of self-cultivation in the way Confucians systematize their own, it is clear in the text that becoming an ideal person in the Zhuangist sense, a *zhen ren* ("true person") who resembles the mad person, in most cases involves agentive deliberation and choices, most often explicitly aimed at undermining agency itself.

If to be like the mad person in the relevant way is to lack propositional knowledge, manifest transgressive (or "wandering") activity, and to be determined by the patterns of nature themselves, this requires deliberate and agentive action on some initial level, aiming at undercutting this very agency. The Zhuangists seem clear that human nature is associated with agency, in terms of the ability and tendency to make *shi-fei* distinctions, and the undermining of that tendency, and the ability to become determined by natural patterns in the way the mad person can (according to the Zhuangist conception of madness) is for most people something that will itself require a great deal of cultivation and sustained effort.

5

Synthesis and Medicalization in Early Han Views of Mental Illness

In this chapter, I discuss the view of madness and mental illness that develops in the "syncretic" texts and medical texts of the early Han. This view, I argue, is the most plausible account of mental illness and self-cultivation of those on offer in early Chinese philosophy. Indeed, this view comes closest to offering an analysis of states like madness as mental illness in the way it is understood in modern-day medicine. This does not entail that the syncretists were the first to have a concept of mental illness in early China. There are two reasons for this: (1) As I have argued previously, mental illness is a natural kind, about which early Chinese thinkers had a variety of things to say, even when they conceived of it very differently than our contemporaries;[1] (2) the discussions of madness and other mental illnesses in pre-Han texts show that these conditions are extensionally the same as concerns behavior and mental states as the new syncretist "medicalized" versions. It would be arbitrarily scientistic to deny the concept of mental illness in the absence of specific etiological accounts of it that come sufficiently close to current-day accounts. This would be akin to denying that medieval people had a concept of malaria when they thought the illness was caused by bad air (*mal aria*), and only gained such a concept when the discovery was made in the late nineteenth and early twentieth centuries that it was transmitted by mosquitoes, and of the parasite responsible. This would be an especially absurd position, given that the symptoms and disorder or illness of malaria were both understood and even fairly effectively treated prior to the discovery of its cause and sufficient understanding of malaria. Prior to the late nineteenth- and

[1] Peter Zachar argues that instead of natural kinds, psychiatric disorders should be taken as "practical kinds," which allow for indeterminate cases. He writes: "in psychiatry, indeterminacy is more than an occasional exception. It exists at the boundary of the normal and the abnormal, and between conventionally recognized symptom configurations and a more extensive, interconnected symptom space" (Zachar 2015). The shift to practical kinds on this basis, however, is unnecessary when we countenance the existence of indistinct or vague natural kinds, such as cluster kinds like species. See Boyd 1999, 67–98.

The Dao of Madness. Alexus McLeod, Oxford University Press. © Oxford University Press 2021.
DOI: 10.1093/oso/9780197505915.003.0006

early twentieth-century developments, no one knew whether malaria was caused by a virus, a parasite, or some other cause of disorder. As with all natural kinds, we can encounter them in nature without understanding much (or anything) about them, and come to increase our understanding of them over time.

This origins of the new "medicalized" view of mental illness can be found in the syncretic texts and texts developing "correlative cosmology," such as *Huainanzi* and *Chunqiu Fanlu*, though the seeds of this view can be found earlier in Warring States material. The syncretists reject both the negative and positive views of mental illness, arguing that a complex of nature, circumstances, and individual activity is responsible for most mental illness, and that the key to avoiding or eliminating mental illness is the undermining of conceptualization and elimination of desires. The key move in these texts is away from that of the moralized conception of mental illness found in both Confucian and Daoist/Zhuangist texts prior to the Han, and toward a more naturalistic view of mental illness, as represented most fully in Han texts such as *Huangdi Neijing*. We see a "naturalistic shift" in the late Warring States and continuing into the Han, with shift in interest from the specifically moral to concern with the natural world and its relationship to the human organism. During this period, we see the beginning of systematized medical literature, such as the medical texts unearthed in the Mawangdui excavation, most likely dating to the third century BCE.[2] There are a number of reasons for this naturalistic shift, including the movement of debates surrounding human nature into characteristics of the person in the late Warring States, as well as the systematization of knowledge in the period and the rise of private literature and concern with method.[3] Interestingly, however, though moral considerations fall mainly by the wayside in Han syncretist considerations of mental illness, there are still elements of the new understanding that can be easily linked to issues of morality and self-cultivation, even if the Han syncretists and medical thinkers themselves were largely silent about this connection.

[2] Harper 1998, 36–41.

[3] Joshua Brown and I discuss these issues in chapter 2 of Brown and McLeod 2020. Donald Harper discusses the rise of medical literature during this period in particular, writing: "Medical literature proliferated in the fourth to third centuries B.C. as new ideas arose and the impetus for committing knowledge to writing grew. The transformation of medicine from an archaic craft dominated by magico-religious belief and practice into a theoretically-grounded discipline was as much a function of the new literacy as it was of the rationalizing tendencies in thought. Medicine became one of many fields of natural philosophy that were defined by the books the specialists transmitted" (Harper 1998, 43).

The syncretic view of mental illness and cultivation also creates crucial groundwork for Buddhist thought in China, which is introduced in the late Han, and adopts numerous elements concerning the mind from the syncretic view that are not present in Indian Buddhism. The conception of "controlled madness" is based on the synthesis of views found in texts such as *Huainanzi*, suggesting that a view like this not only had some influence in later Chinese philosophy, but that it can also help us better understand the connections between illness and agency. The problem is recognized and worked out with an eye to avoid what we might see as the shortcomings of the two approaches discussed in Chapter 3. I consider also whether the Huainanist approach solves the problems with the other two without creating difficult problems of its own. While there are some complications still on the *Huainanzi* account, I argue that it is ultimately an improvement over the other two in terms of making sense of illness and agency, a problem we still have today.

Han Syncretism

In the late Warring States and more fully into the early Han, new methods of philosophical and more generally intellectual pursuit emerged, involving attempts to unify various schools, positions, and themes that were seen as opposed or contradictory in earlier history. Scholars have called this new trend "Han syncretism," and it is generally associated with a number of late Warring States and early Han texts and intellectual trends. Some have engaged in debates concerning the association of new schools or existing schools with syncretistic texts, such as the "Huang-Lao" school, which John Major associates with Han Daoism.[4] Syncretic texts of the Han (and late Warring States), such as the *Lushi Chunqiu*, *Huainanzi*, *Shizi*, and *Chunqiu Fanlu*, do not easily fall into school categories (with some exceptions—the authors of the *Chunqiu Fanlu* seem to explicitly think of their work as Confucian, despite the syncretic content of the work). Despite association with different schools, the Han syncretic texts often consciously attempted to integrate positions of other schools into their overarching systems. This is why we think of them as syncretic, rather than simply as influenced (consciously or

[4] Major 1993, 10. Kidder Smith writes that "Huang-Lao is a combination of the Yellow Thearch (*Huangdi*) and Laozi teachings practiced in the early Han" (Smith 2003, 146). This is easier to accept if Daoism itself is a Han construct, associated with Huang-Lao.

unconsciously) by other schools. These texts show us concerted attempts to integrate and make sense of the teachings of numerous disparate schools and texts of earlier periods as compatible on some fundamental level.

Because of the methodological similarities between the late Warring States and early Han syncretic texts, Ban Gu (32–92 CE) during the Eastern Han created the category of *zajia* 雜家, or "Syncretist School" to classify texts such as *Huainanzi* and *Lushi Chunqiu* engaged in various kinds of conscious methodological syncretism.[5] *Zajia* can thus be taken as a kind of methodological categorization—not a "school" in terms of particular characteristic viewpoints on any given cluster of concepts or practical goals, but in terms of a loosely shared commitment to a synthesis of a variety of diverse positions. As Knoblock and Riegel write, "the classification *zajia* does not mean a miscellaneous compendium that collects diverse views without reconciling them, but rather a work that presents a blending of materials, representing previously distinct positions."[6]

We should not attribute too much to the school categorization of Ban Gu. The syncretic texts of late Warring States and early Han were not bound together by any shared affiliation or commitment to positions. Indeed, though we find commitment to syncretism across these texts, the ways in which the various texts achieve synthesis is often very different and leads to a variety of different (and incompatible) views. Rather than a "school," the syncretic methodological commitments of these texts represented an intellectual trend that began in the late Warring States and peaked in the middle part of the Western Han, interestingly tracking the rise of correlative cosmology.[7] We can consider this trend in light of Huang-Lao, *Zajia*, or other categorizations, but this masks the extent to which the syncretic mode seems to have been a more widely distributed feature of intellectual culture in the early Han than such school-based analysis would suggest.[8]

One of the key features of the syncretism of the late Warring States and early Han was its grounding in large part in the new "naturalism" of the period, connected to the system of correlative cosmology developed in the late

[5] *Hanshu*, 3.10.320–321. Smith 2003, 150. Smith renders *zajia* as "those who weave disparate things together."

[6] Knoblock and Riegel 2001, 43.

[7] R. P. Peerenboom argues that it was commitment to the new naturalism that developed in the early Han that links these intellectual trends, "the notion of causal correlative cosmology—of Zou Yan, present in rudimentary form in the Huang-Lao thought of the *Boshu* and developed by Dong Zhongshu." Peerenboom 1993, 257.

[8] As found in "Confucian" texts such as *Chunqiu Fanlu*.

Warring States and the increasing prominence of *fang* 方 ("method") texts, and presented in fullest flower in texts such as the early Han text *Chunqiu Fanlu*, a syncretist "Confucian" treatise developing two distinct versions of correlative metaphysics based on *yin-yang* and "Five Phases" (*wu xing* 五行).[9] The development of correlative cosmology involved a move away from earlier causal accounts of events in the world involving an often agent-like *tian* (variously understood as Heaven, God, nature), and toward a more mechanistic picture of *dao* as manifest in particular regular patterns, the motions of which could be understood in terms of changes of phase and movement between *yin* and *yang* characteristics.[10] While it is impossible to associate a single particular text with this naturalistic shift and movement toward correlative cosmology, the move is already apparent as early as texts such as the *Xunzi* and the *Lushi Chunqiu*.

The implications of this naturalistic shift and the syncretic trend for madness and self-cultivation specifically are not initially easy to see. In the Han syncretic texts, unlike the *Zhuangzi* or early Confucian texts, the concepts of madness and the mad person are not central considerations or deployed to make broader points about the nature of personhood, knowledge, or self-cultivation. We do, however, find a new and interesting view develop concerning madness, mental illness, and illness more generally, both in Han syncretic texts such as (in particular *Huainanzi* and *Chunqiu Fanlu*) and in the new medical literature developed in the Han, represented by the *Huangdi Neijing* texts, developed further through the rest of the Western and Eastern Han, in texts such as the Eastern Han works *Nan Jing*, *Jingui Yaolue*, *Shang Han Lun*, and *Wen Bing Xue*. In these texts, mental illness (like illness more generally) is seen as linked primarily to naturalistic explanations such as quantity and movement of *qi* and the functioning of specific organs with respect to one another. Illness, according to the new naturalistic views of the Han, comes about through the disordering of certain regular biological processes concerning the body and mind. While aspects of the thought of Confucian, Daoist, and other thinkers is certainly discernable in the Han medical texts and influenced these thinkers, the moralistic consideration of mental illness found in both negative (Confucian) and positive (Zhuangist)

[9] Queen and Major claim argue that the material in the *Chunqiu Fanlu* definitively associated with Dong Zhongshu does not contain discussion of the Five Phases, but only *yin-yang*. Five Phases material in the *Chunqiu Fanlu*, they claim, was "likely written by other authors" (Queen and Major 2015, 451–452).

[10] More on the "naturalistic shift" can be found in Brown and McLeod 2020, 53–54.

senses is absent. In texts such as *Huangdi Neijing*, mental illness is largely no longer a matter of moral self-cultivation, but one of descriptive empirical consideration, of unbalanced properties of organs and mind. This is not to say that moral considerations are absent in texts such as *Huangdi Neijing*. But, unlike in earlier texts, the moral here is reduced to the medical, rather than the medical reduced to the moral. In the Han medical texts, *qi*, operation of the organs, and *yin* and *yang* characteristics are the ultimate explanation for physical and mental function, and insofar as we can understand moral development as relying on a certain balance in mental state, then moral development ultimately relies on naturalistic medicine.

While the syncretism of the early Han is not as obviously on display in medical texts such as *Huangdi Neijing* as it is in broader intellectual texts such as *Huainanzi* and *Chunqiu Fanlu*, the content and methodology of *Huangdi Neijing* can be understood as crucially linked to the syncretism and correlative cosmology of early Han thought. In this section, I look to the topics of mental illness (and madness in particular) in the Han syncretic texts, examining the new views we find of such illness, which will then inform the discussion of the next section, on the move to the naturalistic and medical conception of illness found in the *Huangdi Neijing*.

The *Huainanzi*

The project of the *Huainanzi*, constructed by Liu An, the vassal king of Huainan during the middle part of the Western Han Dynasty, was straightforwardly syncretic. While the scope and diversity of the text (and the fact that it was written and compiled by a large team of scholars with likely numerous views and aims) make it impossible to give a single easy answer to the question of the purpose(s) of the text, one clear overarching aim of Liu An himself was a justification of the system of semi-independent vassal rulership in the Han. Liu was concerned about the increasing centralization of the Han state and its growing direct administration over states which had once been independent national and cultural units before the beginning of the imperial era.[11] The overarching argument of the *Huainanzi*, that the wise ruler does not attempt to impose a single way on all things, but recognizes the inherent usefulness and unity of the vast variety of different peoples, customs,

[11] Vankeerberghen 2001, 13; Major et al. 2010, 11.

ways, teachings, and so on, redounded to Liu's political benefit, at least in theory. To apply the lessons of the *Huainanzi* to imperial government would be to recognize the sense in which the seemingly disparate states could be understood as united on a deeper level, and to make sense of such unification through grasping of the fundamental patterns and principles underlying the operation of all of these states.

In service of this broader message, the authors of the *Huainanzi* attempted to create an even more ambitious synthesis of not only a variety of seemingly disparate states, customs, and people, but of all knowledge and all known aspects of the cosmos. Perhaps even more than the political aim, the main centerpiece of the *Huainanzi* is this syncretic method, and the attempt to unify all human knowledge in an understanding of the foundation or root (*ben*) that the ruler can then use to understand and thus control the world—whether understood in terms of the people or other things in the world. Through much of the text, this synthesis of all knowledge is guided through a seemingly Zhuangist framework, although modified so as to allow compatibility with the host of other teachings and schools of earlier periods.

Donald Harper points out that the *Huainanzi* project included a number of scholars of *fang* ("practical method"), specialists in astronomy, medicine, and other such natural arts. This, according to Harper, is what accounts for the numerous chapters in the text concerning astronomy, geography, and medicine.[12] The *fangshi* 方士, associated with medical practitioners in texts such as *Huangdi Neijing*, if they were part of Liu An's philosophical syncretist project, worked with and influenced a variety of other thinkers, and likely pushed along the "naturalistic shift" in Han thought. The imperial project and systematization of knowledge led to a naturalistic syncretism. As Harper writes, "as a book of natural philosophy, the *Huainanzi* undoubtedly distills the knowledge of Liu An's recipe-and-art gentlemen [*fang shu zhi shi* 方術之士]."[13]

One of the first things we notice when looking to discussions of *kuang* (madness) in the *Huainanzi* specifically is that *kuang* here is more reminiscent of illness in the modern sense than what we find in early Confucian and Daoist/Zhuangist texts. We see here expression of the kind of view we find in

[12] "[*Fangshi*] participated in the compilation of the *Huainanzi* with its several chapters devoted to cosmology, astrology, geography, and the human body" (Harper 1998, 51).

[13] Harper 1998, 51.

Huangdi Neijing. This is perhaps attributable to the influence of the *fangshi* in the project, the combining of philosophical concerns with the practical method concerns of physicians, astronomers, and other experts at Liu An's court. In the first chapter of *Huainanzi*, there is a passage discussing *kuang* that exactly parallels considerations we find in the *Huangdi Neijing* texts, concerning the connection between states like madness and the disordering of *qi* caused by overabundant emotion:

> 夫喜怒者，道之邪也；憂悲者，德之失也；好憎者，心之過也；嗜欲者，性之累也。人大怒破陰，大喜墜陽，薄氣發喑，驚怖為狂。憂悲多恚，病乃成積；好憎繁多，禍乃相隨。故心不憂樂，德之至也；通而不變，靜之至也；嗜欲不載，虛之至也；無所好憎，平之至也；不與物散，粹之至也。
>
> Joy and anger disorder (*xie*) the *dao*. Grief and sorrow eliminate potency (*de*). Being fond of detesting (others) leads the mind astray. Attachment to desires harms one's nature/inborn characteristics. A person's great anger destroys *yin*, and their great joy submerges *yang*. Weak *qi* makes one mute/dull, and alarmed one becomes mad (*kuang*). When one is grieving, sorrowful, or often enraged, illness (*bing*) is completed and accumulated. When one is fond of detesting (others) and complicates things, disaster follows along with it. Thus, having a mind without grief or happiness, one arrives at potency. To pass through it yet not change, one arrives at stillness. Not holding onto attachment to desires, one arrives at emptiness. Not having anything which one is fond of detesting, one arrives at peace. Not being given/prone to scattering things, one arrives at the pure state.[14]

The use of *xie* 邪 here to describe the effect of joy and anger on our understanding of *dao* is reminiscent of medical explanations of the time, as it was understood in terms of causes of illness. We see the term used throughout *Huangdi Neijing* to flag particular causes of illness. This entire passage echoes themes we find in medical texts of the period. Emotions such as grief, sorrow, joy, and anger lead to illness, including madness. This happens through their operation on *qi*. We find here an attempt to explain the causal mechanism

[14] *Huainanzi* 1.16.

behind illness (particularly mental illness) through reference to *qi* and its states, particularly the *yin* and *yang* qualities of *qi*, as well as its quantity and location.

The view of overabundant emotion leading to *kuang* is common in the Han, and it is found in a number of texts. In the *Chunqiu Fanlu*, we find a passage expressing a view similar to that found in the *Huangdi Neijing* and *Huainanzi*, concerning the effects of such emotion on *qi*, which leads to various disorders:

> 怒則氣高，喜則氣散，憂則氣狂，懼則氣懾。
>
> Anger leads to the heightening of *qi*, joy leads to the dissolution of *qi*, grief leads to the madness of *qi*, fear leads to the terror of *qi*.[15]

This view of illness and balance relies on the views of *qi*, *yin-yang*, and Five Phases developed in the correlative cosmology of the early Han. While we find the view that overabundant emotions and desires contribute to or directly cause mental illness in earlier texts, the adoption of *qi* and its states as the mechanism for this development of illness is fully fleshed out only in Han texts, reaching its peak in the medical texts of the later Han.

There is a strong Zhuangist flavor to this passage, as the authors offer a picture of treatment and maintenance of health as involving the "emptiness" achieved through elimination of desires, overabundant emotion, and certain kinds of self-concern. We find this also in the *Huangdi Neijing*, which offers restriction of certain kinds and amounts of emotion as treatment. In order to undermine the illnesses caused by anger and other abundant emotion, we should try to eliminate anger in the mind, according to the *Huangdi Neijing*.[16] While both the *Huangdi Neijing* and the *Huainanzi* make similar claims in this way concerning treatment, neither text offers us a practical method for undermining such mental states, as do more practically focused texts like those of the Buddhists and Neo-Confucians of later generations. This is part of the reason that it appears that Han thinkers (at least in these cases) are more interested in explanation than in practice—undermining the

[15] *Chunqiu Fanlu*, 77.1.

[16] *Huangdi Neijing Suwen* 3.3: 大怒則形氣絕 ("Great anger causes the *qi* of the body to be cut short.") Wang Bing's commentary to the passage reads: "This is . . . warning against unrestrained happiness or anger. Their excessive operation causes disease" (Unschuld and Tessenow 2011, 68).

common position that early Chinese texts in general are more focused on practice and behavioral outcomes than explanation of the world (a general claim often used to support the further claim that early Chinese thinkers had little to no interest in metaphysics).[17]

The connection of illness to *qi* and the states of *yin* and *yang* also ties illness to the issue of proper human functioning and natural patterns. There are certain normative amounts and movements of *qi*, according to the picture developed in the Han, particular ways that *qi* will tend to act, including augmentation and depletion, following a natural and unimpeded pattern, unless it is interrupted through either human agentive activity, or the spontaneous (*ziran*) nonagentive activity of the world. This regular activity can be disrupted in a number of ways—environmental factors, and dysfunction of organs or other places in the body that can store and transfer *qi* (of which more is said in medical texts than texts such as *Huainanzi*). The most commonly discussed disruption of such regular activity in nonmedical texts like *Huainanzi* is problematic mental states. In particular, desires and emotions are accorded the power to disrupt the proper functioning of *qi*, as seen in the earlier passage of the *Huainanzi*. Grief, sorrow, anger, and joy—all of these lead to imbalance in the mind that effects *qi* in negative ways. This raises the question of whether desire and emotion *in general* have the deleterious effect the *Huainanzi* discusses, or whether instead it is a certain type of desire or emotion that has such effect. The examples given of harmful emotions for the most part appear to be among the most extreme or energetic emotions. Anger and grief, for example, are mentioned, but not sadness, amusement, or excitement. It appears that the view here is that certain problematic emotions or overabundant emotions can be problematic in that they disrupt the natural activity of *qi*.

While anger and grief might be expected as examples of such problematic emotions, joy (*xi* 喜) and happiness (*le* 樂) are added to the list in the earlier *Huainanzi* passage. Joy and happiness do not immediately suggest the kind of strong, extreme, and disruptively powerful emotions that might plausibly disrupt the functioning of *qi* and *yin* and *yang* motions. While what we find here may suggest a kind of Zhuangist view involving the elimination of desire and agency, we find something different in the *Huainanzi* as concerns

[17] A number of scholars through the years have argued for this view, including A.C. Graham ("the crucial question for [early Chinese philosophers] is not the Western philosopher's 'What is the truth?' but 'Where is the Way?'" [Graham 1989, 3]) and Chad Hansen (2000, 3). See also Peerenboom's discussion of Hansen in Peerenboom 1993, 59.

emotions such as joy and happiness (and the relationship between the two). One important feature of the passage is that early on it is specifically *great* anger (*da nu* 大怒) and *great* joy (*da xi* 大喜) that have the kind of disruptive effect on *qi* that can lead to madness or illness more generally. Grief, sorrow, and rage are specifically tied to the "completion of illness" (*cheng bing* 成病). While these emotions are linked to illness, achieving balance and potency requires lacking both grief (presumably the complex of negative emotions) and happiness.

The *Huainanzi* contains a number of discussions of joy and happiness in this connection. This view of the problematic nature of overabundant emotion and desire found in the *Huainanzi* and other Han texts stands in stark contrast with a particular strain of thought prevalent in the Warring States, associated with texts such as the *Zhuangzi*, and perhaps influencing the *Mengzi* as well. On this view, emotion and desire are linked to human nature (*xing* 性), and following the natural patterns of *dao* requires embracing, rather than reforming, this nature. The short text *Xing Zi Ming Chu* 性自命出, unearthed in the 1993 Guodian excavation, offers a positive view of emotions (*qing* 情), even the kind of extreme or overabundant emotions that texts such as *Huainanzi* and *Huangdi Neijing* argue lead to illness through disruption of the operation of *qi*. In the *Xing Zi Ming Chu*, the idea seems to be that emotions must be taken as natural and acceptable as part of our *xing* due to the ease and regularity with which they arise in the mind (*xin* 心). There, we find an embrace of overabundant emotion as key to the thriving life, both extreme joy and extreme grief.[18] The text associates the very emotions picked out by the *Huainanzi* as having deleterious effect as being associated with human nature (*xing* 性).

> 喜怒哀悲之氣，性也。
>
> The *qi* of joy, anger, mourning, and sorrow is human nature.[19]

Following a theme of the *Zhuangzi* and *Mengzi*, the *Xing Zi Ming Chu* assumes that the spontaneous, natural, and uncultivated responses and features of our minds are positive, beneficial, and lead to thriving if followed.

[18] Kenneth Holloway discusses this aspect of the text, writing "we can see *qing* [emotions] not merely tolerating, but actually embracing extreme emotional friction at the immanent level" (Holloway 2013, 22).

[19] *Xing Zi Ming Chu* 1.1; see Middendorf 2008, 152.

They reject the idea that allowing free rein to our emotions could lead us to a state of illness or disorder, given that these emotions are themselves part of the inborn characteristics we receive from *tian*. A passage from *Xing Zi Ming Chu* demonstrates this celebration of abundant emotion:

> 凡至樂必悲，哭亦悲，皆至其情也。哀，樂，其性相近也。是故其心不遠。哭之動心也，浸殺，其烈戀戀如也，戚然以終。樂之動心也，浚深鬱陶，其烈則流如也以悲，悠然以思。
>
> in each summative joy there is necessarily sorrow—crying is also grief, and the two together are the summation of your emotions (*qing*). Mourning and happiness are close together in nature, thus in the mind they are not distant. Crying moves the heart, in tears and isolation—you are intensely unable to bear parting, melancholy with the end. Joy moves the heart, reaching deep and making you giddy. If you are intense then you are tearful and in sorrow, and leisurely in contemplation.[20]

Note that this position relies on a view of human agency as independent of the natural patterns, and the view that modification of the patterns of our minds or activities through cultivational effort would then represent a move away from natural patterns. Human agency, as such, is seen as *not* a proper part of nature, and in that sense transcendent.[21] Due to the naturalistic shift in the early Han, we see a move toward a picture of agentive activity involving self-cultivation, reformation, and ritual as itself natural. Both agentive and nonagentive action, the action of persons and the action of nature, are due to the activity of *qi*. And as such, some natural activity (such as restraint of emotions and desires) can facilitate effective operation of *qi*, and some natural activity, such as overabundant emotion and desire, can disrupt effective operation of *qi*. We see that in Han texts such as *Huainanzi* and *Huangdi Neijing*, there is no appeal to nature to demonstrate the value of particular states or things.

Kenneth Holloway, discussing the positive view of emotions (including extreme emotion) in the *Xing Zi Ming Chu*, contrasts this view with what he thinks of as dominant views in the Western tradition, particularly in Greek

[20] *Xing zi ming chu* 11; Holloway 2013, 23, modified.
[21] Joshua Brown and I discuss this at length in Brown and McLeod 2020, 59.

and Roman thought, in much of which overabundant emotion is seen as problematic. Holloway writes:

> In Greece and Rome, anger was seen as something that was dysfunctional, particularly when expressed in public. Private anger was seen as also something that led to the brutalization of others, and certainly had no positive moral attributes. Medieval and early modern scholarship similarly describes a trope where civility involves a break from earlier times when anger was allowed to blossom forth to the immediate detriment of others.

In the view of the *Xing Zi Ming Chu*, however,

> anger is not seen as something to repress, for it is not seen as degenerating into improper expressions of violence. Instead, when we reach such outlier moments in our lives it is an opportunity to stretch our understanding and reach a transcendent level.[22]

While Holloway is surely right here about the evaluation of emotion in *Xing Zi Ming Chu*, a position it shares with the *Zhuangzi*, there is no need to look as far afield as Greece and Rome to find a contrast to this view. As I have shown here, it can be found in the early Chinese tradition itself, most clearly in Han Dynasty texts, in which overabundant emotions and desires are explicitly tied to disorder, and seen as aspects of the mind necessary for us to overcome or undermine if we hope to gain thriving.

Part of what seems problematic about the emotions discussed in numerous passages of *Huainanzi* linked to disruption of proper operation of *qi* is that they are stronger than other emotions. There also seems to be a concern with *overabundance* of emotion here. That is, the *Huainanzi* may not be instructing us to eliminate all desires and emotions—indeed, it is unclear how one could do this while still functioning as a human being. Rather, it may be instructing us to moderate our desires and emotions, avoiding the kinds or strength of desires and emotions or that can have a buffeting effect on the mind. *Huainanzi* 10.19 discusses the differences between three kinds of people with respect to illness: the wise, who can exert

[22] Holloway 2013, 25.

themselves without becoming ill; those of the middling sort, who can exert themselves but thereby become ill; and the lowliest, who are ill and cannot exert themselves.[23] We see from this that overexertion is among the potential causes of illness, which suggests a similar view concerning mental states. The *Huainanzi* does not mean by "exertion" (*lao* 勞) just *any* kind of activity, which would be better captured by *xing* 行, but in particular energetic and exertive activity, of the kind that plausibly leads to exhaustion. Another passage in chapter 10 links illness to lack of restraint.[24] Likewise, strong emotions such as grief or anger, which have a kind of intrinsic intensity that others lack, tend toward disruption of the mind and imbalance of *qi*. Additionally, even emotions not intrinsically intense of themselves can be present overabundantly, in which case they, too, can cause such disruption. The nature of desire is similar. Indeed, this was a key insight of Xunzi's in the late Warring States, and one which may influence the view in the *Huainanzi*. According to Xunzi, desire becomes problematic when unconstrained purely because desire becomes overabundant in such a case, due to its natural tendency to grow ever stronger and more robust. Without putting limitations onto our desires and thus reshaping them, they will simply grow to the point that they become overabundant and thus disruptive.[25] It is not, according to Xunzi, that desire in itself is problematic. Xunzi does not see value in eliminating desires—indeed, he likely would not see it as even *possible* to eliminate desires.[26] We can stop these desires from becoming problematic in just the ways the *Huainanzi* seems to be concerned with through limitation and thus reshaping of desires via ritual. Such reformed desires will not have the deleterious effects of imbalancing and disordering the mind that overabundant desires have.

Notice that while Xunzi's view concerning desire limitation and reformation is consistent with that of the *Huainanzi*, the *Huainanzi*'s reasons for encouraging limitation of desire diverge somewhat from Xunzi's. For Xunzi, the fundamental problem with overabundant or unchecked desire was that it led to interpersonal conflict, due to clashing desires (if I desire infinite wealth, for example, then I will also require the wealth others hold, and thus will necessarily come into conflict with them), and that it undermined the possibility of desire satisfaction (I cannot possibly satisfy a desire for infinite

[23] *Huainanzi* 10.19: 通智得而不勞，其次勞而不病，其下病而不勞。
[24] *Huainanzi* 10.23: 用之不節，乃反為病.
[25] *Xunzi* 19.1.
[26] Hagen 2007, 126.

wealth, since at no point will I actually possess infinite wealth).[27] On the view of the *Huainanzi*, however, the primary problem with overabundant desire is its imbalancing effect on the mind and on the proper activity of *qi*. Such imbalance, according to the *Huainanzi*, leads to illness.[28] Action consistent with ritual, for both Xunzi and the authors of *Huainanzi*, has a salubrious effect on the mind, but for the *Huainanzi* this effect has to do with maintenance (or obtaining, *de*) of the *dao*, in terms of proper balanced activity following the natural patterns. A passage from chapter 2 of the *Huainanzi* puts ritual into this context:

> 是故以道為竿，以德為綸，禮樂為鉤，仁義為餌，投之于江，浮之於海，萬物紛紛孰非其有。夫挾依於跂躍之術，提挈人間之際，撣掞挺挏世之風俗，以摸蘇牽連物之微妙，猶得肆其志，充其欲，何況懷環瑋之道，忘肝膽，遺耳目，獨浮游無方之外，不與物相弊搬，中徙倚無形之域，而和以天地者乎！

> this is why one should use *dao* as a pole, potency as a line, ritual and music as a hook, humanity and righteousness as bait—taking it up and casting it into the river, floating it in the sea. Which of the scattered myriad things will one fail to possess? Those who rely on deviant techniques, who control the realm of persons, who seek profit above and below according to the customs of the age in order to grope for and link together the subtleties of things: even such people will realize their intentions and fulfill their desires. How much more then will this be so of those who cleave to the precious *dao*, forgetting even their liver and gall, abandoning hearing and seeing, along floating and wandering beyond the boundless, not mixed up with things, lingering in the realm of the formless, and harmonizing with heaven and earth?[29]

We see also in this passage an example of the kind of syncretist position early Han texts are known for. The authors of the *Huainanzi* here tie action consistent with ritual and righteousness (Confucian concerns) to the kind of nonintentional "wandering" (*you*) the Zhuangists enjoin, marked by the undermining of desires and self-conception. According to the *Zhuangzi*, commitment to ritual, humanity, and righteousness is ultimately the way to

[27] *Xunzi* 19.

[28] *Huainanzi* 13. 23, for example: 陰陽相捔者也。離者必病 (*yin* and *yang* attack one another. If this is left behind one necessarily becomes ill).

[29] *Huainanzi* 2.7. Major et al. 2010 trans., modified.

achieve something like this Zhuangist state, which then allows the mind to operate in the proper ways, to be balanced such that the activity of its *qi* is not disrupted. Ritual then also plays a role in maintenance of health, as illness is attributed to disruption of the proper activity of *qi* and imbalance.

Because illness (*bing* 病) is understood in a more naturalistic way here, connected to the operation of *qi*, which connects mental and physical activity, illness is always accessible or manifest externally, in ways we can recognize through observation. That is, illness will always have physically observable manifestations, as the disruption of *qi* that leads to illness will also itself have observable features in terms of the dysfunctional physical activity also caused by disruption. A passage from chapter 2 of *Huainanzi* explicitly makes this claim: "When there is illness internally, there will necessarily (*bi*) be a manifestation of it externally" (夫有病於內者，必有色於外矣).[30]

The disturbance of mind associated with mental illness more generally (whether in the form of *kuang* or some other form) is associated with *qi* in a number of other passages of the *Huainanzi*, following this general Han tendency to explain proper operation, disorder, and illness in terms of the activity of *qi*. Given that *qi* is disrupted and buffeted by overabundant emotion and desires, the *Huainanzi* enjoins us to learn to disconnect our emotions and graspings from conditions in the world, as these situations (which are largely outside of our control) would then have the potential to disorder the mind, to drive us mad or cause other problems. The following passage from chapter 1 describes the sage's state with respect to disturbance of the mind:

> 故雖游于江潯海裔，馳要褭，建翠蓋，目觀掉羽、武象之樂，耳聽滔朗奇麗激抮之音，揚鄭、衛之浩樂，結激楚之遺風，射沼濱之高鳥，逐苑囿之走獸，此齊民之所以淫泆流湎。聖人處之，不足以營其精神，亂其氣志，使心怵然失其情性。處窮僻之鄉，側溪穀之間，隱于榛薄之中，環堵之室，茨之以生茅，蓬戶甕牖，揉桑為樞，上漏下濕，潤浸北房，雪霜滾灖，浸潭苽蔣，逍遙於廣澤之中，而仿洋於山峽之旁，此齊民之所為形植黎黑，憂悲而不得志也。聖人處之，不為愁悴怨懟，而不失其所以自樂也。是何也？則內有以通於天機，而不以貴賤、貧富、勞役失其志德者也。

Thus roaming along a riverbank or seashore, galloping with Yao Niao or riding a chariot beneath a kingfisher-feathered canopy, the eyes seeing the

[30] *Huainanzi* 2.14.

"Plumes of the Pheasant" dance or the performance of the "Emblems of King Wu" music, the ears listening to lavishly clear, elegant, and rousing melodies or being stimulated by the licentious music of Zheng and Wey or getting wrapped up in the stirring traditional ballads of Chu or shooting at high-flying birds along the lakeshore or hunting wild beasts in hunting preserves: all these are things that average people find alluring and intoxicating. *Sages experience them but not so much as to dominate their quintessential spirit or to disorder their vital energy, so as to cause their minds to become anxious (chu) and lose their essential natures.* To reside in a remote village on the side of a deep gorge hidden amid dense vegetation in a poor hut with a thatched roof on which grass sprouts up, whose door is overgrown by vines and which has small round windows like the mouth of a jar and a mulberry staff for a hinge, a hut whose roof is leaky and whose floor is damp, whose sleeping quarters are drafty and blanketed by snow and frost so that the grass mats are soaked; to wander in a vast marsh and ramble on the side of mountain slopes: these are things that would make average people develop dark moods and make them anxious and sad and unable to concentrate on anything. Sages live in places like this, but they do not make them worried or angry or make them lose what makes them content on their own. What are the reasons for this? Because they intrinsically have the means to penetrate the mechanism of heaven, and they do not allow honor or debasement, poverty, or wealth to make them weary and lose their awareness of their potency.[31]

The term *chu* 怵 here signifies a disturbance of mind, akin to "anxiety" or "stress." We find the same concept in the Cook Ding passage of *Zhuangzi* 3, where *chu* is understood as a potentially helpful mental state in certain cases. Here, the *Huainanzi* takes a more standard line, associating such mental states with disorder, resulting from (and causing new) disruption of the activity of *qi*.

The understanding of madness (*kuang*) in the *Huainanzi* is in line with that of its view of illness in general, though as in other texts, we find specific focus on *kuang* and some of its features. As in the earlier Confucian and Daoist/Zhuangist texts, we find consideration of the potential positive and negative features of *kuang*. What is interestingly absent, as mentioned earlier, is consideration of *kuang* in moral or value terms. *Kuang* is not linked

[31] *Huainanzi* 1.19, Major et al. 2010 trans. Emphasis is mine.

explicitly to self-cultivation in the way we find in earlier texts, and it is seen as largely independent from issues of agency, rather than as resulting from development of the self through agentive considerations. While there are certain features of *kuang* we might see as beneficial, following the Zhuangist line, the *Huainanzi* does not evaluate the state of *kuang* as either morally positive or negative. Rather, it is a matter of health, of improper functioning of *qi*. In this sense perhaps, *kuang* can be taken as a negative, but it is not a *moral* evaluation that is involved here.

For our purposes, the most important passage in the *Huainanzi* concerning *kuang* comes in the final chapter, *Yaolue*. The *Yaolue* chapter is often understood as a synthetic overview of the contents of the *Huainanzi*, an attempt to draw the connections between the various seemingly disparate parts of the overarching text.[32] We also find in the *Yaolue* brief accounts of what the authors think of as the important themes and messages of each of the individual chapters of the *Huainanzi*. The statements made about particular chapters in the *Yaolue* chapter are often different from those found in the chapters discussed, in order to make clear the connections between chapters. As Judson Murray puts it, *Yaolue* is "an invaluable aid to readers because it makes explicit what is not obvious or easily understood in the text's chapters."[33] In the description of the *Xiuwu* chapter (chapter 19), the authors of *Yaolue* bring up the issue of madness, which does not arise in chapter 19 itself. A crucial passage distinguishes the mad person from the sage on the basis of knowledge, which is attained through the kind of cultivation enjoined in the *Xiuwu* chapter. The passage[34] reads:

> 今夫狂者無憂，聖人亦無憂。聖人無憂，和以德也；狂者無憂，不知禍福也。故通而無為也，與塞而無為也同；其無為則同，其所以無為則異。故為之浮稱流說其所以能聽，所以使學者孳孳以自幾也。
>
> Now, mad persons are without grief, and sages too are without grief. Sages are without grief because they harmonize by means of potency, whereas mad persons are without grief because they do not know [the difference between] bad and good fortune. Thus, the non-action (*wu wei*) of those who fully comprehend [the *dao*] and the non-action of those who are obstructed from [the *dao*] are alike with regard to their non-action but differ with

[32] See Murray 2004.
[33] Murray 2004, 68.
[34] Also discussed earlier in Chapter 2 of this book.

> regard to the means by which they are non-active. Thus on their behalf, what can be heeded has been brought to the surface, declared, circulated, and explained, thereby inspiring scholars to diligently appropriate [these principles] for themselves.[35]

Cultivation, mainly in terms of understanding the patterns inherent in the world and the interconnection of all knowledge, leads to ends that are practically similar to certain features possessed by the mad person. The view of the *Huainanzi*, however, is that such ends are not sufficient to make one a developed person. The sage has something more than the mad person—namely, the knowledge that allows for the contextual understanding of when particular mental states are called for. There are certain potentially positive features that the mad person will have, according to this passage, but having these features alone is not sufficient for proper action, as the *Zhuangzi* seems to claim. Development of knowledge of the reasons behind certain actions, and the agentive performance of those actions through self-development, rather than the agentless *ziran* activity enjoined by the *Zhuangzi*, is what the *Huainanzi* calls for.

Moreover, the sage's knowledge becomes *accessible* through the explanations of the general content and principles underlying this knowledge (fitting into the *Huainanzi*'s structure of root and branches). We can access the knowledge of the sages through texts and follow their thinking so as to generate the kinds of action they were able to create. Because the sage operates from understanding, from a base of knowledge, the sage's actions can be grasped and followed. The mad person's actions, however—spontaneous, wild, and unconstrained (like uncultivated "nature" itself)—cannot be crafted through cultivation or artifice. As the *Zhuangzi* argues (a point accepted here by the *Huainanzi*), the actions of the mad person are not produced from agentive decisions and cultivation, but rather from spontaneous responses to the world and features of mind. The *Huainanzi* points out that not only can one not duplicate such action through agentive means (as it does not derive from cognitive access to anything), but that such action on part of the mad person is also not reliable and insensitive to context, because it is not based in action. The mad person will be without grief not only in cases in which they *should* be without grief, but even in cases where they should. The mad person's lack of knowledge of the difference between misfortune and fortune will lead them *sometimes* to beneficial

[35] *Huainanzi* 21.19, Major et al. 2010, modified.

action, but sometimes to disaster. Action based on knowledge is sensitive to context, while the nonagentive activity of the mad person is not. As we see in the passage from chapter 1, the mental state of the sage does not "depend on things," and it is the knowledge of the sage that allows for this. While the mad person may be buffeted by the world sometimes in ways that are advantageous, carried on the wind to a peaceful clime, such a person can just as easily be carried to a disaster.

Here, we see a distinction between knowledge and action that pushes the two farther apart than what we find in earlier texts such as *Zhuangzi* or the early Confucian texts. Knowledge is not here understood as practical ability, although a certain practical ability may follow from such knowledge—rather, it is understood as propositional and as underdeterminative of activity. Knowledge, that is, is not understood as the ability to act in certain ways, or we would have to conclude that the mad person and the sage discussed in this passage both possess knowledge. Rather, it is a certain cognitive grasp of reasons, of *why* one acts a certain way, and agentive consideration.

This passage echoes a similar passage found in chapter 1, though in this passage this is expressed through consideration of the protection of the "internal" (*nei*). Because of this lack of knowledge, according to the chapter 1 passage, the mad person cannot respond properly to situations, and cannot adjust their activities when differences are called for. The key passage reads:

> 今夫狂者之不能避水火之難，而越溝瀆之險者，豈無形神氣志哉？然而用之異也。失其所守之位，而離其外內之舍，是故舉錯不能當，動靜不能中，終身運枯形于連嶁列埒之門，而蹪蹈於汙壑阱陷之中。雖生俱與人鈞，然而不免為人戮笑者，何也？形神相失也。故以神為主者，形從而利；以形為制者，神從而害。
>
> Now, mad persons cannot avoid the disasters of flood or fire, and cannot cross over the obstacles of ditches and gutters. How could this be, that they are without body, spirit, vital energy (*qi*), or will? Though this is the case, they use them differently. They have lost the relative positions they are supposed to guard, and have left their external or internal dwellings. Thus, they make mistakes and don't hit on the right responses, and they cannot strike a balance between movement and stillness. Throughout their lives they drag their withered bodies along the edge of mountain ridges and embankments, stumbling into filthy ditches and sewage pits. Although they were born the same as other people, they cannot escape condemnation

and ridicule. Why? Because their bodies and spirits have lose their relative positions. Thus when the spirit rules, the body follows and benefits from this. When the body governs, the spirit follows and is harmed by this.[36]

This passage, agreeing with the *Zhuangzi* on one point, locates the activity of the mad person in their complete lack of agency. The mad person's activity, lacking agentive direction based on knowledge, cannot be responsive to situations, cannot be altered to take different features into consideration. While the sage can act in the way things call for, based on understanding of situations, principles, and the effects of action, the mad person is simply dependent on the whims of nature, carried by nonagentive activity, which will not always take one where one wants to go. The Zhuangist image of the "natural patterns" (*tian li*) as determining the activity of the perfect person is here flipped on its head. Relying on the patterns of nature in the Zhuangist sense, undermining our agency, will sometimes take us to the correct place, but will often also lead us to disaster. If we make ourselves like water flowing along with the contours of the land, sometimes we will end up in the sea, but sometimes we will end up in a stagnant waste. To use the image of the earlier passage, through following natural patterns, water finds its way into sewage pits just as naturally as it finds its way into fresh springs. The mistake here is to assume that the natural patterns will always lead to something positive or advantageous. In order to ensure proper results of action, agentive action based on knowledge must play a role.

The distinction between knowledge and activity here is emphasized based on the distinction between body (*xing* 形) and spirit (*shen* 神). The activity of the mad person is associated with body absent the direction of spirit, nonagentive and spontaneous (*ziran* 自然) activity in which the body responds to things without the guidance of knowledge. The same agentless spontaneity and lack of knowledge that leads the mad person to be without grief (as described in the chapter 21 passage) also leads the mad person to stumble into ditches and sewage pits. As we might say, even a broken clock is accurate twice a day.

The view developed on the difference between the mad person and the sage (or even regular people) in the *Huainanzi* requires a conception of knowledge very much connected with an agentive and perspective-bound approach (of the kind rejected in the *Zhuangzi*).

[36] *Huainanzi* 1.22, Major et al. 2010 trans., modified.

To be swayed by or drawn to act by things, rather than through internal agentive impetus, is doubly dangerous, according to the *Huainanzi*. Not only does the kind of spontaneous and nonintentional action prized in the *Zhuangzi* lead to falling into disasters because of the inability to discern between proper and improper activity, but it also makes one susceptible to the power of things in the world to disturb the mind, to create the kinds of overabundant emotions and desires that lead to states like madness. The *Huainanzi* points out that spontaneous action, or action following the natural patterns,[37] is not free of internal and mental implications. A key mistake of the *Zhuangzi*, according to this view, is that action following the natural patterns was taken to be largely free of mental and internal effect. That is, the mind of the individual who achieved a state of spontaneous natural action following the patterns was understood as detached or unmoved by things in the world. In the *Huainanzi*, we find the view that, on the contrary, one who has achieved the kind of nonagentive spontaneous activity understood as following natural patterns will experience the same kinds of shifting of activity and buffeting by things in the *mind* as they will in the body.

不知道者，釋其所已有，而求其所未得也。苦心愁慮以行曲，故福至則喜，禍至則怖，神勞于謀，智遽於事，禍福萌生，終身不悔，己之所生，乃反愁人。不喜則憂，中未嘗平。持無所監，謂之狂生。

Those who do not know the *dao* abandon what they already possess and strive after what they do not yet possess. With a distressed mind and anxious thoughts, they try to realize misguided precedents. When good fortune arises, they feel happy. When bad fortune arises, they feel frightened. Their spirit is exhausted by plans, their intelligence is wearied by affairs. Misfortune and fortune sprout forth, yet to the ends of their lives they are undeterred, for what they themselves have caused, they turn around and blame others. Unhappy and aggrieved, their center is never balanced. They hold to what is unexamined. This is called a life of madness (*kuang*).[38]

One of the keys to this divergence between the Zhuangist and the *Huainanzi*'s view is the development of the naturalistic viewpoint in the early

[37] Unlike in the *Zhuangzi*, there is only a single instance of the term *tian li* 天理 in the *Huainanzi*, in the first chapter (*Huainanzi* 1.5).

[38] *Huainanzi* 14.16. Major et al. 2010 trans., modified.

Han bringing the body and mind into closer alignment, and basing the states in the latter on the former. Once we have a view of *qi* and its operation that takes features of mind to be linked to and caused by certain "psychophysical" states governed by *qi*, then we come to see that states of mind cannot be disconnected from external situations. That is, we cannot inhabit situations without these situations having a particular effect on our minds as well as our bodies. In the *Zhuangzi*, as well as in other early texts such as the Confucian texts *Mengzi* and *Xunzi*, we find the view that one can *disconnect* the mind from situations. One can maintain a certain frame or state of mind even through radically different situations. Indeed, gaining this ability, according to some texts, is the key aim of self-cultivation.[39]

When one does not cultivate the kind of knowledge that enables one to understand situational differences and to transform oneself as called for by the changes in the world, one inevitably ends in disaster. A passage from the *Jingshen* chapter discusses some of the implications of such lack of knowledge in its connection to madness:

> 夫癩者趨不變，狂者形不虧，神將有所遠徙，孰暇知其所為！故形有摩而神未嘗化者，以不化應化，千變萬抮，而未始有極。
>
> The thinking of the leper is not altered; the body of the madman is not impaired. But when their spirits make their far-off journey, who will have time to think about what they did [in their lives]? Thus even though the body disappears, the spirit is never transformed. If you use what does not transform in response to transformations, [even through] a thousand alterations and ten thousand evolutions, you will not have begun to reach a limit.[40]

We find a number of passages in early texts demonstrating the view of the possibility of the disconnection of situations and states of mind. The final chapter of the *Xunzi*, as discussed in Chapter 3, contains a passage that claims Xunzi himself retained the mind of a sage while putting on the "visage" or external appearance (*se*) of a mad person.[41] In chapter 4 of the *Zhuangzi*, Yan Hui floats the possibility of internally retaining his intentions inwardly while

[39] The *heng xin* 恆心 (fixed/constant mind) of *Mengzi* 1A7, for example. Also the "mirror-like" mind (*xin ruo jing* 心若鏡) whose constancy is its ability to follow things, in *Zhuangzi* 7.6.

[40] *Huainanzi* 7.10, Major et al. 2010 trans., 251.

[41] *Xunzi* 32.7.

outwardly conforming with the wishes of the bad ruler.[42] While the *Huainanzi* does advocate severing the link between the mind and external things, in terms of desires that lead to a host of problems, including madness,[43] this undermining of desire and overabundant emotion is very much a result of agentive self-cultivation—indeed, the kind of development of knowledge that aims at discernment of right and wrong action and development of character, akin in this way to Confucian modes of self-development. A description of chapter 2 of the *Huainanzi* in the concluding *Yaolue* chapter reads:

> 《俶真》者，窮逐終始之化，嬴垺有無之精，離別萬物之變，合同死生之形。使人遺物反己，審仁義之間，通同異之理，觀至德之統，知變化之紀，說符玄妙之中，通回造化之母也。

> The *Chuzhen* chapter exhaustively traces the beginnings and endings of the transformations of things, infuses and fills the essence of being and non-being, separates and distinguishes the changes of the myriad things, unifies and equates the forms of death and life. It enables one to disregard things and return to the self (*ji*), to investigate the space of humanity and righteousness, to understand the patterns of same and different, to observe what ties together the utmost potency, to know the strands of changes and transformations, to speak of the core of the deepest mystery, and to understand the mother of creation and transformation.[44]

This discussion of "returning to the self" (*fan ji* 反己) contrasts with both the Confucian "overcoming the self" (*ke ji* 克己)[45] and the Zhuangist view that "the perfected person is without a self" (*zhi ren wu ji* 至人無己).[46] This is perhaps particularly surprising given that the chapter discussed here, *Chuzhen*, is one of the most Zhuangist-influenced of the chapters of the *Huainanzi*, even duplicating whole passages from chapter 2 of the *Zhuangzi* itself. Of course, in its appropriation of Zhuangist material (as in its use of the material of other schools and texts), the *Huainanzi* necessarily departs from the original intentions, as the goal is to ultimately fit together the various

[42] *Zhuangzi* 4.1 然則我內直而外曲.
[43] *Huainanzi* 1.21. Major et al. 2010, 76.
[44] *Huainanzi* 21.3. Major et al. 2010 trans., modified.
[45] *Analects* 12.1.
[46] *Zhuangzi* 2.3.

disparate schools and positions to form a synthesis. We find here in the *Yaolue* passage a description of the Zhuangist-influenced chapter 2 as providing something very non-Zhuangist: a means to return to the self, to make distinctions between things in terms of right and wrong, and to use this to understand the world in ways that lead to proper action.

Another important feature of the *Huainanzi* as concerns madness (and illness in general) can be found in the *Yaolue* chapter. In the discussion of chapter 1 of the *Huainanzi* in that chapter, we find an interesting link between the cosmological and ethical consideration of the *Huainanzi* and the medical thought of texts like the *Huangdi Neijing*. The authors of the *Huainanzi* clearly saw the new medical projects developing in the Han, using concepts of *qi* and *yin-yang* to analyze human physiological function, health and disease, as closely linked to the project of self-cultivation through attaining knowledge. The kind of self-cultivation that we see in earlier Confucian and Daoist/Zhuangist texts as associated with moral development or spiritual thriving is also linked in the *Huainanzi* to medicine and the proper operation of the human body. Explaining the benefits of understanding chapter 1 of the *Huainanzi*, a passage from *Yaolue* reads:

> 執其大指，以內治五藏，瀸濇肌膚，被服法則，而與之終身，所以應待萬方，鑒耦百變也。若轉丸掌中，足以自樂也。
>
> Grasping its main tenets, one can inwardly order the five organs,[47] and enrich the flesh and skin. If you adhere to its models and standards, and partake of them to the end of your days, they will provide the means to respond and attend to the myriad aspects of the world and observe and accompany its manifold changes, as if rolling a ball in the palm of your hand. Surely it is suffices to bring yourself joy![48]

We see here both an appeal to health and to knowledge—that is, understanding and applying the ideas of chapter 1 of the *Huainanzi* will lead to both good physical health and the kind of knowledge that leads to joy (*le* 樂). One way of understanding the second point is in terms of *mental* health. A number of passages in the *Huainanzi* echo the *Huangdi Neijing* in its connection of

[47] The "five organs," the heart, lung, liver, spleen, and kidney, are discussed extensively in the *Huangdi Neijing*.
[48] *Huainanzi* 21.2. Major et al. 2010 trans., modified.

overabundant emotion, disruption of *qi*, and illness. Overabundant emotion, desire, and attachments ultimately cause illness via their disruption of *qi*, as explained in the following passage from the *Jingshen* chapter:

> 人大怒破陰，大喜墜陽，大憂內崩，大怖生狂。除穢去累，莫若未始出其宗，乃為大通。
>
> A person's great anger destroys *yin*, and their great joy submerges *yang*. Great grief ravishes the interior, and great fear gives rise to madness. Yet if you eschew the dust of daily living and relinquish attachments, you will be as calm as if you had never left your Ancestor and thereupon will become grandly pervasive.[49]

Although the *Huainanzi* provides a somewhat similar explanatory structure to what we find in earlier texts regarding the connection between illness and overabundant emotion and desire (yet here newly through the means of *qi*), the place of madness in self-cultivation is explored in the text in a way beyond what we find in any other early text beside the *Zhuangzi*. Unlike the *Zhuangzi*, the *Huainanzi* takes madness to be a negative state, in which one's actions are not properly connected to knowledge which would allow these actions to be well-directed or reliable. While madness can result from overabundant emotion and desire, the authors of the *Huainanzi* also seem to hold that one cannot be held morally responsible for madness. Madness, like other forms of mental illness, is a matter of medicine *rather* than morality. Such mental illness can play a pivotal role in moral self-cultivation, but only insofar as it can get in the way of such self-cultivation. This standing in the way, however, is not always (or perhaps even often) the result of agentive activity. While the proper operation of *qi* can be disrupted by cultivated states of overabundant emotion or desire (which then the agent would presumably be responsible for), there are also myriad other ways *qi* can be disrupted. The appeal to *qi* in discussions of illness in the early Han thus medicalize illness, in the sense that they shield it to some extent from the realm of morality and moral evaluation, even if there is still a close connection between the two.

Chapter 2 of the *Huainanzi* offers a reflection on the nature of the differences between people who gain understanding and those who become mad. The

[49] *Huainanzi* 7.14. Major et al. 2010 trans., modified. *Huainanzi* 1.16 is nearly identical in its first part.

chapter attributes the difference to divergence in features of the *jingshen* 精神 (quintessential spirit) and its connection to the world. One passage reads:

> 肌膚之於寒燠，其情一也；或通於神明，或不免於癡狂者，何也？其所為制者異也。
>
> The instinctive responses are the same in everyone, but some can achieve spiritual intelligence, and some cannot avoid derangement and madness. Why is this? That by which they [these tendencies] are controlled is different.[50]

The means of control mentioned here are discussed in more detail in an earlier passage in the chapter, which describes the sage in terms at first remarkably close to the Zhuangist vision, but later becomes clear as meant quite differently:

> 是故聖人之學也，欲以返性于初，而游心於虛也。達人之學也，欲以通性於遼廓，而覺於寂漠也。若夫俗世之學也則不然，內愁五藏，外勞耳目，乃始招蟯振繾物之毫芒，搖消掉捎仁義禮樂，暴行越智於天下，以招號名聲於世。此我所羞而不為也。
>
> 是故與其有天下也，不若有說也；與其有說也，不若尚羊物之終始也；而條達有無之際。是故舉世而譽之不加勸，舉世而非之不加沮，定於死生之境，而通於榮辱之理。雖有炎火洪水彌靡於天下，神無虧缺於胸臆之中矣。若然者，視天下之間，猶飛羽浮芥也。孰肯分分然以物為事也！
>
> The learning of the sage seeks to return to its origin and to set the mind to roaming in emptiness. The learning of the knowledgeable seeks to connect nature to the great expanse [of the world] and to awaken stillness and quiescence. The vulgar learning of the age is not like this. It tugs at potency and drags at nature. Internally it vexes the five organs, externally it belabors the eyes and ears. Then one begins to pick at the wriggling and curling minutiae of things; moving and swaying with humaneness, righteousness, ritual, and music. You lord your conduct and project your cunning over the world, seeking title, fame, and reputation from the age. This I am ashamed to do. For this reason, having the world does not compare with being content. Being content does not compare with wandering carefree through the ends

[50] *Huainanzi* 2.17. Major et al. 2010 trans., modified.

> and beginnings of things and penetrating the frontier between something and nothing. Those who are thus are not more encouraged if the whole world praises them; are not more melancholy if the whole age contradicts them. They are firm in the boundary between life and death and comprehend the guiding pattern of honor and disgrace. Though raging fires and flooding waters wreak havoc throughout the world, their spirit remains undiminished in their breasts. Those who are like this view the realm of the world as flying feathers and floating twigs. How could they be willing to busily make things their affairs?[51]

The use of Zhuangist language here presents a bit of a puzzle, given that we have seen that the authors of the *Huainanzi* reject much of the Zhuangist view of madness in terms of the embrace of "wandering," "emptiness," and nonagentive action as expressive of the sage. This suggests (if the passages are consistent) a very different view of these concepts taken from the *Zhuangzi* here in chapter 2 of the *Huainanzi*. Attributing such radical reinterpretation of Zhuangist ideas is far from controversial—from the beginning of the chapter, we find quotes from the *Zhuangzi* used to express and endorse ideas almost diametrically opposed to those the Zhuangists held. As Harold Roth notes of the chapter: "All the principal themes of chapter 2 are found in the *Zhuangzi*, although they are not, in all cases, intended to be understood in the same way as in the source text."[52]

We also find here a connection between the learning and cultivation enjoined by the *Huainanzi* and health. Lacking this learning leads to illness, through the disruption of the proper operation of physical components of the body, such as the five organs and the eyes and ears. There seems to be a connection to the kind of considerations of physical and mental health found in the *Huangdi Neijing* and other medical texts. In the early Han, as part of the development of syncretic and pluralistic systems, in concert with the naturalistic shift, the medical and moral are brought together as aspects of a larger holistic project of personal development. Later, I turn to the *Huangdi Neijing* itself to show how the development of this project in that text builds on earlier syncretic ideas of texts like the *Huainanzi*. In it and other Han medical texts, we find the fullest development of the view of madness and mental illness more generally as disconnected from the moral project. It is thus in the

[51] *Huainanzi* 2.16–17. Major et al. 2010 trans., modified.
[52] Major et al. 2010, 77.

Han that we can locate the development of the medicalization of madness—although the moral understandings of the Confucians, Zhuangists, and others do not completely disappear in later years, but develop alongside the view we find in Han syncretist and medical texts. The Han syncretist and medical texts thus give us a "third option" concerning the nature of mental illness and its connection to personhood and self-cultivation.

The *Huangdi Neijing*—Apotheosis of the Medicalization of Mental Illness

The *Huangdi Neijing* understands various mental disorders, including *kuang* 狂, as *bing* 病 (disorder, illness). Indeed, in early China, mental illnesses do not seem to have been treated as a special class of illness distinct from other physical illnesses.[53] Despite common claims to Hippocrates being the first to envision mental disorders as illnesses under the purview of medicine,[54] *Huangdi Neijing* gives us evidence that such positions were accepted from a relatively early date in China.[55] The *Huangdi Neijing*'s date of composition cannot be definitively determined, but most scholars date it to the early Han Dynasty (between the second and first centuries BCE).[56] Some scholars argue for an early date of composition for parts of the text, such as the *Suwen* (素問), one of two texts that comprise the *Huangdi Neijing* (the other being the *Lingshu*).

We see in *Huangdi Neijing* the kind of concern with correlative cosmological explanation that developed in the late Warring States and early Han, though what is most likely is that a store of medical knowledge developed over many years in early China was fused with and organized via new causal explanations concerning *qi*, *yin-yang*, and Five Phases that developed in the late Warring States and early Han. In the *Huangdi Neijing*, illness is treated as a special category of disorder—one to be treated via the techniques of physicians. While it would be incorrect to call this the *beginning* of medical thought in early China (as medical like philosophical thought can exist absent an explicitly systematized theoretical and practical account), it is

[53] York 2012, 167.
[54] Pietikainen 2015, 19.
[55] It is unlikely that the views concerning *kuang* and other mental disorders contained in the *Huangdi Neijing* originated with the writing of that text. The exact antiquity of these views, of course, cannot be known. But it is not a stretch to say that they could date back to at least the time of Hippocrates in Greece (fourth century BCE).
[56] Sivin 1990, 4.

certainly the oldest extant textual systematization of medical thought. In it, we find explanation of many of the discussions of the causes of illness and subsequent treatments for it that I have described throughout this book. According to view found in the *Huangdi Neijing*, understanding the causes of illness is crucial to learning how to treat illness. We must understand what kind of disorder of *qi* leads to a particular illness, so as to be able to restore proper function of the relevant *qi*, whether in terms of movement, location, or quantity.

We find here a two-level explanation of the root of illness. The concepts of illness and disorder are linked, with the latter the explanation for the former. Not all disorder (*luan*) is illness (*bing*), but particular kinds of disorder linked to the human organism and the operation of *qi* within it. A passage from chapter 2 of *Huangdi Neijing Suwen* reads:

> 故陰陽四時者，萬物之終始也，死生之本也，逆之則災害生，從之則苛疾不起，是謂得道。道者，聖人行之，愚者佩之。從陰陽則生，逆之則死，從之則治，逆之則亂。反順為逆，是謂內格。是故聖人不治已病，治未病，不治已亂，治未亂，此之謂也。夫病已成而後藥之，亂已成而後治之，譬猶渴而穿井，鬭而鑄錐，不亦晚乎。

> Thus *yin* and *yang* and the four seasons are the end and beginning of the myriad things, the root of death and life. Turning away from them causes disaster, harming one's life, and following them keeps illnesses from arising. This is called obtaining the *dao*. The *dao* is what the sage practices, and what the doltish person merely wears for decoration. Following *yin* and *yang* leads to life, turning away from them leads to death. Following them leads to order, turning away from them leads to disorder (*luan*). Returning to following from being turned away is called inner investigation. This is why the sage does not put into order those who are already ill, but rather puts into order those not yet ill, does not put into order that which is already disordered, but puts into order that which is not yet disordered. Thus it is said. If an illness is already advanced and then medicine is used to treat it, or if disorder is already advanced and then there is attempt to order things—this is like being thirsty and only then digging a well for water, or going to war and only then casting weapons. Isn't it too late by that point?[57]

[57] *Huangdi Neijing Suwen* 2.3.

A number of mental illnesses are discussed in the *Huangdi Neijing*. In addition to *kuang*, which as we have seen is discussed in a number of earlier texts, we find the earliest mention of the illness *dian* 癲, a mental illness linked with *kuang* in a number of places in the text, in both the *Suwen* and *Lingshujing* sections. The most extensive discussion of *dian*, including its classification with *kuang* in the same category of illness, comes in the *Duankuangbing* 癲狂病 ("The Illnesses of Depression and Madness") chapter. I here translate *dian* as "depression" based on its symptomatic features as described in the *Huangdi Neijing*, but the illnesses of *dian* and what we today call "depression" do not line up perfectly. Given my view of mental illness as of the natural kind discussed earlier, however, I am perfectly willing to identify *dian* with depression, although early Chinese medical scholars did not think about depression in exactly the same way modern-day psychiatry does. But we should expect as much. After all, people in times and places distant from our own thought very differently about all kinds of natural entities and phenomena.

While the *Huangdi Neijing*'s conception of the causes of mental illness, treatment for it, and its role in personhood and the moral development of the individual and community are different than what we see in earlier texts, the text's account of the behavioral aspects of madness itself is largely consistent with earlier understandings. Thus, we can rely on the *Huangdi Neijing*'s clinical description and its general (thin) account of illness as offering widely accepted views in early China, even if the thick theoretical account of illness on offer, as well as the discussion of etiology on offer, is new to the Han.[58]

In the *Huangdi Neijing*, *bing* is understood in terms of improper functioning of the body—functional disorder, in this sense. The causes for these disorders, or illnesses, are described in terms of a number of technical terms, including *fu* 府 and *zang* 藏 (organs, storehouses), *mai* 脈 (vessels),[59] and most importantly, *qi* (vital essence), which stores and travels in the organs and vessels.

Paul Unschuld and Hermann Tessenow, in the introduction to their translation of the *Suwen* of the *Huangdi Neijing*, discuss what they see as

[58] Concerning the distinction between "thin" and "thick" descriptions (and concepts), see Väyrynen 2016.

[59] The *Huangdi Neijing* offers different classifications of *mai*, including *jing* 經, *luo* 絡, *du* 督, and *ren* 任, different collections of vessels.

two distinct uses of the term *bing* in the text, referring to the suffering or symptoms of illness and the underlying causes:

> *Bing* appears in contexts suggesting a meaning of being ill from the perspective of a patient, and it was used in other contexts to denote what medical theory believes to be the pathological change or dynamics in an organism underlying visible or otherwise noticeable signs. These differences could be expressed through translations such as "to suffer from," or "suffering," "ailment," "illness" in terms of the feelings of a patient and the assessment of his status by his lay environment.[60]

Here, *bing* is understood then in the sense of "internal functional disorder," referring to underlying disease, in terms of disordered *qi* or improperly functioning parts of the organism. In addition, the manifestation of this disorder in terms of symptoms represents the externally accessed sense of *bing*. Notice that this conception of *bing* can be (and is) connected with the issue of specifically mental *bing* such as *kuang* in a way similar to contemporary conceptions of mental illness. Mental illness today is understood as manifest in *behavioral* symptoms, where the underlying disease is understood in terms of a combination of brain functioning and social dysfunction. As I discuss later, the issue of the biological versus social basis of mental illness is the basis of much discussion and controversy surrounding the issue. It turns out, though, that illness as a category in general (physical as well as mental) requires both reference to organic functioning and moral/social elements. Though it is much more obvious in the case of mental illness, it is no less present in physical illness.

The *Lingshujing* of *Huangdi Neijing* contains a chapter specifically on the mental illnesses of *dian* and *kuang*. On the topic of illness in general and its causes, both sections have much to say. The *Suwen* opens with a discussion of the general problem that leads them to a consideration of the topics of the text. In a discussion between Huang Di and Qi Bo, there is a revelation that people in the ancient times lived for over one hundred years and their strength remained consistent throughout their lives. People of the current day, however, diminish in strength after about fifty years, and they rarely live to one hundred. Qi Bo explains that the secret of those of ancient times is that they understood and followed the *dao* and acted so as to follow the natural

[60] Unschuld and Tessenow 2011, 20.

patterns (here understood as the transformations of *yin* and *yang*).[61] Right at the beginning of the text, then, there is a claim merging the moral and medical ends of the text. Illness is primarily due to the depletion or improper movement and transformation of *qi*, and this was/is due to improper activity, such as reckless eating, insufficient or irregular sleep, and incorrect work habits. An additional piece of the picture is the variety of desires modern people (in terms of early China) took on, which dissipated their efforts and abilities by misdirecting their *qi*. Qi Bo explains in the first chapter of *Suwen*:

> 以欲竭其精，以耗散其真，不知持滿，不時御神，務快其心，逆於生樂，起居無節，故半百而衰也。
>
> Through their (modern people's) lust they exhaust their vital essence, through their wastefulness they dissipate their true [*qi*]. They do not know how to maintain fullness and they engage their spirit when it is not the right time. They make every effort to please their hearts, but they oppose the true happiness of life. Rising and resting miss their terms. Hence, it is only one half of a hundred years and they weaken.[62]

Here, we see the key claim linking the effects of old age and moral action of persons. Illness, old age, and death, at least as we generally see them in society, are not the result of human nature, but are instead the result of *divergence* from our nature, which is action in concert with natural patterns. Note the similarity between the explanation of human illness and frailty here and in other early texts such as *Huainanzi* and *Zhuangzi* and in the descriptions of the fall and decline of humanity in Abrahamic religious texts. As in those texts, most early Chinese texts imagine a paradisiacal ancient time in which humans acted properly and enjoyed perfect mental, physical, and moral health. Ultimately in both traditions it was *human action* that led to decline in all of these areas. The response to this decline, then, is the realignment of human activity with the *dao*. As with the Abrahamic texts, however, in early Chinese texts there seems to be an acceptance that humanity can never return to the state of perfection we had during the period of "grand purity" (*taiqing* 太清), as the *Huainanzi* describes it,[63] or the days of the ancients, as other texts describe them. We

[61] *Huangdi Neijing Suwen* 1.1; Unschuld and Tessenow 2011, 30.
[62] *Huangdi Neijing Suwen* 1.1; Unschuld and Tessenow 2011, 32.
[63] The text uses a number of other constructions to refer to these beginnings as well, including *taishi* 太始 (grand beginning) and *taichu* 太初 (grand origin). See Major et al. 2010, 266n7.

can, all texts seem to agree, make progress such that the situation for our health and overall well-being becomes better than it is, but there are limits to this. Apparently, the initial decline from perfection is a barrier past which there is no return. It is likely not an accident that such elaborations of the development of humanity as a whole seem to mirror our conception of the development of the individual human organism.

In the *Huangdi Neijing*, the answer to this question of how to move the human closer to this original state of perfection is in large part the reduction or redirection of desires, which are seen as a major piece of the puzzle. In addition, discovering and acting consistently with the natural patterns (which requires undermining of desire) enables the proper movement and transformation of *qi*, which leads to the health of the individual, physical, mental, and moral (with no distinction drawn). Thus, the methods of creating health are ultimately the same as the methods for cultivating moral personhood. This, of course, entails that failures are the same and have the same sources. The sources of madness and other mental illnesses will at least in part be based in human activity. Of course, what level of responsibility we accord to mentally ill or disordered individuals will change depending on the specifics of the views of the thinkers who bring something like this *Huangdi Neijing* view on board.

Desires arise, according to the *Huangdi Neijing*, with dissatisfaction with the state of things, due to the disorder of *qi*. Thus we see here a kind of circular explanation, with *qi* ultimately playing every role. It is unclear from just this whether the circularity is vicious. As *qi* is ultimately responsible for all activity, including that of the mind, particular transformations of *qi* bear responsibility for creating the desires that take us away from following the natural patterns. Disordered *qi*, that is, creates greater disorder in *qi*, which results in illness, which is itself a kind of manifestation of disordered *qi*. We need not see this as vicious—there are simply two levels of explanation at work here. We can discuss things from the level of symptoms and physical and mental functioning, and we can discuss things from the level of *qi* responsible for all of this activity. We most often care about things in terms of the physical and mental way we interact with them—and thus we speak about illness and treatment in this sense. But this does not preclude speaking about illness and treatment in terms of *qi*—or even *completely* in terms of *qi*. This is not dissimilar to contemporary scientific materialist explanation. At the level of explanation of illness with which we as sufferers are concerned, we speak of symptoms, of complaints, of medicines, of the intervention of doctors. We can also consider illness from the level of chemistry, however, in which we focus on the viral, bacterial, interaction of chemicals in cells, and so on. We could even reduce all of this to the level of physics. Indeed, in order to explain the efficacy of certain treatments or why we need to take a certain medicine, doctors must often refer to the deeper level of chemical or physical explanation to describe the process on this level. Reference to these deeper levels count as *explanation* of the disease process at work and its treatment. *Qi* can be understood in a similar way. While on one (most apparent) level of explanation we can speak in terms of desires and the disruption of action consistent with natural patterns leading to physical and mental imbalances, a deeper explanation of this will refer to particular transformations of *qi*, and their disorder.

While illness is understood in the *Huangdi Neijing* in both physical and mental terms, the two are not always clearly distinguished (a particular illness can be characterized by physical and mental effects or symptoms). In certain parts of the *Huangdi Neijing*, there is specific focus on mental illness as a specific category. Both *Suwen* and *Lingshujing* contain informative discussions of mental illness in general, offering explanations of the relationships between various emotions and *qi*. A passage of the *Suwen* reads:

> 余知百病生於氣也，怒則氣上，喜則氣緩，悲則氣消，恐則氣下，寒則氣收，炅則氣泄，驚則氣亂，勞則氣耗，思則氣結，九氣不同，何病之生
>
> I know that the one hundred illnesses are the result of (imbalances) in *qi:* anger results in heightened *qi*, joyousness results in slowed *qi*, sadness results in dissipated *qi*, fear results in reduced *qi*, the feeling of cold results in congealed *qi*, over-excitement results in radiating/flowing *qi*, alarm results in disordered qi, exhaustion results in depleted *qi*, thoughtfulness results in integrated *qi*. These nine types of *qi* fail to be unified. How does illness result?[64]

The text then goes on to explain further how the emotions discussed have their particular effects on *qi*, which can then in turn cause a host of physical and mental illnesses. We see here a wide range of mental states attributed to changes in *qi*, including a number of states we may not expect to see classified as *bing* 病 (illness), such as "joyousness" (*xi* 喜) and "thoughtfulness" (*si* 思), both of which cause certain changes in *qi* and can themselves be caused

64 *Huangdi Neijing Suwen* 39.6.

by such changes. Perhaps what is going on here is a suggestion that joy and thoughtfulness as provoking illness can be understood as *excessive* amounts of these generally unproblematic states. Thus, perhaps we should understand *xi* here as "excessive joyousness," of the kind apparent in manic states, and understand *si* as "excessive thoughtfulness."

About *kuang* 狂 (madness) specifically, the *Huangdi Neijing* has quite a bit to say. Discussing the "five disorders" (*wu luan* 五亂), a passage reads:

> 邪所亂：邪入於陽則狂，邪入於陰則痺，搏陽則為巔疾，搏陰則為瘖，陽入之陰則靜，陰出之陽則怒，是謂五亂。
>
> That in which one is disordered: when one enters into *yang* then one becomes *kuang*, when one enters into yin one becomes indolent. Encountering *yang* then this becomes the illness of *dian* (lethargy/depression), encountering *yin* this becomes complete silence (*yin*). When *yang* enters into *yin* then one becomes mild (*jing*), when *yin* goes out from *yang* then one becomes angry. These are the five disorders.[65]

Kuang is treated in the *Huangdi Neijing* as an illness attributable to an overabundance of *yang* energy (*yang qi*).[66] The *kuang* person is one who is "mad" in the classical sense, acting without restraint, agitated and animated, unconcerned with social convention or repercussion. *Kuang* illness appears to be similar to what we today refer to as *mania*. Indeed, a number of scholars, recognizing the similarity in these concepts, refer to the sometimes paired ailments of *kuang* and *dian* (a depressive state caused by overabundance of *yin qi*) as "bipolar disorder." This seems a fair enough identification. "Madness" is a felicitous translation of *kuang*, as the English term has similar connotations in its early use to this frenetic form of mental illness, which became a more general term to describe various kinds of mental illness before the modern period.[67]

The term can also be a general term to refer to mental illness of all kinds (similar to "madness" in English), and it can sometimes refer to anything seen as wildly outside of the norms of society, and the attitudes and motivations

[65] *Huangdi Neijing Suwen* 23.8. The text calls these *five* disorders, though there are six listed. I take it that the third clause and the fourth are further comments on the second—but if this is the case, that would make only *four* disorders apparent here.

[66] *Huangdi Neijing Suwen* 46.6.

[67] Pietikainen 2015, 7: "'Madness' . . . suggested manic restlessness, wildness, and loss of self-control. Even today, we may describe an angry or enraged person as 'mad.'"

that lead one to act in such bizarre ways. Thought processes themselves can be understood as mad even in the absence of action—though this has to be a lesser kind of madness, rendered invisible. The quintessential example of the "madman" is the person flouting accepted social norms openly, loudly, and in full view of the entire community.

Another passage in *Suwen* attributes *kuang* to disorder of the body:

血泄者，脈急血無所行也。若夫以為傷肺者，由失以狂也。

As for the blood flow, the blood in the vessels has nowhere to travel. If this is taken to be an injury to the lung, this is an error that leads to *kuang*.[68]

Unschuld and Tessenow understand this passage differently, taking the reference to *kuang* here to be about the "confusion" of the practitioner who incorrectly diagnoses the blood blockage discussed. Interestingly, they also cite the nineteenth-century Japanese scholar Mori Risshi's interpretation of the word *shi* 失 in the passage as equivalent to *shi xin* 失心 (losing one's mind), although this construction does not appear in the *Huangdi Neijing*.[69] Either way, this shows us an interesting connection between physical states and mental conditions in the *Neijing*.

Perhaps the most important chapter concerning mental illness in the *Huangdi Neijing* is the *Diankuangbing* ("The Illnesses of Depression and Madness") chapter of *Lingshujing*. The chapter offers descriptions of both *dian* and *kuang*, explanations of their causes, and plans for treatment:

癲疾始生，先不樂，頭重痛，視舉目赤，甚作極，已而煩心。候之於顏。取手太陽、陽明、太陰，血變為止。

癲疾始作，而引口啼呼喘悸者…癲疾始作，先反僵，因而脊痛…

狂始生，先自悲也，喜忘、苦怒. . . 狂始發，少臥不飢，自高賢也，自辯智也，自尊貴也，善罵詈，日夜不休…

狂言，驚，善笑，好歌樂，妄行不休者，得之大恐. . . 狂，目妄見，耳妄聞…狂者多食，善見鬼神…

[68] *Huangdi Neijing Suwen* 76.2.
[69] Unschuld and Tessenow 2011, 661n42.

> When the illness of *dian* begins, first there is unhappiness, one's head is heavy (as in sleep) and pained, one is unable to rise and has bloodshot eyes, grown to the extreme. This ends with a *disturbed mind* (*fan xin*). Later it appears in the face. In the hands there is abundance of *yang*. *Yang* overflowing, there is abundance of *yin*. The blood changes and stops at this.
>
> As the illness of *dian* progresses, one's voice is drawn out and whimpering, one breathes heavily and is fearful. . . . As the illness of *dian* progresses, one first returns to catatonic state, because of a stiff spine. . . .[70] When the illness of *kuang* begins, at first one is sorrowful, and forgets all joy. One is bitter and angry. . . . When *kuang* commences, one sleeps little and goes without eating, and believes oneself to be lofty and important. One believes oneself to be discriminating and wise, to be revered and honored. One blames and insults others, and goes day and night without rest. . . .
>
> The words of madmen are startling, and they laugh and sing songs [for no reason]. They act recklessly and without rest, and through this gain great fear . . . The *kuang* look absurd to the eye, and sound absurd to the ear . . . *Kuang* people eat a large amount, and appear to see the ghosts and spirits.[71]

Here we see the classic list of symptoms for *kuang* and *dian*. Interestingly, while the philosophical texts of the Warring States and Han have much to say about *kuang*, they are almost completely silent about *dian*. *Kuang* seems to be the quintessential example of madness in these authors. While it is impossible to say for sure why this is, one imagines it is due to the visibility of *kuang* in comparison with other mental illnesses (the *kuang* person will be seen and heard in a way the *dian* person is not, for example, even when there is comorbidity of the two in an individual).

The *Huangdi Neijing* also discusses problematic or bothersome mental states such as anxiety (*chu* 怵, *you* 憂) and sadness (*bei* 悲) in alternative ways to what we find in the *Zhuangzi* (as discussed in Chapter 3 of this book). These states are connected to various states of *qi*, facilitating the causal argument concerning disorder of *qi* and illness (including mental illness). The beginning of chapter 66 of *Huangdi Neijing Suwen* reads:

> 黃帝問曰：天有五行，御五位以生寒暑燥濕風，人有五藏，化五氣，以生喜怒思憂恐

[70] To treat *dian*, the chapter suggests observing behaviors and drawing blood to properly direct the *qi*.

[71] *Huangdi Neijing Lingshujing* 22.

> Huang Di asked: "Heaven has the Five Phases, which control the five positions. Thereby they generate cold, heat, dryness, dampness, and wind. Humans have the five organs, which transform the five kinds of *qi*, and generate joy, anger, thoughtfulness, anxiety, and fear."[72]

The key move in the "medicalization" of mental illness (and illness more generally) in the *Huangdi Neijing* is the move to naturalistic explanations of illness that allow for the intervention of medical treatments, and explanation of the efficacy of these treatments. With the focus on *qi*, its quantity, and its movement (connected with other correlative cosmological ideas of the time such as the Five Phases and *yin-yang*), the *Huangdi Neijing* suggests the possibility of treating mental and physical illness through manipulation of the movement of *qi* to our various organs, thus taking mental illness from the realm of morality and self-cultivation to that of medical treatment. It is with this shift that we find the close of consideration of mental illness in connection with self-cultivation and agency in early China.

[72] *Huangdi Neijing Suwen* 66.1.

Conclusion

Madness and Self-Cultivation: Ways Forward

Now that I have provided an account of the development of views of mental illness, agency, and self-cultivation in early Chinese texts, we arrive now at a consideration of the potential implications of these views. While one might focus on intellectual history and explicating the philosophical views of early China, I believe there are important lessons to be learned from early Chinese thinking on mental illness. In this conclusion, I consider some of the lessons we might draw from the discussions of this book, both for related issues in early Chinese thought, and for philosophy, psychiatry, and treatment of mental illness today.

Can we, and *should we*, import aspects of the views discussed in this book to contemporary contexts? Many will, of course, naturally be skeptical that it might prove useful to adopt the medical views of the *Huangdi Neijing* concerning *qi* and adopt techniques from the text, including bleeding and acupuncture, as effective methods for treating illness. Modern medicine, we take it, has developed and advanced beyond what was available to people in early China. However, it would be unwise to conclude on this basis that early Chinese texts contain nothing about mental illness from which we can learn and which might help us to further develop our understanding of illness, its connection to agency and morality, and our methods of treatment. While on the whole modern medicine may be far more effective than early Chinese medicine in certain ways (but not all ways!),[1] the only way we can determine this is to have in mind a particular treatment goal. The only way to measure the success of anything is with respect to our concerns in employing it. As Aristotle recognized, a thing, art, and so on, can only be evaluated as good or bad with respect to its function.[2] And when it comes to human-invented arts,

[1] The National Institutes of Health, among other well-known medical institutions, continues to take seriously and study a number of treatment methods associated with the "traditional Chinese medicine" of ancient texts such as *Huangdi Neijing*. See https://nccih.nih.gov/health/whatiscam/chinesemed.htm

[2] *Nicomachean Ethics* 1.7: "for all things that have a function or activity, the good and the 'well' is thought to reside in the function" (W. D. Ross trans.).

The Dao of Madness. Alexus McLeod, Oxford University Press. © Oxford University Press 2021.
DOI: 10.1093/oso/9780197505915.003.0007

such as medicine, we must measure it with respect to what we intend for such an art to do. Right away, we have somewhat different evaluative standards for the art of *yi* 醫 ("medicine") of the *Huangdi Neijing* and modern medicine, as the two contain much of the same content but blur at the boundaries.

Even given the evaluative standards of modern medicine, however, it would be presumptuous to think that early Chinese medicine has nothing to teach us simply because we have advanced techniques in a number of areas. New discoveries are made every day on the basis of things that were understood in different times and places, but never considered, discovered, or known by scholars or physicians in the West. In addition, our understanding of the bounds of medicine itself is a matter more of philosophy than of science. While contemporary techniques for evaluation and treatment are based on sound principles of scientific medicine (for the most part), our conceptions of disorder, illness, and medicine are still very much loosely formed. What counts as a disease, a malady calling for treatment, and what is a matter of ethics, of self-cultivation and social adjustment, a "problem of living"? Psychiatry in particular is a field of medicine in which these questions take a prominent position.

For example, one question that naturally arises concerning mental illness is whether those with particular mental disorders may simply perceive the world more accurately. While most people understand the world as containing mind in connection with particular activity (that is, activity we deem as human and thus agent-based), others do not see mind anywhere (autistic people who have to learn techniques to discern where mind may be operative), while others see it in a far broader range of cases than usual. While we may be able to determine that particular ways of perceiving the world are more *common* to humans than others, it will be difficult if not impossible to determine that any of these given ways is the *correct* way of perceiving the world—that is, uniquely captures the way the world is, or tracks actual features of the world. There are a host of reasons for human perception being as it is, most of which, on our best scientific account of the world, have to do with helping to ensure survival, whether through enabling use of aspects of our environments, facilitating social interaction and cooperation, or other features enabling us to remain viable in our world. This does not necessarily (or even likely in many cases) track actual features of the world. That is, our perception of the world is not necessarily an accurate guide to the features of the world or what this world (assuming a world independent of observing subjects that can be characterized and is a certain way—not an assumption that all early Chinese thinkers would share!) is actually like. We know, from many years of empirical science, that our general intuitions are not reliable indicators of the way the world is or works. And there are a number of perceptual features humans have that we understand well as operating inaccurately in terms of representing the world, but because they help serve purposes ultimately more important for human survival (which explains their development). For example, certain optical illusions can create the perception of motion in our vision when there is none there, because of particular features of our visual system designed to give us an advantage in our interactions with things in the world. Likewise, there are numerous events and things in the world that we do not perceive, such as electromagnetic fields, in part perhaps because tracking these features of the world would give humans no advantages concerning survival, and thus these abilities never developed (certain abilities, like the ability to sense via echolocation, *did* develop in bats, who developed in very different environments and conditions than humans).

Thus, we cannot take the divergence of a particular perceptual type or conceptual scheme from that of the norm (even built into the nature of humans) as thus giving us an inaccurate understanding of the world (this would be a version of a naturalistic fallacy). It may turn out to be the case that the schizophrenic person who sees mind everywhere has an ultimately more accurate perception of the world. If panpsychism (the view that consciousness permeates the material world) is correct, then the divergence from the human norm that represents symptoms of certain mental disorders such as schizophrenia may be a more accurate perception of the world. Were that to be the case, would it still make sense to refer to schizophrenia and similar conditions as disorders? Perhaps. They could very well be disorders in terms of damaging our ability to survive, while at the same time representing a more accurate perception of the world. We can see here some of the difficulty inherent in understanding the concept of disorder. That is, any concept of disorder has to be grounded in some conception of relevant order. If order is the proper functioning of the human being, how do we understand this proper functioning? Is it to function in a way following from a *design* to maximize chances for survival? Or to simply function in such a way so as to maximize chances for survival? Or to function in such a way as to have an accurate perception of the way the world is independently? Let's consider these. We might be inclined to take proper function in terms of following from function designed to maximize chances for survival. So that functioning in a nonschizophrenic way is linked to certain brain developments that in the past proved vital to our survival. But notice that the problem with this is that it doesn't take *current* conditions into consideration. Though we often speak about evolution as if it is something that happened in the past and culminated in where we are now, it's actually the case that evolution is ongoing and continuous. Thus we cannot think of the features we have today as the "final state" of human features, nor can we completely see past evolutionary developments as giving us the final arbitration on the proper function of the human or any other organism. Take the schizophrenia example again. Our environment could presumably change in such a way as to make schizophrenic character evolutionarily valuable—and in such a case, we would expect to see schizophrenia eventually become a dominant trait among humans over time (given long-term maintenance of the relevant conditions). Conditions can change relatively quickly, even if evolution takes some time to catch up. So the view of proper functioning that takes proper functioning as connected to past evolutionary design is unable to account for the fact that a divergence from a norm that may have diverged from proper functioning based on past design might in fact maximize one's chances for survival in some novel environment, and thus seemingly be a *proper* function in that new environment. Let's consider, then, the next option—that proper function is understood in terms of activity that maximizes chances for survival, independently of whether this activity is designed to do so based on past selection. If this is the case, then proper function will be dependent on not only facts about human constitution and normal tendencies but also on facts about our environment and location. It can be the case that normal human tendencies *do not* correspond with proper functioning, due to recent environmental changes that make it the case that most of us are operating with harmful action selected in the past to deal with different environments that no longer obtain.

Proper functioning, we see, is difficult to pin down. What is implausible, though, given what we know about human development and evolution, is that proper functioning would ever robustly track the truth—that is, that proper human perception is an accurate guide to the way the world is. This is because if proper human perception is linked to evolutionary success, then there are simply too many likely scenarios of useful yet inaccurate perceptions (and ones we have discovered!) to imagine that our perceptual abilities were selected for their ability to track the way things are (given that there is such a thing). The fact that we have discovered unperceived entities and that we have demonstrated that in a number of cases at least our perception is inaccurate shows that proper perception (in an evolutionary sense) does not track the way the world is. And we don't need the exciting or surprising cases to demonstrate this—we have a host of mundane cases, such as our perception of distant objects as small, our perception of converging lines as representing perspective, or our perception of artfully applied oil paint as representing a face or a mountain.

The Zhuangist position can then be seen as a challenge to the idea that the madman or other "disordered" person is disordered at all when viewed from particular perspectives of order. For example, if we take proper functioning and order to be understood in terms of the veridicality of our experience, we may be left with a very different conception of proper functioning than ones we most often use, which render (perhaps) the schizophrenic person more "properly functioning" than those without this condition. That is, we might take proper functioning to be a matter of perceptual and behavioral tendencies that match, mirror, or manifest the state of the world (understood in terms of the "natural patterns" *tian li* 天理). The Zhuangists recognize that the natural patterns are such that things in the world are constantly in flux, never remaining the same. This is one reason that focusing on Confucian ideals like ritual or virtue, like being stuck in the mindset of valuing wealth, fame, or health, often leads us astray. When we insist on one perspective and valuation, we may perform properly or get the world correct in certain situations, but when things change, we will badly misfire. Operating effectively along with the world requires changing along with the world, just as keeping effective track of time requires continual (regular) motion of the clock. And just like even a broken clock is accurate twice a day, those stuck in particular perspectives and with particular valuations are sometimes right about the world and have effective action.

Given that the world is constantly changing, that the myriad things are in constant transformation, the person who accurately perceives the world and acts in ways that follow the natural patterns will also be constantly changing, unfixed, and will resemble a person who most of the world thinks of as "mad." Of course, a crucial question for the Zhuangist is whether such a person is *in fact* mad and we ought to thus reevaluate madness, or whether the Zhuangist is instead making a rhetorical move, in essence claiming that while the Zhuangist sage might appear to society to be mad, they actually are not, and it is simply our inability to recognize the myriad changes and perspectives that leads us to think of such a person as mad. In this case, we are like the cicada and student dove of chapter 1, looking up at the gigantic fish/bird and puzzling in our bewildered confusion.

A key question for us here is that of how madness (and mental illness more generally) and its potential treatments fit into the structure of self-cultivation. Are the mentally ill barred from the cultivation of Confucian virtue, Mohist impartiality, or the kind of broad understanding of the patterns of nature discussed in *Huainanzi* and *Chunqiu Fanlu*? Do the methods of treating madness as such help generate understanding of the patterns of nature? Or, for the Zhuangist, do the mentally ill have special access to understanding of the natural patterns, and thus an advantage in becoming "genuine persons"? Do mental illnesses aid or hinder us in the task of moral self-cultivation and development of the ideal person? Or do they make no difference one way or the other to the project of self-cultivation?

On the Confucian view, mental disorder is linked with vice, connected to failure to cultivate oneself properly. The agent has a key role to play in the etiology of mental disorder and thus takes on moral responsibility for it. At the same time, the Confucian view insists on the pivotal role of community in the construction of character, taking the agent as a complex of individual and community. The community then also holds responsibility for the mental illness of individuals in the community. To ensure the proper operation of the community and proper functioning of individuals, including avoidance of mental disorder, the proper rituals must be enacted in accordance with roles in the community. On the Confucian view, to the extent that there is mental disorder in a society, this shows that the proper moral way is not being followed in some crucial aspect. This is likely the reason that the authors of the *Xunzi* felt it necessary to explain away Xunzi's seeming madness at the end of the final chapter of the text.

A key question facing the Confucian concerns the relationship between mental disorder or illness and agency itself. To what extent can illness be *part* of our agentive states? That is, one of the features of mental illness is that it affects the very aspects of the person that generate agency—the ability to think rationally, to make distinctions, to recognize, to form intentions, to choose, and so on. Insofar as these agentive states are compromised via illness (of whatever cause), is it then possible for the ill person to develop at all, let alone in the ways the Confucians recommend? There does seem to be a sense of the hopelessness of madness in Confucian texts, as well as little on offer in terms of treatment.

On the Zhuangist view, the very idea of mental illness is subverted, and the mad person is rendered a sage. The features of the ideal person, according to the Zhuangist, line up with those of the mad person, and mad persons can be taken as closer to the ideal than "sane" or conventional persons. This view of mental illness seems to amount to a denial that the mad person (or one with similar states) is ill at all. The mad person, on this reading, is certainly not disordered in an objective sense. They are deemed disordered and ill from the perspective of those trapped within narrow ways of thinking about the world—but this determination does not make the mad person actually disordered, actually ill, actually mad. The situation is a bit tricky for the Zhuangist here, as one of the central views of the *Zhuangzi* seems to be that nothing is determinately "this" (*shi*) or "not this" (*fei*) outside of a particular perspective, yet all perspectives are limited and contingent.[3] Thus, the mad person *does* qualify as mentally ill from a particular perspective. We enhance our ability to thrive when we develop the capacity to shift perspectives in response to the transformation of things. The mad person's agentive capacity is compromised, a capacity that reinforces the sense of self and identity that prevents us from being able to shift perspectives. Thus, the mad person is inherently better at engaging in the kind of activity (shifting of perspectives) that leads to thriving.

There are, of course, a number of difficulties facing the Zhuangist view as well. Is it plausible that the mad person and other mentally ill persons thrive in ways that sane people do not? Or that the mad person can truly shift perspectives in the way the Zhuangist claims? The Zhuangist romanticization of madness leaves us with perhaps a very inaccurate picture of both the mental state and behavioral characteristics of the mad person. At the same time, however, it offers a path for the rehabilitation of the mentally ill person in society, a ground for the valuation of such a person, and even the opening of a potential method of treatment for certain kinds of mental illness.

The syncretist/medical account of mental illness takes a large step toward the distancing of the issue of mental illness from that of moral self-cultivation, though the two are still linked in key ways. While madness, depression, and other mental illnesses are understood as disorders with "psychophysical" causes (in terms of *qi*) and amenable to medical treatment, medical texts link mental illness to uncontrolled or imbalanced emotions in

[3] The Zhuangists seem to tiptoe carefully around the potential problem that if this is true, then asserting this claim itself is only so from within a perspective, similar to the way Pyrrhonian skeptics insist that their skeptical position is not itself a dogmatic claim, but rather a suggestion based on appearances.

a similar way to Confucian texts. Perhaps the biggest shift in the Han syncretist and medical texts is the naturalistic shift toward understanding mental illness as ultimately caused by disorders of *qi*. Insofar as *qi* and its operation in the human organism can be manipulated through various physical means (the methods described in *Huangdi Neijing* and other medical texts), it can be addressed (at least to some extent) by physicians, or anyone with the requisite medical knowledge and tools.

The syncretist account removes the issue of mental illness from self-cultivation and moves it into medical consideration, in part because it separates the issues of behavior and knowledge, as we see in the *Huainanzi*'s discussion of the activity of the sage and the mad person. Acting in a particular way is not in itself following natural patterns or acting properly, but having the right *reasons* is required, and the right knowledge, as understood not in a behavioral sense.

Mental Illness and Emotion

If we read early Chinese discussions of mental illness as wholly explanatory and tied to the issues of personhood and agency, there is much we will miss. I have no presumptions in this book to have covered every issue (or even most issues) surrounding mental illness in early Chinese texts, one important feature of these texts. Still, one of the important aims of a number of early Chinese texts was to help readers overcome difficult mental states, break through doubt, depression, or anxiety, and to cultivate positive outlooks that contribute to overall human thriving. This aspect of numerous early texts is an important piece of the puzzle in understanding early Chinese views of mental illness. More than this, however, such aspects of early texts can still be of enormous use today, as the psychological conditions of the past are similar to those of today in many respects, and the therapeutic approaches to handling these conditions in the past, insofar as they were successful, can provide us with tools for dealing with these conditions today as well.

While Daoists texts such as the *Zhuangzi* and *Daodejing*, the *Neiye* chapter of *Guanzi*, and some syncretist texts such as *Huainanzi* are most obviously concerned with such focus on treatment, we find aspects of this in parts of Confucian and Mohist texts as well. There are at least three general techniques for treatment found in a variety of early Chinese texts, which fit into a consideration of self-cultivation and how it might operate in the context of current-day therapeutic approaches: (1) reduction of self-concern; (2) detachment from desires and emotions; and (3) regulation of activity.

In a number of texts, in particular the *Zhuangzi* and early Confucian texts, we find a recommendation that it is possible to reduce or even eliminate various kinds of psychological distress by reducing our self-concern or sense of self. In order to understand what this amounts to, we have to understand what these various texts understand the nature of the "self" to be, in what sense(s) we should reduce our concern with this self, and the means by which we can reduce such concern.

The *Neiye*, a chapter compiled in the text *Guanzi*, offers a manual for the kind of self-cultivation discussed here—namely, a guide to proper and thriving life and avoidance of the kind of disorder represented by madness and illness more generally. Toward the beginning of the text, we find an account of the *xin* (mind) and instruction on how to maintain order and harmony in the mind:

> 凡心之刑，自充自盈，自生自成；其所以失之，必以憂樂喜怒欲利。能去憂樂喜怒欲利，心乃反濟。彼心之情，利安以寧，勿煩勿亂，和乃自成。
>
> The form of the mind is full of itself and replete of itself, born of itself and completed of itself. That in which is loses this form is necessarily grief, happiness, joy, anger, and desire for profit. If one is able to move away from grief, happiness, joy, anger, and desire for profit, then the natural feelings of the heart cleave to rest and calm. Don't trouble them, don't derange then, and harmony will be completed of itself.[4]

This is consistent with advice we find in texts ranging from *Zhuangzi* to *Huangdi Neijing*. While as we have seen earlier that *Zhuangzi* 4 refrains from overarching rejections of *any* mental state, there are certainly mental states that make it more difficult for one to attain the kind of flexibility of the Zhuangist sage. The "fasting of the mind" (心齋 *xin zhai*) discussed in *Zhuangzi* 4 is understood in terms of reduction of reliance on the usual mental states. In *Zhuangzi* 15 the summation of purity (*cui zhi zhi* 粹之至) is associated with the absence of grief and happiness (*you le* 憂樂) in the mind.[5]

[4] *Guanzi* 49.1, Eno trans. modified.
[5] *Zhuangzi* 15.2.

A passage from the *Zhongyong* chapter of the *Liji*, like the earlier *Guanzi* passage, associates harmony (*he*) with the restriction of the emotions.[6] The *Huangdi Neijing*, although its discussion of treatment for illness focuses much more on physical techniques, also stresses the connection between emotion and mental illness, suggesting that restraining the emotions is an important aspect of treatment.[7]

The Social Nature of Madness

The Zhuangists argued that the socially determined nature of mental illness undermines its identity as illness, somewhat similar to contemporary opponents of psychiatry and skeptics. The difference, of course, is that for the Zhuangists it is not the failure of mental illness to resemble physical forms of illness marked by physical disease states, but rather the fact that social norms, expectations, and makeup play a role in the determination of any state as one of mental illness. Following the Zhuangist view on language and reality, the Zhuangist view on illness is that any phenomenon that requires a perspective-bound feature for its existence is not legitimate outside of this perspective, and not something we can attribute to the world itself independently of us and those perspectives. Thus, while it may turn out that there can be mental illness within some perspective, if we can shift perspectives, this illness disappears. For the Zhuangists and others who accept this view, there is no objective perspective-independent reality of mental illness. The proper response to illness in many (perhaps most) cases is not treatment or self-cultivation so as to eliminate or cure this illness, but rather shifting of perspective so as to render this illness nonillness. The Zhuangist response to mental illness, though it rejects the idea of the mentally ill person as truly ill or disordered, differs from that of Szasz and the modern anti-psychiatry movement. While Szasz and the anti-psychiatry movement base their criticism in a commitment to illness as physical and not functional, thus disallowing the category of mind to qualify (a position I criticized in Chapter 2), the Zhuangist position requires no such commitment to either physicalism, reductionism or eliminativism about mind, or an implausible rejection of functional illness. While the Zhuangist view is

[6] *Liji*, *Zhongyong* 1.

[7] Unschuld and Tessenow 2011, 594. "When anger abounds and does not end, then it will harm the mind."

ultimately more plausible than that of Szasz (and does not make the mistake of associating illness with particular kinds of physical disease state), it is still problematic, in part due to failure to consider social context adequately. Even if we concede to the Zhuangist that an individual can accurately consider a particular mental state or tendency as nonillness and valuable given a shift of perspective, such perspectives will be incompatible with those of other members of society, in such a way as to make social interaction and community impossible or at least incredibly difficult. This is a more general problem for the Zhuangist position.[8]

The Confucian self-cultivational response to mental illness also necessarily involves a communal element. While the focus in most Confucian discussion of madness is on individual failure, we might salvage a more positive aspect of the view. Given the Confucian view of communal personhood, discussed in Chapter 1, it turns out that communities will bear responsibility for the mental illness of individuals as much, or perhaps to an even greater extent, than the ill individual.

Is there some sense in which moral self-cultivation might form part of a treatment program for such illness? We tend not to take this seriously today, in part because of the separation we have made in contemporary society between morality and medicine, but perhaps we should consider this more carefully. While the Confucian view is perhaps ultimately too harsh in its acceptance of mental illness as *completely* governed by agentive considerations, we have good reason to think that moral and spiritual self-cultivation *can* play a role in the management and treatment of mental illness, and the disanalogies between mental and other forms of illness are just what makes this possible.

As contemporary psychologists argue, mental illness is often due to a combination of genetic predisposition and situational features.[9] What calls for anxiety, anger, joy, or other responses will almost always be in large part dependent on communal norms, of the kind integrated into the expectations and behavioral tendencies of individuals from a young age, through interaction with the community. This is why, for example, certain unfilial actions or disrespect of a parent or elder will cause enormous shame in certain East Asian cultures, while not doing so in many Western cultures. It is also argued that cultural factors make certain groups, such as Asian

[8] See Fraser 2015, 55.
[9] https://www.ncbi.nlm.nih.gov/pmc/articles/PMC1940091/

Americans, less likely to seek psychiatric health care than other ethnic groups in the United States.[10]

None of this would have been news to ancient Chinese scholars such as the early Confucians, who recognized that the behaviors and attitudes of individuals are not due solely to individual character and decisions. This is the reason Confucius taught that if one wishes to become virtuous, one must be careful about who they are around.[11] He advised that we should take as friends only those who are at least as morally good as we are.[12] Being part of harmonious and virtuous communities is necessary for the development of healthy behaviors, attitudes, and emotions. If we are in bad, vicious, or unhealthy communities, our beliefs, emotions, expectations, and attitudes (among other things) will be disordered in critical ways.

This is relevant when it comes to mental illness, because such illness is at least in part a matter of behavioral and emotional norms governed by society. Confucians would likely have said of our own modern world that the alienation created by the self-centeredness required for modern economic and consumer culture plays a major role in driving mental illness. Tu Weiming writes that according to the Confucian view, "self-centeredness easily leads to a closed world . . . to a state of paralysis."[13] The kinds of community that promote self-centeredness and self-concern (which can range from the seemingly innocuous concern with "defining oneself" via various individual and consumer choices to the corrosive lack of empathy or care for others in the community) are likely to inculcate in individual members the kind of behavioral and attitudinal traits that contribute to mental illness.

While we may disagree with ancient Chinese scholars on the exact nature of the connection between mental illness and emotions such as anger, joy, or anxiety, work in modern psychiatry suggests that we should take to heart their point about how communally influenced features of our behavior and attitudes can contribute to causing mental illness and must play a role in treatment.

As we try to address the widespread and seemingly increasing problem of mental illness in our modern world[14] (the Centers for Disease Control and Prevention estimates that more than 50 percent of the US population will be

[10] https://www.ncbi.nlm.nih.gov/pmc/articles/PMC1071736/
[11] *Analects* 4.1.
[12] *Analects* 1.8.
[13] Tu 1985a, 114.
[14] https://www.ncbi.nlm.nih.gov/pmc/articles/PMC5316795/

diagnosed with a mental illness or disorder within their lifetimes, and that as many as 4 percent of the population lives with serious mental illness[15]), we should take heed of the Confucian view. There is evidence that mental illness is increasing in younger members of society, along with increases in suicide and attempted suicide.[16] Such increases in mental illness may say less about individual traits than they do about certain alienating and corrosive features of our society. As Confucius himself said: "the faults of an individual are in each case attributable to their group."[17] While many efforts, including providing greater access to professional mental health treatment, should be part of our response to the problem of mental illness, we should also carefully and seriously consider which aspects of our shared cultures may be contributing to the rise of mental illness. A healthy community is also a thriving community.

[15] https://www.cdc.gov/mentalhealth/learn/index.htm
[16] https://psycnet.apa.org/doiLanding?doi=10.1037%2Fabn0000410
[17] *Analects* 4.7.

Bibliography

All primary source material from Chinese texts have been cited from the Chinese Text Project, unless otherwise listed:

Agren, Hans. (1982). "The Conceptual History of Psychiatric Terms in Traditional Chinese." In G. Li, M. Zheng, and T. Cao, eds., *Explorations in the History of Science and Technology in China*. Shanghai: Chinese Classics Publishing House, 573–581.

Allan, Sarah. (2017). *The Heir and the Sage: Dynastic Legend in Early China* (revised and expanded edition). Albany: SUNY Press.

Ames, Roger. (2011). *Confucian Role Ethics: A Vocabulary*. Hong Kong: The Chinese University Press.

Ames, Roger, and David Hall. (1998). *Thinking from the Han: Self, Truth, and Transcendence in Chinese and Western Culture*. Albany: SUNY Press.

Arneson, Richard. (1994). "Autonomy and Preference Formation." In J. Feinberg, J. Coleman, and A. Buchanan, eds., *In Harm's Way: Essays in Honor of Joel Feinberg*. Cambridge: Cambridge University Press, 42–75.

Balan, Luminita. (2001). "Wandering in the World of Zhuangzi." *The Romanian Journal of Chinese Studies* 1(1), 14–18.

Barnes, Corey. (2016). "The Social Nature of Individual Self-Identity: Akan and Narrative Conceptions of Personhood." *Comparative Philosophy* 7(1), 1–19

Barnwell, Scott. (2011). "Classical Daoism—Is There Really Such a Thing?" https://baopu81.wordpress.com/2011/10/16/classical-daoism-is-there-really-such-a-thing-part-1/

Berger, Douglas. (2016). *Encounters of Mind: Luminosity and Personhood in Indian and Chinese Thought*. Albany: SUNY Press.

Berkson, Mark. (2005). "Conceptions of Self/No-Self and Modes of Connection: Comparative Soteriological Structures in Classical Chinese Thought." *Journal of Religious Ethics* 33(2), 293–331.

Berkson, Mark. (2016). "Xunzi as a Theorist and Defender of Ritual." In E. Hutton, ed., *Dao Companion to the Philosophy of Xunzi*. Dordrecht: Springer, 229–267.

Boyd, Richard. (1999). "Kinds, Complexity, and Multiple Realization: Comments on Millikan's 'Historical Kinds and the Special Sciences.'" *Philosophical Studies* 95(1/2), 67–98.

Brindley, Erica. (2010). *Individualism in Early China: Human Agency and the Self in Thought and Politics*. Honolulu: University of Hawaii Press.

Brooks, Bruce, and Taeko Brooks. (2001). *The Original Analects: Sayings of Confucius and His Successors*. New York: Columbia University Press.

Brown, Joshua, and Alexus McLeod. (2020). *Transcendence and Non-Naturalism in Early Chinese Thought*. London: Bloomsbury.

Bruya, Brian. (2001). "Qing and Emotion in Early Chinese Thought." Ming Qing Yanjiu 10(1), 151–176.

Carnap, Rudolf. (1956). "Empiricism, Semantics, and Ontology." *Revue International de Philosophie* 4, 20–40.

Carr, Karen, and Philip J. Ivanhoe. (2000). *The Sense of Antirationalism: The Religious Thought of Zhuangzi and Kierkegaard*. New York: Seven Bridges Press.

Chai, David. (2019). *Zhuangzi and the Becoming of Nothingness*. Albany: SUNY Press.

Chan, Joseph. (2002). "Moral Autonomy, Civil Liberties, and Confucianism." *Philosophy East and West* 52(3), 281–310.

Chen Hongbing. (2008). 莊子僧肇人生觀比較研究——基於道家哲學與 佛教中國化關係的研究. *Guanzi Xuekan* 管子學刊 1, 85–91.

Chiu, Martha Li. (1986). *Mind, Body, and Illness in a Chinese Medical Tradition*. PhD diss., Harvard University.

Chong, Kim-chong. (2010). "Zhuangzi and Hui Shi on Qing." *Tsinghua Journal of Chinese Studies* 40(1), 21–45.

Chong, Kim-chong. (2016). *Zhuangzi's Critique of the Confucians: Blinded by the Human*. Albany: SUNY Press.

Christman, John. (2020). "Autonomy in Moral and Political Philosophy." In E. Zalta, ed., *Stanford Encyclopedia of Philosophy*. https://plato.stanford.edu/entries/autonomy-moral/

Churchland, Paul. (1981). "Eliminative Materialism and the Propositional Attitudes." *The Journal of Philosophy* 78(2), 67–90.

Collins, Steven. (2014). "Madness and Possession in Pali Texts." *Buddhist Studies Review* 31(2), 195–214.

Connolly, Tim. (2011). "Perspectivism as a Way of Knowing in the *Zhuangzi*." *Dao: A Journal of Comparative Philosophy* 10(4), 487–505.

Cook, Constance, and John Major. (2004). *Defining Chu: Image and Reality in Ancient China*. Honolulu: University of Hawaii Press.

Cottingham, John, Robert Stoothoff, and Dugald Murdoch, trans. (1991). *The Philosophical Writings of Descartes*, Vol. III. Cambridge: Cambridge University Press.

Coutinho, Steve. (2014). "Conceptual Analyses of the *Zhuangzi*." In X. Liu, ed., *Dao Companion to Daoist Philosophy*. Dordrecht: Springer, 159–191.

Cyranoski, David. (2010). "China Tackles Surge in Mental Illness." *Nature* 468(7321), 145.

De Bary, William Theodore, ed. (2011). *Finding Wisdom in East Asian Classics*. New York: Columbia University Press.

Doris, John. (2002). *Lack of Character: Personality and Moral Behavior*. Cambridge: Cambridge University Press.

Drescher, Jack. (2015). "Out of DSM: Depathologizing Homosexuality." *Behavioral Science* 5(4), 565–575.

El Amine, Loubna. (2016). *Classical Confucian Political Thought: A New Interpretation*. Princeton, NJ: Princeton University Press.

Ellis, Havelock. (1900). *Studies in the Psychology of Sex, Vol. 2: Sexual Inversion*. Watford: The University Press.

Feinberg, Joel. (1986). *Harm to Self: The Moral Limits of the Criminal Law*, Vol. 3. Oxford: Oxford University Press.

Foucault, Michel. (1988). *Madness and Civilization: A History of Insanity in the Age of Reason*. New York: Vintage Books. (Reprint of 1965).

Franke, William. (2018). *Apophatic Paths from Europe to China*. Albany: SUNY Press.

Fraser, Chris. (2015). "Zhuangzi and the Heterogeneity of Value." In L. Kohn, ed., *New Visions of the Zhuangzi*. St. Petersburg, FL: Three Pines Press, 40–58.

Freud, Sigmund. (1918). *Three Contributions to the Theory of Sex*. 3rd ed. New York: Nervous and Mental Disease Publishing Company.

Freydberg, Bernard. (2005). *Imagination in Kant's Critique of Practical Reason*. Bloomington: Indiana University Press.

Gardner, Daniel. (2003). *Zhu Xi's Reading of the Analects: Canon. Commentary, and the Classical Tradition*. New York: Columbia University Press.

Goldin, Paul. (1999). *Rituals of the Way: The Philosophy of Xunzi*. Chicago: Open Court.

Goldin, Paul. (2011). "Persistent Misconceptions About Chinese 'Legalism.'" *Journal of Chinese Philosophy* 38(1), 88–104.

Goldin, Paul. (2015). "The Consciousness of the Dead as a Philosophical Problem in Ancient China." In R.A.H. King, ed., *The Good Life and Conceptions of Life in Early China and Graeco-Roman Antiquity*. Berlin: De Gruyter, 59–92.

Graham, Angus. (1967). "The Background of the Mencian Theory of Human Nature." *Tsinghua Journal of Chinese Studies* 6(1–2), 215–271.

Graham, Angus. (1989). *Disputers of the Tao: Philosophical Argument in Ancient China*. Chicago: Open Court.

Graham, Angus. (2001). *Chuang-Tzu: The Inner Chapters*. Indianapolis: Hackett.

Graham, George. (2013). *The Disordered Mind: An Introduction to Philosophy of Mind and Mental Illness*. Abingdon: Routledge.

Hacking, Ian. (1995). "The Looping Effects of Human Kinds." In D. Sperber, D. Premack, and A. Premack, eds., *Casual Cognition: A Multidisciplinary Debate*. Oxford: Oxford University Press, 351–394.

Hagen, Kurtis. (2002). "Xunzi's Use of *Zhengming*: Naming as a Constructive Project." *Asian Philosophy* 12(1), 35–51.

Hagen, Kurtis. (2003). "Xunzi and the Nature of Confucian Ritual." *Journal of the American Academy of Religion* 71(2), 371–403.

Hagen, Kurtis. (2007). *The Philosophy of Xunzi: A Reconstruction*. Chicago: Open Court.

Hansen, Chad. (1983). *Language and Logic in Ancient China*. Ann Arbor: University of Michigan Press.

Hansen, Chad. (1995). "Qing (Emotions) in Pre-Buddhist Chinese Thought." In R. Ames, C. Solomon, and J. Marks, eds., *Emotions in Asian Thought: A Dialogue in Comparative Philosophy*. Albany: SUNY Press, 181–211.

Hansen, Chad. (2000). *A Daoist Theory of Chinese Thought*. Oxford: Oxford University Press.

Hansen, Chad. (2014). "Zhuangzi." In E. Zalta, ed., *Stanford Encyclopedia of Philosophy*. https://plato.stanford.edu/entries/zhuangzi/

Harper, Donald. (1998). *Early Chinese Medical Literature: The Mawangdui Medical Manuscripts*. London: Kegan Paul International.

Holloway, Kenneth. (2013). *The Quest for Ecstatic Morality in Early China*. Oxford: Oxford University Press.

Honeychurch, William. (2015). *Inner Asia and the Spatial Politics of Empire*. Dordrecht: Springer.

Hooker, Evelyn. (1957). "The Adjustment of the Male Overt Homosexual." *Journal of Projective Techniques* 21, 18–31.

Hu Shaohua. (2000). *Explaining Chinese Democratization*. Santa Barbara, CA: Praeger.

Hutton, Eric. (2016). *Xunzi: The Complete Text*. Princeton, NJ: Princeton University Press.

Ing, Michael. (2012). *The Dysfunction of Ritual in Early Confucianism*. Oxford: Oxford University Press.

Inwood, Brad, and L. P. Gerson, eds. (1998). *Hellenistic Philosophy: Introductory Readings*. 2nd ed. Indianapolis: Hackett.

Ivanhoe, Philip. (1993). "Zhuangzi on Skepticism, Skill, and the Ineffable *Dao*." *Journal of the American Academy of Religion* 61(4), 639–654.

Jochim, Christian. (1998). "Just Say No to 'No-Self' in Zhuang Zi." In R. Ames, ed., *Wandering at Ease in the Zhuangzi*. Albany: SUNY Press, 35–74.

Kim, Sungmoon. (2014). *Confucian Democracy in East Asia: Theory and Practice*.

Kim, Sungmoon. (2016). *Public Reason Confucianism: Democratic Perfectionism and Constitutionalism in East Asia*. Cambridge: Cambridge University Press.

Kinsey, Alfred. (1948). *Sexual Behavior in the Human Male*. Philadelphia: W.B. Saunders.

Kjellberg, Paul, ed. (1996). Essays on Skepticism, Relativism, and Ethics in the Zhuangzi. Albany: SUNY Press.

Klein, Esther. (2011). "Were There 'Inner Chapters' in the Warring States? A New Examination of Evidence about the *Zhuangzi*." *T'oung Pao, Second Series* 96(4/5), 299–369.

Knechtges, David, and Taiping Chang, eds. (2010). *Ancient and Medieval Chinese Literature: A Reference Guide, Part One*. Leiden: Brill.

Knoblock, John, and Jeffrey Riegel. (2001). *The Annals of Lu Buwei*. Palo Alto, CA: Stanford University Press.

Kupperman, Joel. (2004). "Tradition and Community in the Formation of Character and Self." In K. Shun and D. Wong, eds., *Confucian Ethics: A Comparative Study of Self, Autonomy, and Community*. Cambridge: Cambridge University Press, 103–123.

Kuriyama, Shigehisa. (1999) *The Expressiveness of the Body and the Divergence of Greek and Chinese Medicine*. New York: Zone Books.

Lee, Janghee. (2005). *Xunzi and Early Chinese Naturalism*. Albany: SUNY Press.

Lewis, Mark Edward. (2006). *The Construction of Space in Early China*. Albany: SUNY Press.

Li, Chenyang. (2014a). "The Confucian Conception of Freedom." *Philosophy East and West* 64(4), 902–919.

Li, Chenyang. (2014b). *The Confucian Philosophy of Harmony*. London: Routledge.

Li, Chenyang, and Peimin Ni. (2014). *Moral Cultivation and Confucian Character: Engaging Joel Kupperman*. Albany: SUNY Press.

Liu, JeeLoo. (2014). "Chinese Qi-Naturalism and Liberal Naturalism." *Philosophy, Theology, and the Sciences* 1(1), 59–86.

Liu, JeeLoo. (2015). "In Defense of Chinese Qi-Naturalism." In C. Li and F. Perkins, eds., *Chinese Metaphysics and Its Problems*. Cambridge: Cambridge University Press, 33–53.

Liu, Xiaogan. (1994). *Classifying the Zhuangzi Chapters*. Ann Arbor: Center for Chinese Studies, University of Michigan.

Loewe, Michael. (2011). *Dong Zhongshu, a "Confucian" Heritage and the Chunqiu Fanlu*. Leiden: Brill.

Loy, Hui-Chieh. (2003). "*Analects* 13.3 and the Doctrine of 'Correcting Names.'" *Monumenta Serica* 51(1), 19–36.

MacIntyre, Alasdair. (1981). *After Virtue*. Notre Dame: University of Notre Dame Press.

MacIntyre, Alasdair. (1988). *Whose Justice? Which Rationality?* Notre Dame: University of Notre Dame Press.

MacIntyre, Alasdair. (1991). "Incommensurability, Truth, Virtues: Conversation Between Confucians and Aristotelians about the Virtues." In E. Deutsch, ed., *Culture and Modernity*. Honolulu: University of Hawaii Press, 104–122.

MacKenzie, Matthew. (2007). "The Illumination of Consciousness: Approaches to Self-Awareness in the Indian and Western Traditions." *Philosophy East and West* 57(1), 40–62.

MacKenzie, Matthew. (2008). "Self-Awareness without a Self: Buddhism and the Reflexivity of Awareness." *Asian Philosophy* 18(3), 245–266.

Mair, Victor. (2000). *Wandering on the Way: Early Taoist Tales and Parables of Chuang Tzu*. Honolulu: University of Hawaii Press.

Mair, Victor. (2012). "What Is *Geyi*, After All?" *China Report* 48(1–2), 29–59.

Major, John. (1993). *Heaven and Earth in Early Han Thought*. Albany: SUNY Press.

Major, John, Sarah Queen, Andrew Meyer, and Harold Roth. (2010). *The Huainanzi: A Guide to the Theory and Practice of Government in Early Han China*. New York: Columbia University Press.

Makeham, John. (1994). *Name and Actuality in Early Chinese Thought*. Albany: SUNY Press.

Mattice, Sarah. (2019). "Confucian Role Ethics: Issues of Naming, Translation, and Interpretation." In A. McLeod, ed., *The Bloomsbury Handbook of Early Chinese Ethics and Political Philosophy*. London: Bloomsbury, 25–44.

Mark, Zvi. (2003). "Dybbuk and Devekut in the Shivhe ha-Besht: Toward a Phenomenology of Madness in Early Hasidism." In M. Goldish, ed., *Spirit Possession in Judaism: Cases and Contexts from the Middle Ages to the Present*. Detroit: Wayne State University Press, 257–301.

McLeod, Alexus. (2011). "In the World of Persons: The Personhood Debate in the *Analects* and *Zhuangzi*." *Dao: A Journal of Comparative Philosophy* 11(4), 427–457.

McLeod, Alexus. (2012). "*Ren* as a Communal Property in the *Analects*." *Philosophy East and West* 62(4), 505–528.

McLeod, Alexus. (2015). *Theories of Truth in Chinese Philosophy*. London: Rowman and Littlefield International.

McLeod, Alexus. (2018a). *The Philosophical Thought of Wang Chong*. London: Palgrave Macmillan.

McLeod, Alexus. (2018b). "Xunzi and Mimamsa on the Source and Ground of Ritual: An Analogical Argument." *Philosophy East and West* 68(3), 737–761.

McLeod, Alexus. (2018c). *Philosophy of the Ancient Maya: Lords of Time*. Lanham, MD: Lexington Books.

McLeod, Alexus. (2019). "The Problem of Anxiety in the *Zhuangzi* as Contrasted With Indian and Hellenistic Views." In A. McLeod, ed., *The Bloomsbury Research Handbook of Early Chinese Ethics and Political Philosophy*. London: Bloomsbury, 225–246.

Middendorf, Ulrike. (2008). "Again on 'Qing': With a Translation of the *Xing zi ming chu*." *Oriens Extremus* 47, 97–159.

Mou, Bo. (2008). "Searle, Zhuang-Zi, and Transcendental Perspectivism." In B. Mou, ed., *Searle's Philosophy and Chinese Philosophy: Constructive Engagement*. Leiden: Brill, 405–430.

Mou, Bo. (2017). "The Perspective and Perspective-Transcending Dimensions of Consciousness and Its Double-Aboutness Character: Bridging Searle and Zhuang Zi." *Comparattive Philosophy* 8(1), 114–128.

Murray, Judson. (2004). "A Study of 'Yao Lue', 'A Summary of the Essentials': The Huainanzi from the Point of View of the Postface." *Early China* 29, 45–109.

Ng, Vivien. (1990). *Madness in Late Imperial China: From Illness to Deviance*. Norman: University of Oklahoma Press.

Ni, Peimin. (2013). "The Philosophy of Confucius." In V. Shen, ed., *Dao Companion to Classical Confucian Philosophy*. Dordrecht: Springer, 53–80.

Nivison, David. (1996). "'Virtue' in Bone and Bronze." In D. Nivison and B. Van Norden, eds., *The Ways of Confucianism: Investigations in Chinese Philosophy*. Chicago: Open Court, 17–30.

Nolan, Lawrence. (2015). "Cartesian Trialism on Trial: The Conceptualist Account of Descartes' Human Being." In P. Easton, ed., *The Battle of the Gods and Giants Redux: Papers Presented to Thomas M. Lennon*. Leiden: Brill, 137–174.

O'Dwyer, Shaun. (2015). "Epistemic Elitism, Paternalism, and Confucian Democracy." *Dao: A Journal of Comparative Philosophy* 14, 33–54.

Olberding, Amy. (2014). "Perspectives on Moral Failure in the *Analects*." In A. Olberding, ed., *Dao Companion to the Analects*. Dordrecht: Springer, 199–221.

Pankenier, David. (2015). *Astrology and Cosmology in Early China: Conforming Earth to Heaven*. Cambridge: Cambridge University Press.

Peerenboom, R. P. (1993). *Law and Morality in Ancient China: The Silk Manuscripts of Huang-Lao*. Albany: SUNY Press.

Phillips, Michael R., Jingxuan Zhang, Qichang Shi, Zhiqiang Song, Zhijie Ding, Shutao Pang, Xianyun Li, Yali Zhang, and Zhiqung Wang. (2009). "Prevalence, Treatment, and Associated Disability of Mental Disorders in Four Provinces in China during 2001–05: An Epidemiological Survey." *Lancet* 373(9680), 2041–2054.

Pietikainen, Petteri. (2015). *Madness: A History*. Abingdon: Routledge.

Puett, Michael. (2004). "The Ethics of Responding Properly: The Notion of Qing in Early Chinese Thought." In H. Eifring, ed., *Love and Emotions in Traditional Chinese Literature*. Leiden: Brill, 37–68.

Puett, Michael. (2015). "Constructions of Reality: Metaphysics in the Ritual Traditions of Classical China." In C. Li and F. Perkins, eds., *Chinese Metaphysics and Its Problems*. Cambridge: Cambridge University Press, 120–129.

Queen, Sarah, and John Major. (2015). *Luxuriant Gems of the Spring and Autumn*. New York: Columbia University Press.

Rey, Georges. (1983). "A Reason for Doubting the Existence of Consciousness." *Consciousness and Self-Regulation* 3, 1–39.

Rey, Roselyne. (1998). *The History of Pain*. Cambridge, MA: Harvard University Press.

Ripstein, Arthur. (1999). *Equality, Responsibility, and the Law*. Cambridge: Cambridge University Press.

Rosemont, Henry. (2004). "Whose Democracy? Which Rights? A Confucian Critique of Modern Western Liberalism." In K. Shun, ed., *Confucian Ethics: A Comparative Study of Self, Autonomy, and Community*. Cambridge: Cambridge University Press, 49–71.

Rosemont, Henry. (2015). *Against Individualism: A Confucian Rethinking of the Foundations of Morality, Politics, Family, and Religion*. Lanham, MD: Lexington Books.

Roth, Harold. (1991). "Who Compiled the Chuang Tzu?" In H. Rosemont, ed., *Chinese Texts and Philosophical Contexts: Essays Dedicated to Angus C. Graham*. Chicago: Open Court, 79–128.

Sakauye, Kenneth. (2005). "Cultural Influences on Pain Management in the Elderly." *Comprehensive Therapy* 31, 78–82.

Sauer, Sebastian, Siobhan Lynch, Harald Walach, and Niko Kohls. (2011). "Dialectics of Mindfulness: Implications for Western Medicine." *Philosophy, Ethics, and Humanities in Medicine* 6(10), 6–10.

Schneider, Laurence. (1980). *A Madman of Ch'u: The Chinese Myth of Loyalty and Dissent*. Berkeley: University of California Press.

Seiwert, Hubert. (2018). "Health and Salvation in Early Daoism: On the Anthropology of the Taiping Jing." In A. Baumgartner, ed., *Self, Soul and Body in Religious Experience*. Leiden: Brill, 256–275.

Shun, Kwong-loi. (1997). "Mencius on *Jen-Hsing*." *Philosophy East and West* 47(1), 1–20.

Simonis, Fabian (2010). Mad Acts, Mad Speech, and Mad People in Late Imperial Chinese Law and Medicine. PhD Dissertation, Princeton University.

Sivin, Nathan. (1990). "Science and Medicine in Chinese History." In P. Ropp, ed., *Heritage of China: Contemporary Perspectives on Chinese Civilization*. Berkeley: University of California Press, 164–196.

Slingerland, Edward. (2003). *Confucius Analects, With Selections from Traditional Commentaries*. Indianapolis: Hackett.

Slingerland, Edward. (2016). "Interdisciplinary Methods in Chinese Philosophy: Comparative Philosophy and the Case Example of Mind-Body Holism." In S. Tan, ed. *The Bloomsbury Research Handbook of Chinese Philosophy Methodologies*. London: Bloomsbury, 323–352.

Slingerland, Edward. (2019). *Mind and Body in Early China: Beyond Orientalism and the Myth of Holism*. Oxford: Oxford University Press.

Slingerland, Edward, and Maciej Chudek. (2011). "The Prevalence of Mind-Body Dualism in Early China." *Cognitive Science* 35(5), 997–1007.

Small, Sharon. (2018). "A Daoist Exploration of *Shenming*." *Journal of Daoist Studies* 11.

Smith, Kidder. (2003). "Sima Tan and the Invention of Daoism, 'Legalism,' *et cetera*." *The Journal of Asian Studies* 62(1), 129–156.

Song Hongbing. (2016). 論司馬談之"道家"概念與司馬遷之"黃老"概念. *Guoxue Xuekan* 國學學刊.

Stalnaker, Aaron. (2009). *Overcoming Our Evil: Human Nature and Spiritual Exercises in Xunzi and Augustine*. Washington, DC: Georgetown University Press.

Stoljar, Daniel. (2010). *Physicalism*. Abingdon: Routledge.

Sturgeon, Donald. *Chinese Text Project: A Dynamic Digital Library of Premodern Chinese*. https://ctext.org

Sturgeon, Donald. (2015). "Zhuangzi, Perspectives, and Greater Knowledge." *Philosophy East and West* 65(3), 892–917.

Szasz, Thomas. (2003). *The Myth of Mental Illness: Foundations of a Theory of Personal Conduct*. New York: Harper. (Reprint of 1973).

Tiwald, Justin. (2015). "Well Being and Daoism." In G. Fletcher, ed., *The Routledge Handbook of Philosophy of Well-Being*. London: Routledge, 56–69.

Tiwald, Justin, and Bryan Van Norden. (2014). *Readings in Later Chinese Philosophy*. Indianapolis: Hackett.

Tu Weiming. (1985a). *Confucian Thought: Selfhood as Creative Transformation*. Albany: SUNY Press.

Tu Weiming (1985b). "Selfhood and Otherness in Confucian Thought." In A. Marsella, G. DeVos, and F. Hsu eds., *Culture and Self: Asian and Western Perspectives*. New York: Tavistock, 231–251.

Tu Weiming. (1986). "An Inquiry on the Five Relationships in Confucian Humanism." In W. Slote, ed., *The Psycho-Cultural Dynamics of the Confucian Family: Past and Present*. Seoul: International Society of Korea 175–196.

Unschuld, Paul. (2003). *Huang Di Nei Jing Su Wen: Nature, Knowledge, and Imagery in an Ancient Chinese Medical Text*. Berkeley: University of California Press.

Unschuld, Paul, and Hermann Tessenow. (2011). *Huang Di Nei Jing Su Wen: An Annotated Translation of Huang Di's Inner Classic- Basic Questions*. Berkeley: University of California Press.

Van Norden, Bryan. (2007). *Virtue Ethics and Consequentialism in Early Chinese Philosophy*. Cambridge: Cambridge University Press.

Van Norden, Bryan. (2011). *Introduction to Classical Chinese Philosophy*. Indianapolis: Hackett.

Van Oudenhoven, Jan Pieter, Boele de Raad, Carmen Carmona, Anne-Kathrin Helbig, and Meta van der Linden. (2012). "Are Virtues Shaped by National Cultures or Religions?" *Swiss Journal of Psychology* 71(1), 29–34.

Vankeerberghen, Griet. (2001). *The Huainanzi and Liu An's Claim to Moral Authority*. Albany: SUNY Press.

Vayrynen, Pekka. (2016). "Thick Ethical Concepts." In E. Zalta, ed., *Stanford Encyclopedia of Philosophy*. https://plato.stanford.edu/entries/thick-ethical-concepts/

Wakefield, Jerome. (1992). "Disorder as Harmful Dysfunction: A Conceptual Critique of DSM-III-R's Definition of Mental Disorder." *Psychological Review* 99(2), 232–247.

Watson, Burton (1968). *The Complete Works of Chuang Tzu*. New York: Columbia University Press.

Watson, Burton. (2003). *Xunzi: Basic Writings*. New York: Columbia University Press.

Wen Haiming. (2012). "Confucian Co-Creative Ethics: Self and Family." *Frontiers of Philosophy in China* 7(3), 439–454.

Winter, Michael. (2012). *Rethinking Virtue Ethics*. Dordrecht: Springer.

Wong, David. (2004). "Rights and Community in Confucianism." In K. Shun and D. Wong, eds., *Confucian Ethics: A Comparative Study of Self, Autonomy, and Community*. Cambridge: Cambridge University Press, 31–48.

Wong, David. (2009). *Natural Moralities: A Defense of Pluralistic Relativism*. Oxford: Oxford University Press.

Xiao, Yang, and Yong Huang, eds. (2014). *Moral Relativism and Chinese Philosophy: David Wong and His Critics*. Albany: SUNY Press.

Xu Fuguan. (1976). 兩漢思想史. Taipei: Taiwan xuesheng shuju

Yao, Xinzhong. (2006). *Wisdom in Early Confucian and Israelite Traditions*. London: Routledge.

York, William. (2012). *Health and Wellness in Antiquity through the Middle Ages*. Westport, CT: Greenwood.

Zachar, Peter. (2015). "Psychiatric Disorders: Natural Kinds Made by the World or Practical Kinds Made by Us?" *World Psychiatry* 14(3), 288–290.

Zhang, Zailin. (2011). 中國古代哲學中的身心一體論. *Zhongzhou Xuekan* 中州學刊.

Zhao, Dingxin. (2015). *The Confucian-Legalist State: A New Theory of Chinese History*. Oxford: Oxford University Press.

Zheng, Yujian. (2008). "Unconscious Intentionality and the Status of Normativity in Searle's Philosophy: With Comparative Reference to Traditional Chinese Thought." In B. Mou, ed., *Searle's Philosophy and Chinese Philosophy: Constructive Engagement*. Leiden: Brill, 379–399.

Zhou Guidian. (2006). 秦汉哲学. Wuhan: Wuhan Publishing 武汉出版社.

Zimbardo, Philip. (2008). *The Lucifer Effect: Understanding How Good People Turn Evil*. New York: Random House.

Ziporyn, Brook. (2009). *Zhuangzi: The Essential Writings*. Indianapolis: Hackett.

Ziporyn, Brook. (2013). *Ironies of Oneness and Difference: Coherence in Early Chinese Thought; Prolegomena to the Study of Li*. Albany: SUNY Press.

Zufferey, Nicolas. (2003). *To the Origins of Confucianism: The Ru in Pre-Qin Times and During the Early Han Dynasty*. Bern: Peter Lang.

Index